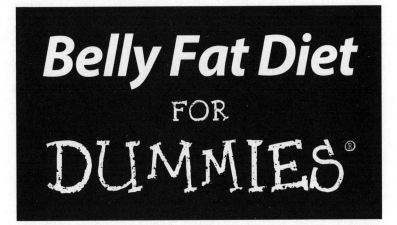

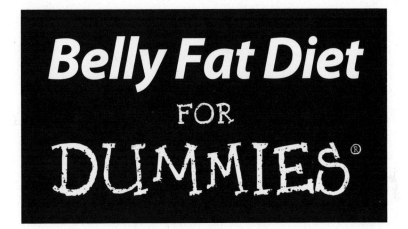

Belly Fat Diet
FOR
DUMMIES®

by Erin Palinski-Wade, RD, CDE

WILEY

John Wiley & Sons, Inc.

Belly Fat Diet For Dummies®

Published by
John Wiley & Sons, Inc.
111 River St.
Hoboken, NJ 07030-5774
www.wiley.com

For general information on our other products and services, please contact our Customer Care Department within the U.S. at 877-762-2974, outside the U.S. at 317-572-3993, or fax 317-572-4002.

For technical support, please visit www.wiley.com/techsupport.

Wiley publishes in a variety of print and electronic formats and by print-on-demand. Some material included with standard print versions of this book may not be included in e-books or in print-on-demand. If this book refers to media such as a CD or DVD that is not included in the version you purchased, you may download this material at http://booksupport.wiley.com. For more information about Wiley products, visit us at www.wiley.com.

Library of Congress Control Number: 2012948925

ISBN 978-1-118-34585-6 (pbk); ISBN 978-1-118-43184-9 (ebk); ISBN 978-1-118-43206-8 (ebk); ISBN 978-1-118-43208-2 (ebk)

Manufactured in the United States of America

10 9 8 7 6 5 4 3 2

WILEY

About the Author

Erin Palinski-Wade, RD, CDE, and "America's Belly Fat Fighter!" is a nationally recognized nutrition and fitness expert who has contributed her expertise to media outlets such as the *CBS Early Show, The Doctors, ABC News, CBS News, News 12, Fox News, Fitness Magazine, Consumer Reports, Chicago Tribune,* and *Prevention Magazine.* She is the author of two weight loss curriculums for health professionals including the "Healthy 'n' Fit Pediatric Weight Management Program" and the "Healthy Resolutions Weight Management Program."

Erin runs a private practice in New Jersey, the Vernon Nutrition Center, where she provides in-office as well as telephone and Internet-based nutrition counseling and coaching. She also frequently serves as a media spokesperson and motivational and keynote speaker, and often partners with food companies and corporations as a nutrition consultant.

Erin is a Registered Dietitian, Certified Personal Trainer, and Certified Diabetes Educator. She currently serves on the Dietetic Internship Advisory Board for the College of Saint Elizabeth and has been appointed to the ZiggityZoom.com advisory board as the nutrition and obesity expert. Erin focuses on providing practical, realistic advice that allows you to not only start seeing results instantly but more importantly, maintain results permanently!

Dedication

This book is dedicated to all those individuals who have ever struggled with their weight and have shown through hard work, dedication, and perseverance that you can achieve your goals.

This book is also dedicated to my incredibly loving and supportive family — without your constant support and belief in me, this book would not have been possible.

Author's Acknowledgments

Writing this book has been an incredible journey, but I could not have done it without the help and support of the terrific people around me. First, I want to thank my wonderful and loving husband who has always believed in me and has given me the confidence and encouragement needed to complete this book. I also want to thank my incredible parents, my sister, my brothers-in-law and sisters-in-law, my niece and nephew, my husband's parents, and all of my extended family including my aunts, uncles, and cousins who have been my cheerleaders throughout this process. I appreciate your constant positive feedback and encouragement more than you could ever know! I am so blessed to have a family as wonderful as you.

I also want to thank nutrition professionals Tara Guidus, RD, and Cindy Heroux, RD, for your guidance and support throughout this process. And special thanks to everyone who made this book possible, including my literary agent Margot Hutchison, acquisitions editor Tracy Boggier, project editor Tim Gallan, copy editor Jessica Smith, technical editor Rachel Nix, art coordinator Alicia South, photographer Matt Bowen, recipe tester Pam Mitchell, nutritional analyst Patti Santelli, and exercise models Jodi Bratch, Constance Coleman, Brandon Hooks, and Chad Martin. I can't tell you how much I have appreciated all of your support, patience, and knowledge.

Publisher's Acknowledgments

We're proud of this book; please send us your comments at http://dummies.custhelp.com. For other comments, please contact our Customer Care Department within the U.S. at 877-762-2974, outside the U.S. at 317-572-3993, or fax 317-572-4002.

Some of the people who helped bring this book to market include the following:

Acquisitions, Editorial, and Vertical Websites

Senior Project Editor: Tim Gallan

Acquisitions Editor: Tracy Boggier

Copy Editor: Jessica Smith

Technical Reviewer: Rachel Nix

Recipe Tester: Pam Mitchell

Nutritional Analyst: Patti Santelli

Assistant Editor: David Lutton

Editorial Program Coordinator: Joe Niesen

Editorial Manager: Michelle Hacker

Editorial Assistants: Rachelle S. Amick, Alexa Koschier

Cover Photos: © iStockphoto.com / dashek

Art Coordinator: Alicia B. South

Cartoons: Rich Tennant (www.the5thwave.com)

Composition Services

Project Coordinator: Sheree Montgomery

Layout and Graphics: Carrie A. Cesavice, Joyce Haughey, Corrie Niehaus, Erin Zeltner

Photographer: Matt Bowen

Proofreaders: Debbye Butler, Rebecca Denoncour

Indexer: Steve Rath

Special Help: Christine Pingleton

Publishing and Editorial for Consumer Dummies

Kathleen Nebenhaus, Vice President and Executive Publisher

David Palmer, Associate Publisher

Kristin Ferguson-Wagstaffe, Product Development Director

Publishing for Technology Dummies

Andy Cummings, Vice President and Publisher

Composition Services

Debbie Stailey, Director of Composition Services

Contents at a Glance

Table of Contents

Chapter 8: Meal Plans 127

Chapter 9: Easing Yourself into Exercise.......................153

Introduction

· ·

*H*ow many people do you know who are 100 percent satisfied with
how their stomach looks? Not many, right? Who wouldn't want a flatter stomach, defined abs, and a slim, toned appearance? In today's society,
waistlines are expanding at epidemic proportions. And although folks give
belly fat cutesy names like "muffin-top" or "beer-belly" or "love handles,"
there's nothing cute about it!

Belly fat not only looks less than desirable, but it also can have very real
and very dangerous health implications. The latest research links belly fat
to everything from heart disease and type 2 diabetes to certain cancers and
even an increased risk of dementia. And, sadly, more individuals today are
overweight than not, so something needs to change.

What if you could quickly and effectively shed this excess belly fat and keep
it off for good? And what if you were able to eat delicious food while doing it?
Sound too good to be true? Well, it isn't!

Throughout *Belly Fat Diet For Dummies,* I show you simple, yet incredibly
effective, strategies to shrink belly fat, improve your health and dietary
habits, increase your physical activity, and have you looking and feeling great
in no time. I help you break through common misconceptions and myths and
show you what really works in the fight against belly fat. Whether you have
more than 100 pounds to lose or just need to shed that last 5 pounds, I show
you what works best for you so you can be successful for life. Get ready to
say bye-bye to belly fat forever!

About This Book

Just as no two individuals are exactly alike, no two individuals lose weight in
the exact same way either. So fad diets and cookie-cutter weight loss plans
usually don't work for most people. But *Belly Fat Diet For Dummies* solves this
problem! Throughout this book, I help you discover exactly what caused you
to gain your belly fat and what customized plan is best for you to lose your
belly fat, achieve your ideal body weight, and keep the weight off permanently!
I don't include any one-size-fits-all plans here. Instead, I offer realistic, practical,
and individualized advice that can have you achieving your goals in no time.

What also sets this book apart from other weight loss plans is the attention
given to weight maintenance. Have you lost weight before only to regain it?

You're not alone! In fact, most dieters don't maintain the weight they have lost for more than a year. But in this book, I show you why most people regain their weight and what steps you need to take to permanently keep your weight (and belly!) off.

The cherry on top is that this book contains more than 40 delicious and easy-to-make recipes as well as individualized meal plans, detailed maintenance plans, and extensive exercise routines to blast away belly fat for everyone from the couch potato to the advanced exerciser.

My guess is that if you have tried unsuccessfully to lose belly fat in the past, you may struggle with specific areas, such as food cravings or eating out. Instead of reading this book in order page by page, you can instead skip right to the areas you need to focus on the most. That's right, you don't have to start with Chapter 1 and read straight through to get the benefits. This book is set up so you can read it in any order that appeals to you and still get all the information you need to achieve the flat belly of your dreams.

Conventions Used in This Book

Although I hear the word repeatedly throughout the day, I really hate the word "diet." A diet is something you go on and off again. But going back to your old habits gets you nowhere. It just helps you gain back all the weight you lost, which is bad for your health (maybe even worse than being overweight in the first place). Even though the word "diet" is used in this book title and throughout the book, I want you to think of it in a different way than you normally would. The Belly Fat Diet isn't a diet to go on and off; it's a lifestyle.

Because the Belly Fat Diet is something you put into effect for life, I stress throughout this book that slip-ups and occasional splurges are fine. I even encourage them! If you don't deal with slip-ups every now and then, you won't learn how to successfully maintain your weight loss in the long term. So when you see the word "diet" throughout this book, remember that it refers to a lifestyle change, not the unrealistic goal of eating perfectly (which can't be maintained).

Here are a few other conventions that I also put to use throughout this book:

- New or technical terms appear in *italics* and are followed by a definition.
- **Bold** indicates the action part of numbered steps and highlights the key words in bulleted lists.
- Web addresses are set in `monofont` so you can easily spot them.
- The tomato icon to the left of this paragraph appears next to the titles of vegetarian recipes in the "Recipes in This Chapter" lists at the beginning of chapters that include recipes.

When this book was printed, some web addresses may have needed to break across two lines of text. If that happened, rest assured that I haven't put in any extra characters (such as hyphens) to indicate the break. So when using one of these web addresses, just type in exactly what you see in this book, pretending as though the line break doesn't exist.

What You're Not to Read

I've packed this book full of helpful information on losing belly fat, maintaining weight loss, and making healthy lifestyle changes. However, throughout the book, I include some additional reference material, fun facts, and technical info. These tidbits are highlighted as sidebars (gray shaded boxes) or are marked with the Technical Stuff icon. This information helps to enhance your overall understanding of belly fat and provide you with more background information, but you can skip over it without missing anything essential.

Foolish Assumptions

I didn't want this book to be overweight, so when I sat down to write it, I made some assumptions about you, the reader, so I could narrow the focus and give you only what you need. Here are the assumptions I made:

- I assume that you have excess belly fat you want to lose.

- I assume that you're ready to get in the best shape of your life and that you're committed to making some lifestyle changes to get you there.

- I assume that, like me, you love food and want a book that provides you with recipes for great-tasting meals, snacks, and desserts that can also help you lose your gut.

- I assume that like most people you have a hectic lifestyle and, even though you're serious about wanting to lose your belly and get healthy, you don't have hours and hours every day to commit to it, so you want simple plans that are easy to implement and stick with.

How This Book Is Organized

Belly Fat Diet For Dummies is organized into five specific parts to help make it easy for you to find the information you're looking for. Here's a brief description of what you can find in each part of the book.

Part I: The 4-1-1 on Belly Fat and the Skinny on the Diet

Part I starts by breaking down what belly fat is, what causes an excess of it, and what impact it can have on your health. In this part, I also help you identify your body type, which is vital to knowing exactly how to effectively shrink your belly. I also show you how to determine whether you have excess belly fat (even if you're at a healthy body weight!) and how to know when you've achieved a healthy waistline. I wrap up the part by outlining the principles of the Belly Fat Diet plan and whom it's appropriate for.

Part II: Working Your Way to a Flatter Belly

I start this part by helping you get prepared for your Belly Fat Diet plan so you can be as successful as possible. Next, I describe the key components of your plan and outline the various plans, including how to determine what plan is most appropriate for your needs. This part also provides you with specific meal plan guidelines and sample meal plans.

This part closes with a chapter on belly-blasting workout routines. First I explain the impact that exercise has on belly fat and provide you with simple strategies to help you get moving, regardless of your exercise history. Then I provide you with a detailed workout plan and effective exercises (complete with detailed descriptions and pictures) that blast belly fat and tone and tighten your abs.

Part III: Cooking Up Some Healthy and Tasty Recipes

What's the point in trying to lose weight and shrink your belly if you can't enjoy yourself while you do it? Right. There is no point in that. Part III starts off by helping you understand how to stock and prepare your kitchen and pantry so you can be successful while saving time, money, and energy.

The remaining chapters in the part provide you with delicious and easy-to-prepare recipes that you're sure to love. The best part is that the recipes are great for your whole family, so you won't have to prepare separate meals to be successful.

Part IV: Overcoming Obstacles and Managing Your Progress

Losing weight is never easy, but keeping it off can be even more difficult. That's why Part IV addresses the most common challenges and pitfalls that can throw you off track when following your Belly Fat Diet plan. This part addresses specific dietary concerns, such as dealing with cravings and emotional eating, handling boredom with your meals, and losing belly fat while following a vegetarian or vegan lifestyle.

This part also discusses how to eat at restaurants, at social gatherings, and on food-centered holidays while still losing weight and keeping it off. The part concludes with a detailed plan for permanent weight loss and strategies on exactly what steps you need to take if you start to see yourself regaining any weight you have lost so you can keep your flat belly for life!

Part V: The Part of Tens

Part V provides a quick breakdown of helpful and fun information to allow you to achieve and maintain a flat belly. You find chapters that list the ten foods that can bloat your belly. I also list the ten nutrients that pack a powerful fight against belly fat.

Icons Used in This Book

As you read through this book, you see icons — small images in the margins — that are designed to call your attention to specific pieces of information. Here are the icons I use along with a description of what they mean:

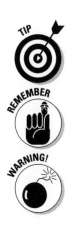

When you see this icon, you know you're about to get helpful tips and practical advice to help shrink your belly and promote effective weight loss.

The text next to this icon typically contains important information that helps you stay on track with your long-term weight loss goals.

I use this icon as a red flag. It draws your attention to common weight loss obstacles that can sidetrack your progress.

This icon identifies helpful information that increases your background knowledge about belly fat; however, this information isn't essential to your basic understanding of belly fat and how to effectively lose it. You can skip these bits of text without missing any information vital to your Belly Fat Diet plan.

Where to Go from Here

If you aren't quite sure what belly fat is and how to identify whether you have too much of it, I recommend starting in Chapter 2. If you already know all about belly fat, its health dangers, and your body type, skip to Chapter 4 to begin understanding the basic principles of the Belly Fat Diet. If you have already lost your belly but need help maintaining your results, head to Part IV to check out the customized maintenance plan to achieve a flat belly for life. No matter what topic you're interested in, you can flip through the table of contents or index to find what you're looking for.

One last thing: This book has a companion website at www.dummies.com/go/bellyfat. Here, you can find additional information that I wasn't able to squeeze into the book.

Part I

The 4-1-1 on Belly Fat and the Skinny on the Diet

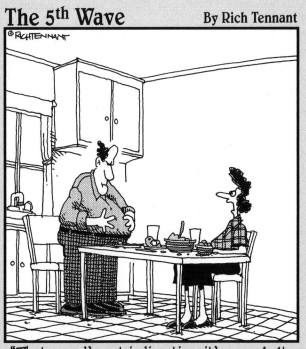

The 5th Wave   By Rich Tennant

"That sound's not indigestion, it's your belt screaming for mercy."

In this part . . .

Obesity rates are steadily climbing, and with them, so are the inches around our waistlines. In this part, I show you how to determine whether you have too much belly fat. I also explain exactly what belly fat is and why it's so dangerous to your health. Every body is different, and so is every belly. I help you gain an understanding of your unique body type so you can determine what led to your excess belly fat and figure out how to shed it for good! Finally, this part outlines the principles of the Belly Fat Diet plan, who it's appropriate for, and how it works, so you can start on your way to achieving the flat belly of your dreams (and keeping it that way!).

Chapter 1

Taking Control of Your Waistline and Your Health

*T*he next time you're in a public place, look around. What do you see? Almost everywhere you look you can see expanding waistlines and bellies protruding over belts. In fact, it's harder to spot a person at a healthy body weight than it is to find one who isn't. The United States is in the midst of a very real and very dangerous epidemic. According to the National Center for Health Statistics, 35.7 percent of Americans over the age of 20 are now obese, and another 33.3 percent are considered overweight. That's the majority of the country! And since 1980, the prevalence of obesity in children and teens has tripled! The scariest part is that so many people are now overweight that it almost appears normal and can be difficult to tell what a truly healthy body weight even is.

The excess weight that these people have is only half the battle, however. When folks are overweight and obese, they often have an increased amount of visceral fat, or belly fat, deep inside their abdominal walls. This fat is extremely dangerous to their health. In this chapter, I help you understand belly fat and get you on the right path to losing fat and weight the healthy (and permanent!) way.

Exploring the Dangers of Belly Fat

The concern about being overweight or obese isn't just about looks. Sure everyone wants to look great in a bathing suit, but your health is more

Throughout this book, I stress that your Belly Fat Diet plan isn't a diet that you go on and off. Instead, it's a lifestyle change. If you make quick, dramatic changes and then go right back to your old behaviors after a few weeks or months, you'll pack on the pounds all over again. Instead, I show you how to make gradual, practical, and doable lifestyle changes that you can implement for life.

Choosing a plan

As I mention earlier, no two bellies are exactly alike. So the same program to reduce belly fat and body weight won't work for everyone. I have designed three individualized programs in the Belly Fat Diet so you can follow the one that works best for you and helps you achieve your ultimate health and weight loss goals. These individualized programs make the Belly Fat Diet unique. The three plans you can choose from include the following:

✔ **The Turbo-Charged plan:** This plan is perfect for the person who wants quick and permanent results. It's also great for the person who has seen few or no results from prior failed dieting attempts. I like to call these folks "resistant dieters." It's the strictest of the meal plans, but it also provides you with the most rapid results.

✔ **The Moderation plan:** This plan is designed for the individual who wants consistent, steady weight loss without feeling terribly deprived. It provides a great balance of healthy nutrients that help you feel satisfied while shedding those unwanted pounds.

✔ **The Gradual-Change plan:** This plan works best for the individual who's at a healthy body weight but has a waist circumference that indicates a risk for health conditions associated with excess abdominal fat. It's also ideal for those who don't want to go headlong into weight loss or who have medical conditions that require them to lose weight more slowly. The Gradual-Change plan allows you to make small changes over time that lead to big results.

Chapter 7 outlines these plans in detail and provides tips on planning and preparing for your plan. Chapter 8 provides menus for each of the plans.

Getting some exercise

After you determine which Belly Fat Diet plan is most approximate for your situation, you need to start considering the best exercises to burn up belly fat. The truth is that you can lose belly fat and body weight through dietary changes alone. However, even when you're at an ideal body weight and have achieved an ideal waist circumference, exercise is still vital to your health. So regardless of whether you want to lose weight, you still need to add physical activity to your daily routine.

The Belly Fat Diet workout plan isn't difficult. You don't need any fancy equipment, and you don't have to join a gym. You just have to commit to putting a few minutes aside a few times a week to get active. In addition to the health benefits, getting active and staying active (in addition to following your Belly Fat Diet plan) will have you achieving your flat belly results quicker than you ever thought possible! And if you need more motivation, think of this: Multiple studies have shown that even without dietary changes, individuals who moderately exercise a few times per week showed significant losses in visceral fat.

The belly-blasting exercises outlined in Chapter 10 target belly fat, burning it up and toning your midsection for a sleeker, slimmer you. And I provide exercises for everyone. If you've never exercised before, the Phase 1 exercises can help you strengthen your midsection and reveal muscles you didn't even know you had. If you're an avid exerciser, the Phase 2 exercises challenge your muscles in new and unique ways, helping you achieve amazing results.

Preparing Meals to Flatten Your Belly

What good would a weight loss plan be if you couldn't eat foods that tasted good? Luckily, you don't have to worry about that issue with your Belly Fat Diet plan. The recipes you can make while losing weight will surprise you and have your taste buds rejoicing. And the best part is that they can be simple and easy to make! You don't need to purchase hundreds of ingredients you've never heard of or slave away over the stove for hours in order to make food that will help melt away belly fat. In Part III, I show you more than 40 recipes you can experiment with.

But first, before you get down to business with the recipes, you need to stock up your kitchen and pantry so you have everything you need on hand to cook for your Belly Fat Diet plan. Chapter 11 helps you tackle this preparation. I provide you with simple tips and tricks to make planning and preparing meals as quick and easy as possible. After all, if your meal plan is too time consuming or takes too much effort, it isn't practical and won't be something you stick with.

In Chapters 12 through 15, I provide you with tasty recipes for breakfast, lunch, dinner, and even snacks and desserts. That's right — the Belly Fat Diet plan encourages you to snack and have dessert! Does it get much better than that? All the recipes I include in this book taste great and are loaded with belly-shrinking nutrients. For instance, seasonings like cayenne pepper, cinnamon, and turmeric are proven belly fat fighters and are incorporated in great-tasting ways into many recipes. Nutrients like omega-3 fatty acids, monounsaturated fats, and fiber also find their way into many of the recipes throughout this book for a powerful fat-fighting punch!

Fighting Through Challenges to Achieve and Maintain a Flat Belly

Achieving your ideal body weight and a flat belly isn't always easy. You may hit some roadblocks along the way, which can cause you to get off track with your Belly Fat Diet plan. But don't worry. In Part IV, I help you identify the most common obstacles you may encounter. I also provide you with the tools you need to overcome these challenges so you can stay on track and reach your weight loss and health goals and keep the weight off permanently!

In Chapter 16, I outline some of the most common pitfalls and slip-ups that may occur as you follow your Belly Fat Diet plan. I show you the best ways to avoid these challenges in the first place and also how to fix them and get right back on track with your plan if they do occur.

A big concern for those trying to lose weight and improve health is eating away from home. Whether you're going out to your favorite restaurant for a nice meal or eating at Grandma's house for a holiday dinner, you have to make smart choices so you don't get off track. After all, you aren't going to eat every meal at home for the rest of your life. In Chapter 17, I outline strategies you can use to stay on track whenever you eat away from home.

Maintaining your losses long term

A huge struggle that many dieters face is maintaining their losses. Losing weight and belly fat mean nothing if you don't make those results permanent. Fad diets are particularly problematic in this regard. You lose weight quickly with these diets, but because you don't implement lifestyle changes, you go right back to old habits and regain the weight.

I don't want you to set yourself up for failure, so I devote an entire chapter to maintaining your weight loss and belly fat losses. In Chapter 18, I show you how to identify when you've reached your weight loss goals, how to know whether you've hit a true plateau, and what to do to break through. I also explain the strategies you can implement daily to make sure your results last permanently. I even include a detailed meal plan to help you maintain your weight as well as instructions on how to adjust if you notice your weight beginning to creep back up.

Chapter 2

The Truth about Belly Fat

In This Chapter

▶ Becoming familiar with your belly fat

▶ Determining the causes of increased belly fat

▶ Identifying the health risks associated with increased belly fat

Did you wake up one morning, start getting dressed, and notice your pants were a bit snug around the waistline? Or did you look in the mirror one day and notice a bit of a "spare tire" around your midsection and wonder where it came from? This extra layer can happen to anyone. Slowly over time, without your realizing it, poor dietary choices, increased stress, and certain lifestyle choices can make your body begin to store an increased amount of fat in and around your waistline. At first, this fat may just seem less desirable physically, and you may start dressing to bring less attention to your stomach. But the issues with belly fat can be far greater than that. In fact, your life may depend on reducing your belly fat and shrinking your waistline!

If you're holding onto excess fat in your abdomen, you can be putting yourself at a much greater risk for many diseases, including heart disease, stroke and even certain cancers. In fact, studies have shown that even if you're at a healthy body weight, storing a high percent of fat around your abdominal area can cause your disease risk to be just as high as that of someone who's overweight.

In this chapter, I show you how dietary and lifestyle habits, along with hormone changes, can affect your level of belly fat. I also explain exactly what belly fat is, how to identify if you have too much, and why this particular fat can be so detrimental to your health.

Judging the Jiggle: What Is Belly Fat?

Belly fat, also known as *visceral fat,* is considered the most harmful form of fat in your body. This type of fat has been linked with everything from insulin resistance, metabolic syndrome, heart disease, and type 2 diabetes to an increased risk for certain cancers.

You may be surprised to find out that even if you're relatively slim, you can still have a high percentage of body fat, particularly in your midsection. Also, if you're overweight, you need to understand that belly fat truly is different from other fat that's distributed to other areas of your body. In general, you need to work on reducing the fat all over your body, especially in your midsection, to decrease your risk of obesity-related diseases and disorders.

In this section, I take a deeper look into what belly fat is and why it's so bad for you.

Distinguishing belly fat from the other types of fat

Your body contains the following three types of fat:

- ✓ **Triglycerides:** This type of fat circulates in your bloodstream. It makes up about 95 percent of the fat within your body.

- ✓ **Subcutaneous fat:** This fat is the layer that lies directly below the skin's surface, between the skin and the abdominal wall.

- ✓ **Visceral fat:** Otherwise known as the dangerous belly fat, visceral fat is the kind located deep within your belly.

Visceral fat hangs beneath the muscles in your stomach. This placement is what makes the fat so damaging to your health. Because this fat is so close to your internal organs, it becomes their best energy source. Think about it this way: If you could buy food from the corner store or the store clear across town, which would you pick? The nearby corner store, of course! Your body thinks in the same way. Why would it pull fat stores from subcutaneous fat in your arms if it can get energy right next door in your abdomen? The visceral fat provides a constant, steady stream of energy to your internal organs, which is where the major health risks lie (see the upcoming section "What belly fat does to your body" for details).

You're probably wondering how you can tell what part of your belly is subcutaneous fat and what part is visceral fat. As you can see in Figure 2-1, the subcutaneous fat is the outermost layer of fat; it's the fat you can pinch between your fingers. This layer sits on top of the abdominal muscle tissue. Below the muscle tissue, where you can't see with your eyes or pinch with your fingers, lays the visceral fat. As you can see in this figure, the visceral fat surrounds all the organs in the abdominal cavity.

If you can pinch a good amount of subcutaneous fat, chances are you have a large amount of visceral fat lurking underneath your abdominal muscles.

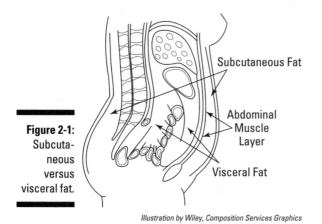

Figure 2-1:
Subcuta-
neous
versus
visceral fat.

Illustration by Wiley, Composition Services Graphics

What belly fat does to your body

It was once thought that fat was just a passive substance; folks thought it just hung around as stored energy. But, in fact, fat is more active than first thought. The latest research shows that fat cells, including both subcutaneous and visceral fat cells, are metabolically active, secreting hormones and chemicals that can impact every organ in your body. When you're at an ideal weight, the hormones and chemicals secreted by fat cells are actually healthy. They do a number of positive things, such as regulate insulin, help to regulate appetite by allowing you to feel satisfied after eating, and even help burn stored fat.

The problem arises when you have more and larger fat cells than normal, which often occurs in an individual who's overweight. These larger fat cells produce more hormones and chemicals than your body needs, which can impact your health over time and place you at risk for diseases like diabetes, stroke, heart attack, and even certain cancers.

 What makes visceral fat cells more dangerous than other fat cells is that they're thought to produce an even greater amount of harmful chemicals, such as excessive hormones and toxins. And because this fat is so close to all your organs, especially the liver, it can be damaging to all your body's systems.

For example, here's how this fat can affect your liver: After blood circulates through the visceral fat, it's directly transported to the liver. The dangerous substances produced by the visceral fat are constantly being rapidly transported to your liver throughout the day (unlike subcutaneous fat stores in your legs and arms, which wait to be called on for energy before releasing fat stores and their byproducts). This increased fat processing in the liver can lead to the development of fatty liver disease and elevated LDL cholesterol levels (the "lousy," or damaging cholesterol).

The Causes of Belly Fat Accumulation

Does it seem like you're hearing more and more about belly fat and its effects on health in the news lately? The reason is not only because we're finding stronger correlations between belly fat and health risks. It's also because, as a whole, the folks in this country are getting heavier and their bellies are expanding rapidly.

Where is this obesity epidemic coming from? Belly fat doesn't just come from one place or one cause. In fact, a number of reasons cause you to start accumulating visceral fat. Surprisingly, they aren't all due to just what you put in your mouth (although that can be part of it)! Your lifestyle, stress level, hormones, and age all play a role in belly fat accumulation.

In the following sections, I break down some of the most common triggers of belly fat, including why they cause fat accumulation and what you can do about it.

The only way to achieve a flat belly is to know exactly what's stopping you from having one and how to go about fixing it!

Physiological causes

Numerous hormones cycle through your body every day. Some of these hormones, when out of balance, trigger your body to begin storing fat, especially in your belly, leading to an increase in both subcutaneous fat and visceral fat. In the following sections, I discuss the biggest hormone culprits of belly fat, how they work, and how you can get them to stop storing fat in your belly.

Insulin

Whenever you eat, the food you consume is broken down in your digestive system into small particles that can be used for energy. Carbohydrates are broken down first in the stomach into the simple sugar known as glucose. *Glucose* is actually the primary source of energy for all the cells in your body. After food has been broken down into glucose, it's absorbed into the bloodstream where it causes a rise in blood sugar levels. *Insulin* is a hormone secreted by the pancreas that allows the cells in your body to take glucose from the bloodstream (as well as glucose stored in the liver, muscles, and fat tissue) for energy.

I like to use this analogy to picture how insulin works: Insulin is the "taxi," glucose is the "passenger," and your body's cells are the "stores" the "passenger" wants to go to. The taxi (insulin) picks up the passenger (glucose) and drives it to the store (cell), where it can then be used for energy immediately or stocked on the store shelves for later use.

When you eat a meal that's converted into glucose (or sugar) quickly, your body experiences a rapid rise in blood glucose followed by a rapid rise in insulin. At this point, the insulin is transporting more and more sugar rapidly into your body's cells. Because you don't need all this energy right away, the extra is stocked away as fat stores for when energy is needed in the future. The problem is that if you store too much of this extra energy and never burn it, you end up with larger and larger fat stores. Because much of this excess energy is transported to cells in the abdomen, you can start to see an increase in abdominal fat stores.

Insulin reacts differently depending on the foods you choose to eat. Foods rich in refined carbohydrates and simple sugars, such as white bread, white rice, and sugary cereals, cause a rapid rise in blood sugar and insulin levels, leading to an increase in belly fat storage. On the other hand, foods high in protein, healthy fats, and fiber slow the breakdown of sugar into the blood- stream, helping blood sugar levels remain fairly consistent during the day and preventing spikes in insulin. So throughout this book, I focus on helping you choose high-fiber whole grains, lean proteins, and healthy fats to promote steady levels of sugar and insulin in your bloodstream, helping to prevent increased storage of belly fat.

Stress hormones

Stress plays a significant role in your control of belly fat. So in order to be successful with your Belly Fat Diet plan and get flat abs once and for all, you must get your stress levels under control.

When you're under stress, your body increases the production of adrenaline, which signals fat cells to release their stores of fatty acids into the body where they're used as energy. This release occurs to provide you with a sudden burst in energy (which is called the *fight or flight response*) to help you fight off or run away from a physical stress. This response was great in the days of the Stone Age when you had to escape from the clutches of a hungry beast or fight a fellow caveman for food, but today's stress mostly comes from work deadlines, long commutes, and overscheduled calendars.

Because your stress occurs due to mental stressors rather than physical stressors, the free fatty acids that are released aren't burned off as energy. As a result, your adrenal glands release the hormone cortisol to help collect and store the unused fatty acids. This help from the cortisol wouldn't be so bad if the cortisol brought the stray fats back to their original homes. However, cortisol loves your abdomen, so it tends to deposit fat there versus in other body cells. So the more often you're stressed, the more this stress response occurs and the more fat is mobilized and deposited into your belly.

Don't stress out over stressing out though. By performing some of the stress management techniques that I cover in Chapter 5, you can reduce your stress and lose that gut.

Lifestyle factors

Several lifestyle factors are contributing to this country's ever-growing weights and waistlines. Schedules are getting busier, stress levels are getting higher, and folks aren't taking the time to properly care for their bodies and minds.

In the upcoming sections, I discuss some of the most common lifestyle factors that increase belly fat. These sections can help you identify the factors that may be holding you back from achieving the flat belly of your dreams.

Societal pressures

When the economy takes a dive, stress levels skyrocket. Those who are out of work suffer the stresses of trying to make ends meet, pay the bills with limited funds, and search for new employment. Those lucky enough to have work may be putting in longer hours with company cutbacks or struggling with long commutes, tight deadlines, and difficult bosses. These daily work and financial stressors lead to the release of the stress hormones cortisol and adrenaline over and over, mobilizing more and more fat into the abdomen. (Check out the earlier section "Stress hormones" for details.)

No matter what the economy is like, however, modern-day living is fast-paced. If you look around at your friends, family, or even your kids, you may notice that they're always rushing to get from one place to the next because they're constantly scheduled for the next work or social event, meeting, or sporting practice. It may feel as though you can never just sit and relax for a minute.

This overscheduling not only increases your stress levels (especially when you're running late), but it also leaves little time to properly care for yourself. You may find you have so much on your to-do list that you struggle to find the time to fit in any exercise or prepare nutritious food. These factors lead to a mostly sedentary lifestyle filled with quick convenience foods that may include belly-busting choices like fast food, frozen meals, or takeout.

Worst of all, these stress-inducing behaviors can start to impact your sleep schedule. You may stay up late with racing thoughts about paying the bills, or you may stay up until 1 a.m. finishing a report for work. Whatever the reason, inadequate sleep not only causes an increased production of the stress hormones I discuss earlier, but it can also start to slow your metabolism and even cause you to feel hungrier. These are all behaviors that can make attaining a flat belly quite difficult.

Poor food choices that can increase belly fat

The food choices you make can either help or hurt your efforts to attain a flat stomach. By transitioning away from belly-bloating foods and instead consuming the majority of your meals and snacks from belly-flattening foods, you can get on track to a smaller waistline and a healthier life. Consider the following eating practices that are poor choices for your midsection:

- ✔ **Consuming refined carbohydrates:** Grains, breads, pastas, and cereals are a common component to many meals, and depending on the variety you choose, you could be sabotaging your efforts to flatten your belly. Refined carbohydrates, such as white pasta and white bread, are quickly converted into glucose in your body, spiking insulin levels and setting off the insulin response that stores abdominal fat (refer to the earlier section "Insulin" for more on this process).

  Instead of these refined products, choose whole grains, which are less processed, leaving more of the outer layers of grain. When choosing a grain product, look to see whether the package says it's 100 percent whole grain or whether it has a whole grain, such as whole wheat or oat, listed as the first ingredient. Chapter 6 provides information on selecting whole grains.

- ✔ **Opting for unhealthy fats:** People often have a misconception that eating fats translates to getting fat. Luckily, the opposite is true! You just have to choose the right fats. Certain fats — especially monounsaturated fats (found in olive oil, nuts, and seeds) and omega-3 fatty acids (found in walnuts and fish) — have actually been shown to help reduce abdominal fat. However, less healthy choices, such as the saturated fat found in high-fat animal products, have been found to store themselves as fat deposits more than other forms of fat.

  One study done by Johns Hopkins University found that the quantity of saturated fat in your diet may be directly proportional to the amount of fat surrounding your abdomen. So aim to choose plant-based fats over animal fats for a leaner, flatter, and sexier midsection.

- ✔ **Downing too many fluid calories:** Sure they may seem harmless, but fluid calories may have a serious impact on your belly. These calories come from drinks mainly made up of sugar (sodas or juices) or saturated fats (creamers in coffee and full-fat milk in specialty coffee drinks). Not only can these drinks trigger an increased insulin response, leading to increased fat storage, but they also leave you feeling unsatisfied. They don't keep you full in the same way calories from solid foods do. Research shows that fluid calories don't provide the same level of satiety as foods, which require you to chew them.

✔ **Low HDL cholesterol levels:** HDL, also known as the "healthy" cholesterol, levels for men should be greater than 45 mg/dL. They should be 50 mg/dL or above for women.

✔ **Elevated blood pressure levels:** Normal blood pressure is considered 120/80 mmHg.

✔ **Elevated fasting blood sugar:** Normal fasting blood sugar is measured as 80 mg/dL–100 mg/dL.

Cardiovascular disease

Research has shown that visceral fat cells in the abdomen can produce proteins that can be damaging to the body in many ways. One of the proteins produced by these cells constricts blood vessels, causing blood pressure to rise. Additional proteins can trigger low levels of chronic inflammation, which can promote clogging of arteries, leading to increased risk for heart attack and stroke.

Increased cancer risk

Increased belly fat can increase cancer risk in both men and women of all ages, but the risk may be even higher for postmenopausal women. After menopause, estrogen production dwindles in the ovaries, leaving the fat tissue to become the main source of this hormone. The larger the fat cells and the more fat cells present, the more hormone that's produced.

Because women who are overweight have more fat cells (and bigger fat cells) than women of a normal body weight, they have increased levels of estrogen circulating throughout their bodies. This extra level of estrogen can promote the growth of tumors in the breast.

Men aren't in the clear though. The extra hormone levels circulating from excessive fat tissue can increase the risk of colorectal cancer in both men and women.

Chapter 3

Step Away from the Scale: Examining Your Health and Body Type

. . . .

In This Chapter

▶ Calculating your BMI and other health-related numbers

▶ Identifying your body type and working with it

. . . .

*I*n the same way you may research your family medical history to determine whether you're at risk for certain health conditions, you also need to research your current health and physical body type to identify whether your body size, composition, and proportions are increasing your risk for future medical complications. After all, if you solely focus on your weight on the scale, you may be missing the bigger picture.

For instance, someone who is of a normal weight can still have a large amount of visceral fat, in some instances, more than another person who is slightly overweight. And the same goes for someone who's "overweight" on a scale. That person may have a large amount of muscle mass or a heavy bone structure, but he may have a low percentage of body fat.

Think about an NFL football player. If you were to just look at his body weight on the scale versus his height, without seeing him, it may seem as though he is overweight or even obese. However, if you were to just look at him with the naked eye, he may look trim and toned. This seeming discrepancy is because a highly conditioned athlete has a large amount of muscle, which weighs more on the scale. The number on the scale tells nothing of his amount of visceral fat or risk for medical complications.

The point is this: Belly fat can be dangerous to your health, and you don't have to be overweight to have too large a percentage of it. You have to consider the whole picture no matter what your scale says. So in this chapter, I show you how to calculate your body's numbers, including body mass index (BMI), waist-to-hip ratio, and health levels like cholesterol, blood pressure, and blood glucose. Finally, I help you determine exactly what body type category you fall into so you can be on your way to losing that stubborn belly fat for good!

Determining Your Body's Health Numbers

Relying solely on your scale or mirror to determine whether you're healthy isn't a good idea. Neither of these methods examines how much visceral fat you have and how it may create complications down the road. Although you don't want to disregard the scale entirely, you do want to be aware that it's not telling you the whole story. Other numbers — such as your BMI, waist-to-hip ratio, and your cholesterol, blood pressure, and blood glucose — are much more important for you to focus on. I explain each of these numbers and how to calculate and analyze them in the following sections.

Assessing your BMI

Your body mass index (BMI) is a formula that takes into account your height versus your weight to determine whether you're at a healthy weight. Although BMI can be a fairly reliable indicator of body fat in most people, some exceptions exist. For instance, the NFL player (or other top athlete) with a very high level of muscle mass may have an elevated BMI without actually having a high level of body fat.

Although BMI doesn't measure body fat directly, research has indicated that it does correspond with direct measures of body fat, which include underwater weighing and dual-energy X-ray absorptiometry (DXA). Because it isn't practical for you or your regular clinician to weigh you underwater or perform a DXA scan, BMI is an easy, inexpensive way to see whether you're overweight or have a high percentage of body fat.

To determine your BMI, use the chart in Figure 3-1. The numbers on the left-hand side correlate with your height in inches. The numbers within the chart correlate with your body weight in pounds. To determine your BMI, find your height in inches, and then move your finger to the right until you reach your approximate weight in pounds. After you find where your height and weight intersect, move your finger upward to the top of the chart to see what your BMI is. For instance, if you are 67 inches in height and weigh 185 pounds, your BMI is 29. If your exact weight isn't listed, simply go to the closest one.

You can also use an online BMI calculator to get your exact BMI. The calculator on the Centers for Disease Control and Prevention (CDC) website is reliable and easy to find. Simply go to www.cdc.gov and search for BMI calculator in the search box on the homepage. You may be able to find a BMI calculator app for your smartphone or tablet as well.

BMI (kg/m^2)	19	20	21	22	23	24	25	26	27	28	29	30	35	40
Height (in.)	Weight (lb.)													
58	91	96	100	105	110	115	119	124	129	134	138	143	167	191
59	94	99	104	109	114	119	124	128	133	138	143	148	173	198
60	97	102	107	112	118	123	128	133	138	143	148	153	179	204
61	100	106	111	116	122	127	132	137	143	148	153	158	185	211
62	104	109	115	120	126	131	136	142	147	153	158	164	191	218
63	107	113	118	124	130	135	141	146	152	158	163	169	197	225
64	110	116	122	128	134	140	145	151	157	163	169	174	204	232
65	114	120	126	132	138	144	150	156	162	168	174	180	210	240
66	118	124	130	136	142	148	155	161	167	173	179	186	216	247
67	121	127	134	140	146	153	159	166	172	178	185	191	223	255
68	125	131	138	144	151	158	164	171	177	184	190	197	230	262
69	128	135	142	149	155	162	169	176	182	189	196	203	236	270
70	132	139	146	153	160	167	174	181	188	195	202	207	243	278
71	136	143	150	157	165	172	179	186	193	200	208	215	250	286
72	140	147	154	162	169	177	184	191	199	206	213	221	258	294
73	144	151	159	166	174	182	189	197	204	212	219	227	265	302
74	148	155	163	171	179	186	194	202	210	218	225	233	272	311
75	152	160	168	176	184	192	200	208	216	224	232	240	279	319
76	156	164	172	180	189	197	205	213	221	230	238	246	287	328

Figure 3-1:
A BMI
chart.

After you've determined your waist-to-hip ratio, use Table 3-2 to check your level of risk.

Table 3-2	Waist-to-Hip Ratio and Risk	
Male Waist-to-Hip Ratio	*Female Waist-to-Hip Ratio*	*Health Risk*
0.95 or below	0.80 or below	Low risk
0.96–1.0	0.81–0.85	Moderate risk
1.0+	0.85+	High risk

Checking your cholesterol, blood pressure, and blood glucose levels

Besides knowing your external size numbers, such as your BMI and waist-to-hip ratio (discussed earlier in the chapter), you also want to know your internal numbers when evaluating your health risk. These numbers include your cholesterol, blood pressure, and blood glucose levels. If you have an increased amount of belly fat, you may be more at risk for diseases like type 2 diabetes and heart disease. To assess your risk and start taking action to improve your health, schedule an appointment with your physician to determine your cholesterol, blood pressure, and blood glucose levels. I discuss each in detail in the following sections.

Cholesterol

Cholesterol is a waxy, fatlike substance produced by the liver and found in all the body's cells. It's also found in many of the foods you eat. Cholesterol is needed to make vitamin D as well as many hormones. In your body, substances called *lipoproteins* package and transport cholesterol to your cells.

Two kinds of lipoproteins carry cholesterol in your body: *High-density lipoproteins* (HDL) and *low-density lipoproteins* (LDL). Having a healthy ratio of these lipoproteins is important to your health.

- **HDL cholesterol:** Otherwise known as the "happy" or good cholesterol, HDL cholesterol is the one you want to have a high amount of. This form of cholesterol is like a garbage truck, picking up and transporting cholesterol back to the liver. The liver then removes the cholesterol from your body.

- **LDL cholesterol:** This cholesterol, referred to as "lousy" or bad cholesterol, is the one you want to have less of. High levels of this cholesterol can lead to a buildup of cholesterol in your arteries, which over time may lead to deadly blockages. Because elevated levels of cholesterol may increase your risk of heart disease, you need to monitor your levels.

In addition to knowing your levels of HDL and LDL cholesterol, you also want to assess the following two additional blood lipids:

- ✔ **Total cholesterol:** *Total cholesterol* is a measurement of HDL cholesterol, LDL cholesterol, and other lipid components. Elevated total cholesterol levels are also an indicator of heart disease, so you want to aim to keep this level within an optimum range.

- ✔ **Triglycerides:** *Triglycerides* are the fats flowing through your bloodstream from the food you eat. Elevated levels of triglycerides are linked with an increased risk of heart disease as well as type 2 diabetes, so it's essential to lower elevated triglyceride levels.

You should aim to have your levels of total cholesterol, LDL, HDL, and triglycerides checked annually or more often if elevated. Your doctor checks your cholesterol by taking a fasting blood sample. Refer to Table 3-3 to see what your cholesterol levels should be.

Table 3-3	Cholesterol Levels and Their Risks	
Blood Lipid	*Range*	*Risk Category*
Total cholesterol	<170 mg/dL	Very Low
	<200 mg/dL	Low
	200–239 mg/dL	Moderately high
	240 mg/dL or higher	High
LDL cholesterol	<100 mg/dL	Very Low
	100–129 mg/dL	Low
	130–159 mg/dL	Borderline high
	160–189 mg/dL	High
	190 mg/dL or higher	Very high
HDL cholesterol	<40 mg/dL (men)	High
	<50 mg/dL (women)	High
	40–59 mg/dL (men)	Low
	50–59 mg/dL (women)	Low
	>60 mg/dL (men and women)	Very Low
Triglycerides	<150 mg/dL	Low
	150–199 mg/dL	Moderate
	200–499 mg/dL	High
	500 mg/dL or higher	Very high

Blood pressure

Blood pressure is just what it sounds like: It's the measurement of the blood's force against the wall of the arteries. Two numbers make up your blood pressure: systolic pressure and diastolic pressure. *Systolic pressure* is a measurement taken as the heart beats, whereas the *diastolic pressure* is the measurement as the heart relaxes in between beats. The measurement is written as the systolic number over the diastolic number.

Elevated blood pressure (also known as *hypertension*), if not controlled, can increase risk for heart disease, stroke, and even kidney disease. So it's important to have your blood pressure checked at least once annually and more often if elevated.

Table 3-4 shows the categories for blood pressure in adults. The systolic and diastolic measurements are considered separately, so it's important to note that if one number is normal and the other is elevated, you're still at an increased risk.

Table 3-4	Categories of Blood Pressure in Adults
Category	*Blood Pressure (Systolic or Diastolic)*
Normal	<120 mmHg or <80 mmHg
Pre-hypertension	120–139 mmHg or 80–89 mmHg
Stage 1 hypertension	140–159 mmHg or 90–99 mmHg
Stage 2 hypertension	160 mmHg or above or 100 mmHg or above

Source: National Heart, Lung, and Blood Institute

Blood sugar

Elevated blood sugar (glucose) is a sign of insulin resistance, a precursor to type 2 diabetes. High amounts of glucose in the bloodstream can lead to serious health consequences, including diabetes, heart disease, and kidney disease.

Having your blood glucose checked on a regular basis is key to preventing and controlling diabetes. If your blood glucose is found to be elevated, dietary changes, exercise, and decreasing belly fat have been shown to help reverse insulin resistance and lower blood glucose levels. Have your glucose levels checked annually or more regularly if they're elevated. Your doctor checks your blood sugar levels by taking a fasting blood sample. Table 3-5 shows the normal range for blood glucose when fasting.

Table 3-5	Fasting Blood Glucose Levels
Glucose Levels	*Category*
Normal	70–99 mg/dL
Pre-diabetic levels	100–126 mg/dL
Diabetic levels	>126 mg/dL

Pulling the info together: Determining your risk for health complications

After you've assessed your BMI, waist circumference, waist-to-hip ratio, blood pressure, and blood levels of cholesterol and blood sugar (all discussed earlier in the chapter), you can determine your risk of health consequences like heart disease and diabetes. Knowing which of these areas is placing you at risk allows you to begin addressing these areas and start making changes to improve your levels and your health.

To determine your current health risk level, count up the number of health assessment levels that are above normal, including your BMI, waist circumference, waist-to-hip ratio, total cholesterol, LDL-cholesterol, HDL-cholesterol, triglycerides, blood pressure, and blood sugar levels. Then use Table 3-6 to see which category you fall into.

As you begin following your Belly Fat Diet, revamping your meal plan, making healthy lifestyle changes, and decreasing your waistline, these levels will begin to improve, and you can decrease your health risks dramatically.

Table 3-6	Health Assessment Levels
Number of Health Assessment Levels Above Normal	*Health Risk*
0	Low
1–2	Moderate
3–4	High
5 or more	Very high

Identifying Your Body Type

If you look at the people around you, you'll notice many different body shapes. Some people tend to carry weight in their legs and hips, some hold more weight in their stomachs, and still others tend to gain weight all over. You'll also notice that almost any person who's above an ideal weight carries at least some excess weight in the belly. However, how this excess weight makes its way to the belly varies depending on the person, his genetics, and his situation.

It's important to understand what body type you are in order to start losing your belly fat once and for all. In the following sections, I show you the most common body types and how to deal with your type.

Apple versus pear type

An *apple-shaped* person is someone who holds a large amount of fat in the abdomen, has a large waist, and has generally slimmer legs and arms. If you're an apple-shaped person, you tend to have a large amount of visceral fat, increasing your risk for heart disease.

A *pear-shaped* body type tends to have a smaller waist with larger hips and legs. Although an overweight pear-shaped person may still have higher than ideal levels of visceral fat, her risk for heart disease tends to be lower because she stores more fat in her extremities. As a result, she has less toxic fat surrounding her organs and producing dangerous hormones and byproducts. You can see what each of these body shapes looks like in Figure 3-3.

Although it's important for every body type to maintain a healthy weight and lose abdominal fat, it's even more critical for you to lose weight to prevent future disease risks if you're an apple-shaped type. The Belly Fat Diet plan is perfect for you and your type, because the weight loss in this plan is specifically geared toward losing your excessive belly fat.

Genetically you may always have thinner arms and legs when compared to your midsection, but, if you're an apple shape, it's critical you strive to keep your waist circumference below the recommended levels (which are less than 35 inches in women and less than 40 inches in men).

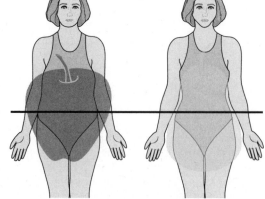

Figure 3-3:
Apple-
versus
pear-
shaped
body types.

Illustration by Wiley, Composition Services Graphics

Slim type

The slim type can be a surprisingly dangerous type. If you're a slim person and at a normal weight for your height, you may not think you have excessive abdominal fat. The truth is that even slim people can have too high a percentage of visceral fat, putting them at risk for complications associated with this excess weight around the middle.

If you're already at or close to an ideal weight, be sure to assess your body proportions. Take out a tape measure and determine your waist-to-hip ratio (see the earlier section "Measuring your waist circumference and waist-to-hip ratio") and use Table 3-2 to see whether you're at risk. If you're at risk even though you're already thin, following the Belly Fat Diet plan can be beneficial to you because it can help you reduce body fat in your abdominal area, helping to improve your waist-to-hip ratio.

After-pregnancy type

If you just had a new baby and are stressing over your bulging stomach, take heart. It can take time after delivery for your belly to go back to normal. Remember that not only is normal weight gain associated with pregnancy, but stomach muscles have been stretched and expanded for nine months. The Belly Fat Diet can help you return to your pre-baby body in an appropriate amount of time.

Even though the Belly Fat Diet can be beneficial to after-pregnancy types, you must be aware of some precautions:

✔ **If you just gave birth and are breastfeeding, don't reduce your food intake too much or lose weight too quickly.** Doing so can reduce your milk production for your baby. Allow yourself time to establish a breastfeeding schedule with your baby before implementing a weight loss routine. Make sure to consult your physician before making changes to your diet while breastfeeding. I generally recommend waiting between six to eight weeks after delivery before starting a weight loss plan.

Choosing the belly-burning foods recommended in the Belly Fat Diet is terrific for both you and your baby, because they're packed with essential nutrients. When choosing a Belly Fat Diet plan, follow the Gradual-Change plan, which provides adequate calories to prevent a decrease in milk production. (See Chapter 7 for details.)

✔ **If you just had a baby but aren't breastfeeding, you can aim for a faster rate of weight loss, but you must have realistic expectations.** A new baby brings along multiple challenges, such as lack of sleep, decreased meal planning, and even stress-related eating. To help you maximize your Belly Fat Diet efforts, focus on behaviors other than just

First Things First: Getting an Overview of the Belly Fat Diet

Visceral fat is true fat in the abdomen. It causes your waistline to expand over time, and it can have dangerous health implications. This type of fat isn't gained or lost overnight. You must transition yourself to a belly-flattening lifestyle to gradually lose visceral fat and keep it off for good. In this section, I show you the most basic ideas that the Belly Fat Diet implements to eliminate visceral fat around your midsection.

Treating the plan as a lifestyle, not another diet

The Belly Fat Diet isn't really a diet. In fact, I strongly dislike the word "diet." Why? Because to me it represents something you're going to go "on" and then go "off," reverting to the old habits that caused you to gain weight in the first place. So from now on, don't think of this plan as a diet; think of it as the Belly Fat Lifestyle.

Lifestyle changes are just what they sound like — changes you make and keep for life. This little secret of the Belly Fat Diet sets it apart from most of the other diets out there. This diet isn't a short-term fix. In other words, you don't keep a one-month commitment and go back to your old habits. If you just want to drop weight quickly in a few weeks (and then regain it all plus more the next month), this plan isn't for you.

If you start out making too many changes at once or being too restrictive, you may find that the changes become almost impossible to stick with, causing you to go back to your old habits. So slow and steady always wins the race. If you start out of the gate sprinting, you'll burn out before you reach the finish line. Rather than burning out, I want you to gradually adjust your eating habits to promote health along with weight loss for life. What good does it do if you lose 20 pounds this month just to gain it back plus more next month? You're better off taking three months to lose 20 pounds if that means you can stick with the changes you have made and can keep that weight off for good.

If you follow the Belly Fat Diet the way it's designed, you aren't going to feel restricted, and you aren't going to give up all your favorite foods permanently. However, you are going to figure out how to make simple changes to your current diet that will provide you with fantastic, long-term results!

Fighting belly fat by eating the right foods

As you transition into a belly-flattening lifestyle, you need to make a few key dietary changes. You can make these changes gradually over time. The more regularly you stick with these changes, the better your results. The following are some general guidelines to follow:

- ✔ **Consume an adequate amount of fiber per day.** Aim for a minimum of 30 grams of fiber daily. Fiber provides you with a sense of satiety without any calories. Increasing your fiber intake helps stabilize blood sugar, control cravings, and prevent overeating — all things that help promote weight loss and flatten your belly.

- ✔ **Consume an adequate amount of healthy fat each day.** Don't worry. Dietary fat doesn't equal belly fat. In fact, it's actually the opposite! Healthy fats in the diet, mainly monounsaturated fats and omega-3 fatty acids, have been shown to help promote a decrease in belly fat. But portion control is still key here. Even though these fats are healthy, they're still rich in calories. So make sure to stick within your recommended fat servings per day, which is outlined in the meal plan guidelines in Chapter 7.

- ✔ **Consume an adequate amount of lean protein.** Lean proteins — which include animal proteins like chicken breast and fish as well as plant-based proteins like tofu and beans — are what make up the majority of your muscle. Without enough dietary protein each day, you may begin to lose muscle mass as you lose weight, which can slow your metabolism. Protein, like fats and fiber, is a nutrient that is slowly digested, helping to regulate appetite and control hunger. I recommend including a source of lean protein at each meal to help you feel satisfied and avoid cravings.

- ✔ **Increase your intake of whole fruits and vegetables.** Vegetables and fruits are not only rich in filling fiber, but they're also loaded with antioxidants and phytochemicals. Certain antioxidants, such as vitamin C, have been linked with reducing belly fat by helping to regulate stress hormones in the body. They're also rich in minerals like potassium, which helps to expel excess water from the body, slimming the belly.

- ✔ **Drink up!** Drinking at least 8 cups of water per day helps keep you hydrated, gives you increased energy, and helps prevent water retention that can bloat your belly. Drinking adequate amounts of fluid also helps with appetite regulation, promoting weight loss.

Keep in mind that some foods can cause belly bloat. This bloat can come on overnight or even after eating just one meal full of belly-bloating foods. Bloat isn't true belly fat, but it can distend your stomach, making your waistline appear larger. Some foods have an instant belly-bloating effect due to their capability to introduce added gasses to the body, causing stomach distension.

Other foods instantly bloat the belly by causing your body to hold on to fluid, giving you that puffy look and feel.

You especially want to avoid belly bloat when you're trying to look your best, such as for an upcoming event like a wedding or party.

Some instant belly-bloating foods to avoid include the following:

- **Carbonated beverages:** These gassy drinks fill your belly with air, causing your stomach to look distended and bloated. Instead, drink water or calorie-free beverages that are rich in antioxidants, such as unsweetened green tea with a squeeze of fresh lemon.

- **Gassy vegetables:** Vegetables that increase gas production, such as cabbage, broccoli, and Brussels sprouts, can cause your stomach to look and feel distended due to a buildup of gas in the gastrointestinal (GI) tract. But you don't have to give up these vegetables entirely. If you slowly increase your portions of these vegetables over the course of a few weeks, versus all at once, it allows your body to adjust to them, helping to produce less gas during digestion. When eating these gassier options, also be sure to cook them thoroughly (raw vegetables can produce even more gas).

- **Gum:** Chewing gum may trigger you to swallow air, which can bloat your belly and cause it to look distended. And even though sugar-free gum may sound like a better choice, it actually contains a high amount of sugar alcohols. These alcohols are only partially digested in your body, so they can lead to gas, bloating, and GI upset — all things that cause your belly to look and feel bloated. If you do want to chew gum, try to limit yourself to only one or two pieces per day.

- **High-sugar drinks:** Drinking a large amount of simple sugars through drinks can lead to spikes in insulin levels. Because an increase in insulin promotes increased fat storage in the abdominal area, you want to avoid these high-sugar drinks. Instead, choose calorie-free beverages, such as water or unsweetened green tea.

  Or try my favorite trick for a lightly flavored, belly-slimming beverage: Freeze 100 percent fruit juice in an ice cube tray. After the juice cubes are frozen, you can pop one into 12 ounces of water. The juice will slowly melt, infusing the water with all-natural flavor with none of the bloat and only a small number of calories.

- **Trans fats:** Studies have shown that the intake of trans fats can promote an increase in belly fat. So carefully screen your foods by looking for the words "partially-hydrogenated oil" in the ingredient list. If you see this term, the food you're selecting contains a source of trans fats. It's best to avoid foods with trans fats or partially-hydrogenated oils. Foods most likely to contain these belly-busting ingredients include baked goods and pastries, commercially fried foods, snack foods like chips and microwave popcorn, and some instant coffee drinks.

Be sure to look at the ingredient list, not just the number of grams of trans fats listed on the Nutrition Facts Panel. Foods can list 0 grams of trans fats if they contain less than half a gram per serving. Less than half a gram sounds fairly harmless, but if you eat multiple servings, you're still taking in a significant source of trans fats. In fact, research has shown that as little as 2 grams of trans fats can be detrimental to your health, so read those ingredient lists carefully!

✔ **White flour:** Foods that list white flour or enriched flour as the first ingredient are mainly made up of refined carbohydrates. These carbs are digested very quickly, causing spikes in both insulin and blood sugar levels, promoting increased fat storage in the abdominal area. Choose whole-grain options instead. Make sure the first ingredient listed is a whole grain, such as oats or whole wheat.

Be cautious when reading labels. Even if a label says "enriched wheat flour" or "wheat flour," it's still a refined flour. You want to see the word "whole" in front of the ingredient, such as "whole-wheat flour," to ensure you're getting a true whole grain.

Knowing that slip-ups are part of the process

When transitioning to a belly-flattening lifestyle, you want to keep in mind that slip-ups are unavoidable. No one is perfect with food intake every day (and those who are tend to burn themselves out over time, which can lead to even more poor food choices). So if you get off track at times, just relax. You won't undo all your hard work with just one meal or in just one day. Simply investigate why this slip-up occurred (maybe you waited too long to eat and caused a poor food choice, for example), and then pick right back up where you left off.

Making lifestyle changes takes time and hard work, but if you pull yourself back together when you get a bit sidetracked, you can achieve your goals not only for a short period of time, but for life!

I want you to be successful for life (and I'm sure you do too!). That's why I help you come up with belly-friendly substitutes for many of your favorite junk foods, such as pizza, french fries, and desserts. You can't deprive yourself. Deprivation doesn't work; it just leads to cravings, hunger, and eventually binges on the wrong foods. Instead, I show you how any food can be adjusted just a little to make it a belly-friendly treat! Check out Chapter 15 for a whole chapter of recipes for satisfying snacks and desserts.

Why the Belly Fat Diet Works

I always like to know why I'm doing something and how it works, and you may feel the same way. So in this section, I explain the main reasons that the Belly Fat Diet works and allows you to not only lose weight but also keep it off permanently!

How it reduces insulin response

Have you tried to lose weight before but struggled with constant hunger and cravings, which made it impossible to continue your diet? If so, you have experienced cravings as a result of *insulin response,* which is the insulin/blood sugar cycle that occurs after eating and is even stronger after eating carbohydrate-laden foods.

Here's how this response works: When you eat a food, especially a food rich in carbohydrates, your body converts it into sugar (glucose) for energy. Insulin transports glucose from the bloodstream into the cells for energy. So when you eat foods that cause a spike in blood sugar, you experience a spike in insulin levels as the insulin rushes into your bloodstream to transport the excess sugar into your body's cells. After the excess sugar is out of your bloodstream, the excess insulin stays there. Your brain, sensing an increased level of insulin, realizes you need more sugar in your bloodstream to prevent your blood sugar from dropping too low. Your body makes you feel hungry and crave sugar, so you eat and get more sugar back into the bloodstream. If you give in to the cravings and consume more simple sugars, the cycle continues to repeat itself over and over. You may find yourself eating a refined carbohydrate, craving more soon after, eating again, and on and on. This cycle can lead to weight gain, and, most importantly, increased levels of dangerous visceral fat. (You can read more about insulin and its connection to belly fat in Chapter 2.)

Luckily, the Belly Fat Diet can help reduce this response. By following the diet, you discover the sources of simple carbohydrates and begin transferring away from these toward whole grains, fresh produce, lean proteins, and healthy fats. This lifestyle change helps to keep your insulin levels balanced, thereby stopping the hunger/sugar craving cycle.

How it regulates blood sugar

When your blood sugar fluctuates rapidly, you can experience intense cravings and hunger. Think about the last time you were very hungry and craving something. What did you want to eat? Most likely it wasn't a steamed vegetable. When you allow yourself to get too hungry, cravings for something high in refined carbohydrates or something heavy, such as a fatty, fried food, sneak in. And if you're eating in a way that allows you to get too hungry on a regular basis, you'll continually experience an increase in food cravings, which can make choosing healthy, belly-friendly foods quite challenging.

The Belly Fat Diet recommends foods that keep you feeling satisfied for hours, not just minutes. These same foods trigger a very small blood sugar response, preventing a spike and fall in blood sugar and insulin levels, which can help keep cravings at bay. By following the diet, you also get in the habit of planning out healthy meals and snacks to eat frequently during the day. Doing so not only keeps blood sugar levels consistent, but it also helps give your metabolism a boost.

How it decreases stress hormones

Stress hormones can be triggered due to emotional and physical stressors. These hormones can, in turn, cause your body to store abdominal fat. Luckily, getting specific foods and nutrients into your diet can actually help to decrease the stress hormones flowing through your body, helping to prevent that belly fat storage. And that's where the Belly Fat Diet comes in.

While following the Belly Fat Diet, you increase your intake of antioxidants, such as vitamin C and healthy fats like omega-3 fatty acids, which help to limit your body's exposure to stress hormones. You also transition to whole grains and make sure to eat at regular intervals throughout the day. All of this helps regulate the neurotransmitters in your brain.

Neurotransmitters, or brain chemicals, transfer signals within your nervous system. Some of these neurotransmitters impact mood, and the foods you eat can directly impact the neurotransmitters. So if you're eating the wrong foods in the wrong amounts, your mood, and in turn your stress levels, may be impacted. Limiting or overconsuming a particular food can trigger imbalances in neurotransmitters that may lead to irritability, moodiness, thinking problems, and even sleeping issues. But, by following the Belly Fat Diet, you take in the right foods (in the right amounts) to help balance your neurotransmitters, feel great, and reduce stress.

The Principles of the Belly Fat Diet

After you understand why the Belly Fat Diet is so successful (see the earlier section "Why the Belly Fat Diet Works"), you're ready to discover the main steps you can take to shrink your waistline and become a healthier version of yourself. This section lists the lifestyle principles you must keep in mind.

Eat more to lose more

One of the main principles of the Belly Fat Diet is that you have to eat more. That's right; you have to eat more to lose more weight! And who doesn't want to eat more? I know I do! But you can't just start eating more of all foods. In fact, that type of uncontrolled eating would be a great way to end up gaining more weight and belly fat. Instead, you want to focus on eating more of the foods that help you get rid of belly fat.

For example, vegetables are an unlimited food. And you actually need to eat more of these to promote weight loss. Foods, such as vegetables, that are rich in nutrients, high in fiber, and low in calories, fill you up without filling you out. Because these foods keep you satisfied, they help control hunger and cravings, which can lead you to make poor food choices. (See Chapter 6 for more on the foods that make up the Belly Fat Diet plan.)

With the Belly Fat Diet, you eat more food than you were likely eating before, but this time you'll see the scale start moving in the right direction. And the best part of all? You won't be hungry! In fact, you may even think that you can't eat the amount of food that I tell you to. That's what makes the Belly Fat Diet so successful: You aren't hungry. And when you don't get hungry, you tend to have fewer food cravings, allowing you to stay on track.

Don't believe me? Visualize this: Imagine that I put two snack options in front of you: three small pieces of caramel or 6 cups of air-popped popcorn. Which one looks more satisfying? Which one takes longer to eat? Which one curbs your appetite longer? Both of these snacks provide the same number of calories, but one gives you so much more food! The Belly Fat Diet works the same way: You choose the foods that provide you with the larger, more satisfying portions but that are actually good for you and promote weight loss.

Properly time your meals

When you commit to the Belly Fat Diet, make sure to eat on a regular basis. If you wait too long in between meals or skip a meal or snack, you can sabotage your weight loss efforts. If you wait too long to eat, you may start to get too hungry. And, of course, excessive hunger is what leads to strong food cravings — and usually for the wrong types of foods. (See the earlier section "Why the Belly Fat Diet Works" for info on why.) Getting overly hungry also leads you to eating too quickly.

The last time you were *very* hungry, did you a) cut the food you finally scrounged up into small bites, chewing each bite thoroughly and stopping when you reached the point of feeling satisfied but not stuffed, or did you b) wolf it down so fast you barely tasted it, leaving you feeling unsatisfied, which led to you looking for something else to eat, and before you knew it, you had eaten so much you felt stuffed or even sick? If you're like most folks, you went with option b. We have all been there, myself included. Thankfully, the Belly Fat Diet can show you how to prevent this.

Excessive hunger can be avoided by eating on a regular basis. Not only do small, frequent meals and snacks control appetite, but they also help boost your metabolism (a great perk)! I recommend not waiting more than three to four hours between meals and snacks. You may be saying "that doesn't work for my schedule," or "I don't have time to sit and eat that often." Before you drop the book, let me explain. Eating every few hours doesn't have to entail elaborately prepared meals and snacks. It also doesn't have to involve sitting down to long meals. A simple snack, such as grabbing a handful of almonds in between breakfast and lunch or munching a few raw vegetables in the after-noon, will suffice. The key is to simply prevent hunger from sneaking up on you.

During the day, you may be busy with work, caring for children, or rushing from one activity to the next. When you're distracted and busy, you often ignore your body's subtle hunger cues. It isn't until you stop or slow down that you realize that you're starving. You want to avoid this situation where you ignore your body until your body can't be ignored anymore. When you get sucked into this routine, you end up reaching for the wrong foods, eating too much, and eating too fast.

Aim to eat within an hour of waking up and then have a light meal or snack every three to four hours. For instance, if you wake up at 6:30 a.m. daily, your schedule may look like this:

- ✔ 7 a.m. Breakfast
- ✔ 10 a.m. Snack
- ✔ 1 p.m. Lunch
- ✔ 4 p.m. Snack
- ✔ 7 p.m. Dinner
- ✔ 9 p.m. Evening snack (if needed)

The evening snack isn't always necessary. It really depends on how late you stay up. Whatever you do, try not to eat within about an hour of going to bed. You won't gain weight from eating late — that's a myth. However, eating too close to bed can affect digestion, cause heartburn, and disrupt your sleep cycle.

Eat fat to fight fat

It takes fat to fight belly fat. Sounds like an oxymoron, doesn't it? But it's true. However, it's only true if it's the good fat. Both good fats and bad fats exist.

Bad fats include saturated fats and trans fats. Saturated fats are mostly found in high-fat animal products, such as butter, red meats, and full-fat dairy. Trans fats, as I mention earlier in this chapter, can be identified in foods by looking for the words "partially-hydrogenated oil" in the ingredient list.

Good fats are those that protect your heart, decrease disease risk, and even promote loss of belly fat. The two best sources of fat are

- ✓ **Monounsaturated fats:** Found in olive oil, nuts, seeds, and avocado
- ✓ **Omega-3 fatty acids:** Found in fish, walnuts, and flaxseed

Multiple studies have found that a diet rich in monounsaturated fats prevents belly fat from accumulating when compared to a high-carbohydrate and high-saturated-fat diet. This may sound like a no-brainer, but the surprising part is that this prevention of belly fat occurred even when both diets delivered the same number of daily calories! Other research has found that monoun-saturated fats may help you lose more belly fat even without changing your normal caloric intake or adding additional exercise. Omega-3 fatty acids have been found in several studies to help reduce the output of stress hormones. Because stress hormones promote the storage of belly fat, consuming a nutri-ent that helps reduce these hormones can in turn help to reduce abdominal fat storage. (Refer to the earlier section "How it decreases stress hormones" for more on how the Belly Fat Diet affects stress hormones.)

Another benefit of fat is that it's filling. Fat provides a longer period of satiety after eating than carbohydrates do. So consuming a meal that contains an ade-quate amount of healthy fat helps you stay full longer, helping to prevent that excessive hunger you know can lead to cravings and overeating. The Belly Fat Diet shows you how to take in around 25 percent of your daily calories from these healthy, belly-flattening fats. (See Chapter 7 to determine how many servings of fat per day are right for you on the Belly Fat Diet.)

Go whole grain

The Belly Fat Diet focuses on transitioning away from refined carbohydrates and consuming only whole-grain starches. Doing so is an essential step in flattening your belly, because refined carbohydrates spike blood sugar and insulin, leading to more and more storage of stubborn belly fat. In fact, research has shown that people who eat a diet rich in whole grains lose more abdominal fat.

So what is a whole grain? A *whole grain* is a grain that hasn't been stripped of its outermost layer. This layer contains the highest amount of fiber and nutrients. *Refined carbohydrates,* like white bread, are grains that have been stripped of their fiber and nutrients. Refined carbohydrates are often *enriched,* meaning that vitamins and minerals have been added back into these foods. However, fiber is rarely added. As a result, these grains are rapidly digested, triggering increases in blood sugar and insulin levels.

To make sure you're selecting a whole grain, look at the ingredients on the food label of any grain product. The first ingredient should always be a whole grain. Whole grains to look for include the following:

- ✔ Bean flour
- ✔ Brown rice flour
- ✔ Oat bran
- ✔ Rye
- ✔ Whole wheat

Foods that list "enriched flour" as the first ingredient are refined and should be avoided.

Because whole grains have a higher fiber content, they help you stay satisfied for a longer period of time than refined grains would. Staying full helps you to control your appetite and portions, thereby promoting further weight loss.

Limit your salt intake

Salt doesn't cause your body to gain fat, but it can still expand your belly. The major problem with sodium isn't its calorie content but the fact that it causes water retention.

Your body contains many electrolytes, with one of the major ones being sodium. Electrolytes help control your body's functions by carrying electrical impulses. The concentration of electrolytes must remain constant if your body is to function correctly. So when your body has a high concentration of sodium due to an increased intake from the foods you eat, the kidneys retain more water in your bloodstream to help regulate your electrolyte levels. Water in the bloodstream moves into your skin through osmosis, giving you that puffy look and feeling. If you've ever eaten a salty meal and had trouble removing your rings the next day, you've experienced this movement of water into your skin. Excessive fluid retention can also cause your stomach to look and feel bloated, making it difficult to have a flat belly.

Excessive sodium intake can do more damage than just making you look bloated. A high intake of sodium can also increase your blood pressure. And studies have shown that your arteries can actually stiffen within just 30 minutes after eating a high-sodium meal, increasing your risk of a cardiac event.

Due to the negative impact of sodium on your health as well as your belly, try to keep your daily sodium intake to 2,000 milligrams or less per day (keep it under 1,500 milligrams per day if you have high blood pressure). While staying within this amount may seem easy enough, you have to be careful. When you start examining food labels, you'll notice how much sodium everyday foods contain! The average American consumes around 3,300 milligrams of sodium per day, which is almost double the recommended amount.

The main culprits to be aware of are table salt added to meals as well as processed foods. Think adding a sprinkle of salt to your dinner is harmless? Think again. Just 1 teaspoon of table salt contains 2,300 milligrams of sodium, which is more than your entire daily intake!

Not only do you want to nix the table salt, but you also want to carefully look at food labels and limit high-sodium foods. Whole, unprocessed foods like fresh produce are naturally low in sodium. So the more you stick to these foods and avoid adding salt at the table (or stove), the easier it is to keep your total daily sodium intake within the recommended amount. *Tip:* If you must eat canned and processed foods, try to select those that are labeled "low sodium" or "sodium free." Become a label watcher!

Sodium is essential to maintaining many body functions. Your body needs sodium daily to exist. So don't avoid all sodium. Having too little sodium can be dangerous to your health as well. Just aim to keep it to less than 2,000 milligrams or less per day. Keep it under 1,500 milligrams per day if you have high blood pressure.

The Health Benefits of a Flatter Belly

The results you get from following your Belly Fat Diet won't just be on the scale and in the mirror. Your insides will thank you as well! Transitioning to a belly-fat-fighting lifestyle helps improve your energy levels and overall health. Doing so truly benefits you from the inside out!

Because visceral fat increases the risk of insulin resistance, it also increases your risk of developing type 2 diabetes. An elevated waist circumference is also associated with increased heart disease risk. So decreasing your belly fat helps prevent both of these diseases. Losing weight, reducing your sodium intake, and increasing your intake of fruits and vegetables also helps to decrease blood pressure and cholesterol levels, providing an added layer of protection for your heart.

As you can see, losing belly fat is more than just looking better; it's about improving your health and quality of life! The following sections focus on the main two benefits you'll achieve with a smaller amount of belly fat: the reversal of metabolic syndrome and the protection of your heart.

Reversing metabolic syndrome

Metabolic syndrome is the name for a group of risk factors that identify whether you're at high risk for developing heart disease, diabetes, and stroke. The more risk factors you display, the higher your disease risk. The risk factors that determine metabolic syndrome are

- ✔ Increased waistline
- ✔ Elevated blood sugar levels
- ✔ Elevated blood pressure
- ✔ Elevated blood lipids

Research has shown that an increased level of visceral fat, because it's metabolically active, can create a chain of chemical reactions in the body that increase all the characteristics of metabolic syndrome.

As you begin to make lifestyle changes following your Belly Fat Diet, your percentage of body fat, including unhealthy visceral fat, will begin to decrease. The less visceral fat you have, the less chemically active this fat becomes in your body. The loss of visceral fat helps reverse insulin resistance, decrease waist circumference, and improve blood lipids — all the things that together create metabolic syndrome.

Maintaining a healthy heart

The lifestyle changes you make while following the Belly Fat Diet help protect your heart. The most important lifestyle change to help your heart is increasing your intake of fruits and vegetables. Because they're loaded with nutrients and fiber but low in calories, your belly-busting meal plan can help you increase your intake of these power foods each day. Consider the following benefits of increasing your intake of fresh produce:

- ✔ **You increase your intake of soluble fiber, which binds to cholesterol and transports it out of the body.** As you likely know, bad cholesterol, referred to as LDL, increases your risk of heart disease and other cardiac problems.

- ✔ **You increase your intake of many nutrients that are protective to your heart.** Because produce is rich in magnesium and potassium, for example, taking in an increased amount of these minerals helps regulate and decrease blood pressure, which allows less strain on the heart. Also, powerful antioxidants, such as lycopene and beta carotene, are rich in many plant-based foods and protect the heart by helping shield cell membranes and molecules from oxidation. Eating produce rich in vitamin C, such as citrus fruits and bell peppers, helps protect the heart by decreasing the levels of stress hormones in the body.

What are you waiting for? Go grab a veggie-packed salad!

The Link Between Inflammation and Belly Fat

When you get a cut, you've probably noticed that as it starts to heal, the skin around it becomes red, puffy, and warm to the touch. These symptoms are referred to as *inflammation,* which is your body's healing response to an injury, illness, or infection. The inflammation you get when you cut yourself or get another type of wound is known as *acute inflammation.* It's localized to one spot and helps the wound heal. *Chronic inflammation* is another condition, which causes your body to become inflamed internally due to stresses from internal or external factors.

In the following sections, I discuss chronic inflammation in more depth, showing you what it is, what causes it, what can prevent it, and how it affects your belly.

What is inflammation?

Inflammation is a complex response of the systems in your body to fight off harmful pathogens, irritants, or even damaged cells. It's your body's way of protecting itself by removing damaging substances and initiating the healing process. It's really part of the immune response.

Think of inflammation as a war in your body. A foreign body, pathogen, or mutated cell enters the body and threatens it by risking damage or disease. To prevent damage, the body unleashes white blood cells to attack the invader. These cells either destroy the invader or wall it off to prevent it from spreading to other areas of the body. The body also releases proteins containing fluids to the area under invasion. The dilation and constriction of blood vessels to move protein and fluid to the area are what contribute to swelling. As nerve endings are compressed from swelling, pain can result.

When inflammation occurs in your body on a regular basis, such as from constant introduction of unhealthy food substances, your body can become chronically inflamed. Chronic inflammation is an autoimmune disease. Your body's defense system switches from protecting you and starts to attack itself and slowly leads to a metabolic breakdown, which can lead to serious, long-term health consequences.

Some individuals with chronic inflammation display symptoms like joint pain and chronic fatigue. Even *gingivitis,* inflammation of the gums, may be an indication of inflammation or impending inflammation in other parts of your body. However, inflammation can also be a silent disease, with few to no symptoms until it causes other serious health conditions.

Poor dietary habits and lifestyle choices, such as cigarette smoking, excessive alcohol intake, and sedentary lifestyle, can increase the risk of chronic inflammation. So if your diet isn't the greatest and you make some of these poor lifestyle choices, you may have underlying inflammation. To be safe, everyone should assume she has a low level of inflammation in her body and should work at preventing it.

The causes of inflammation

Can you guess what one of the biggest contributors to inflammation is? If you said "belly fat," you're right! Fat tissues in your body secrete hormones that help regulate your immune system (which inflammation is a part of). The more fatty tissue you have, the more hormones your body secretes. And when these hormones become out of balance, inflammation can result.

Poor dietary choices can lead to chronic inflammation. Many nutrients and added ingredients, when consumed in excess, can contribute to inflammation in the intestines, which therefore can increase inflammation throughout the body.

Here are some of the biggest inflammation triggers:

- ✔ **Excessive intake of sugar and refined carbohydrates:** Simple sugars, such as added sugar or white flour, can trigger an increase in insulin response, which, over time, can increase inflammation. (You can read more about the insulin response in the earlier section "How it reduces insulin response.") Instead, aim to reduce your intake of sugar by avoiding sugar-sweetened beverages, limiting sugar-packed desserts, and choosing whole-grain starches over their white counterparts.

- ✔ **Trans fats:** These fats are doubly bad in the body because they not only raise unhealthy LDL cholesterol levels, but they also lower healthy HDL cholesterol levels. Research has found that individuals with a high dietary intake of trans fats have more visceral fat. These fats also further increase inflammation in the body.

- ✔ **Vegetable oils:** These oils, such as corn oil, are rich in omega-6 fatty acids and low in omega-3 fatty acids. A diet with a ratio of fats high in omega-6s and low in omega-3s has been linked to increased inflammation. Why? Because a diet rich in carbohydrates, especially refined carbohydrates, has been shown to, when combined with omega-6 fatty acids, increase production of pro-inflammatory hormones called *eicosanoids*. Instead, use oils rich in omega-3 fatty acids or monounsaturated fats, which include flaxseed oil (great source of omega-3s) and olive oil (monounsaturated fat).

✔ **Sodium:** Excessive dietary sodium can stiffen arteries, helping to promote inflammation and increase the risk of a cardiovascular event. Avoid adding table salt to foods, and select whole, unprocessed foods as much as possible to help reduce your sodium intake. (You can read more about sodium in the earlier section "Limit your salt intake.")

✔ **Excessive alcohol:** In moderate amounts (one glass of alcohol per day for women and two glasses per day for men), alcohol can be beneficial and may have mild anti-inflammatory properties. However, increased intake of alcohol has been shown to elevate inflammation markers in the body, which is a sign of chronic inflammation. Excessive alcohol can also increase the storage of visceral fat, further increasing inflammation risk.

✔ **Food sensitivities unique to you:** Do certain foods make you feel sick after you've eaten them? Do you tend to get stomach pains or indigestion after eating them? Have you noticed a change in bowel habits or even a skin rash or hives after eating some foods? If so, you may have a food allergy or intolerance. Consuming a food that your body can't tolerate can cause inflammation because your body views this food as an intruder.

If you notice symptoms of a potential food allergy, see a food allergy specialist to be tested. If you do have multiple food allergies or intolerances, you need to meet with a Registered Dietitian to assess your food intake and ensure you're meeting your body's nutrient needs while eliminating these allergens from your diet.

Food intolerances aren't always easy to diagnose. The best thing to do is to keep a detailed food record of what you eat and how you feel after eating it. Then eliminate the potential food irritant from your diet for two weeks. Add it back in a small amount one day, and then monitor your response. If you notice any symptoms return, eliminate this food from your diet for good. Follow this procedure for any possible food irritant to help you decrease inflammation.

Foods that fight inflammation

When eaten on a regular basis, foods with anti-inflammatory properties can help reduce inflammation in the body, helping to prevent the long-term health consequences associated with it — but only if you also eliminate the foods that cause inflammation (see the preceding section). When inflammation is under control, not only will you have more energy and feel better overall, but you'll also find that weight loss and reduction of belly fat both become easier!

The following foods and nutrients can fight inflammation:

✔ **Fruits and vegetables:** All fruits and vegetables, due to their rich nutrient and fiber content, help to combat chronic inflammation, so make sure to include adequate amounts of these foods daily (see Chapter 7 for the recommended daily servings of fruits and vegetables). Some types of fresh produce, however, are even more potent than others. Some terrific anti-inflammatory fruits and vegetables to include in your meal plan include the following:

- **Apples:** These crunchy fruits contain a high level of *quercetin,* a flavonoid with powerful anti-inflammatory properties.

- **Berries:** These sweet fruits are jampacked with inflammation-busting antioxidants. They also have been found to protect against diseases like cancer and dementia.

- **Broccoli:** This powerful veggie is rich in many phytonutrients, including *sulforaphane,* which helps eliminate potentially carcinogenic compounds in your body, helping decrease inflammation and boost your immune system.

- **Mushrooms:** Rich in immune-boosting compounds, these tasty vegetables are a great way to combat inflammation and disease.

- **Papaya:** This delicious fruit is rich in vitamin C and vitamin E as well as an enzyme called *papain.* Together these help to decrease inflammation and improve digestion.

- **Pineapple:** Rich in the enzyme *bromelain,* this sweet, tart fruit aids in healing and decreases swelling. Bromelain is so powerful, in fact, that research has found extracts of the enzyme to be almost as effective in treating arthritis inflammation as some nonsteroidal anti-inflammatory drugs (NSAIDs)!

- **Spinach:** This vegetable is loaded with flavonoids and carotenoids that help decrease inflammation and oxidative damage in your body's cells.

✔ **Green tea:** This mild beverage is great for helping shrink your waistline as well as for decreasing inflammation. The flavonoids in this tea have natural anti-inflammatory properties. And the compound EGCG in green tea has been shown to help reduce body fat.

✔ **Monounsaturated fats:** These heart-healthy fats help raise your healthy HDL cholesterol levels and reduce overall inflammation. Great sources include olive oil, almonds, and avocado.

✔ **Omega-3 fatty acids:** Research has shown that a diet with a high percentage of omega-3 fatty acids and a low percentage of omega-6 fatty acids has been linked with decreased inflammation. Food sources of omega-3s include walnuts, flaxseed, and fish, such as wild Alaskan salmon.

✔ **Spices:** Certain spices, including garlic, turmeric, cinnamon, ginger, and chili peppers, have potent inflammation-reducing capabilities, so try adding them to meals as often as possible.

✔ **Water:** Staying hydrated is essential to flushing inflammation-causing toxins out of your body. Aim for 64 ounces of water per day. *Remember:* Add an additional 8 ounces of water for every 30 minutes of exercise as well.

✔ **Whole grains:** Rich in fiber, whole grains help control the insulin response in your body. The high B vitamin content of whole grains also helps reduce the inflammatory hormone *homocystine* in the body.

Try adding these anti-inflammatory foods into your meal plan on a daily basis. The more often you eat these foods, the less inflammation that will be present in your body.

Part II
Working Your Way to a Flatter Belly

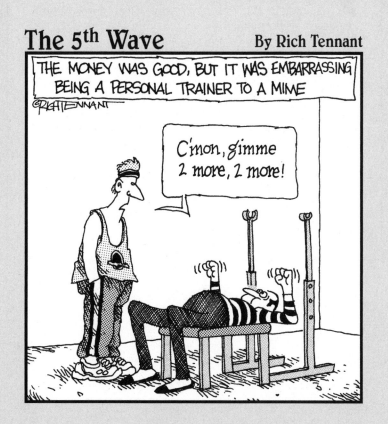

The 5th Wave   By Rich Tennant

THE MONEY WAS GOOD, BUT IT WAS EMBARRASSING BEING A PERSONAL TRAINER TO A MIME

C'mon, gimme 2 more, 2 more!

In this part . . .

You may have heard it said before: "Failing to plan is planning to fail." Planning is key to losing weight and keeping it off permanently.

In this part, I show you how to prepare for success on the Belly Fat Diet plan. I outline the plan's key components and introduce the individualized Belly Fat Diet plans. I help you determine which plan is most appropriate for you so you can start shedding belly fat quickly and easily. You also get specific meal-plan guidelines as well as sample meal plans to get you started.

This part also focuses on exercise, providing belly-blasting workout routines that tone and tighten your tummy to give you results you never dreamed possible! I also share simple strategies to help you get moving and stay moving, even if you've never exercised a day in your life.

Chapter 5

Preparing Yourself for the Belly Fat Diet

In This Chapter

▶ Understanding the philosophy of the Belly Fat Diet

▶ Recognizing the role stress can play in losing belly fat

▶ Adding belly-slimming foods and nutrients to your diet

*Y*our Belly Fat Diet plan isn't just another fad diet to go on and off. Many folks have been on fad diets that have failed them. Diet failure often happens because people think that diets require only temporary habit changes. The Belly Fat Diet plan is different. This plan isn't a quick fix that allows you to lose weight only to gain it right back (plus some!) in a short period of time. This plan is a lifestyle. By following this plan, you discover how to incorporate all your favorite foods while improving not only your waistline but also your health.

Throughout this chapter, I arm you with the tools you need to get started with your Belly Fat Diet lifestyle. I show you step-by-step how to begin so you can transition smoothly and easily away from unhealthy, belly-fat storing habits to habits that blast belly fat and improve your energy levels and over-all well-being. I also point out some of the biggest contributors to belly fat — and they aren't always food! I show you how to recognize these problem areas and some simple strategies to manage them so you stay looking and feeling fantastic!

For additional information on recruiting the support of your family and friends as you embark on the Belly Fat Diet lifestyle, check out www.dummies.com/go/bellyfat.

Understanding the Belly Fat Diet Lifestyle

As I mention earlier, the Belly Fat Diet isn't your typical temporary diet — it's a lifestyle. If the changes you make while following your Belly Fat Diet plan become a lifestyle, those changes become ingrained within you. You won't begin a pattern of yo-yo dieting, where you lose weight only to regain it rapidly. Instead, when you focus on making small, gradual changes that you can stick with, these changes become part of your typical routine — or lifestyle — and you won't be tempted to revert to your old behaviors. Your new habits become your new way of life, and they will likely stick around for good.

In the following sections, I help you understand what you're getting into by giving you an overview of the steps involved in the Belly Fat Diet plan.

Deciding on a plan that fits your personality

Everyone has a different mindset and personality when it comes to weight loss. Some people have the "all or nothing" mindset and want to change everything overnight. Others feel overwhelmed by this approach and need to make only a few changes at once. This flexibility is the magic of the Belly Fat Diet plan. You can follow it in three different ways:

✔ **The Turbo-Charged plan:** If you're someone who wants to dive right in, make many changes at once, and see fast results, the Turbo-Charged plan may be the best fit for you.

✔ **The Moderation plan:** If you need to lose a significant amount of weight, but need to make small changes over time to prevent burnout, the Moderation plan is your best bet.

✔ **The Gradual-Change plan:** If you only have a small amount of belly fat to lose and prefer to make changes over the course of a few weeks rather than days, the Gradual-Change plan is for you.

Regardless of what plan type best fits your needs, the specific meal plans along with the lifestyle changes I discuss throughout this chapter can help you to shed weight and unpleasant belly fat and provide the tools you need to successfully maintain your results for years to come. I discuss each of these three plans in more detail in Chapter 7.

Losing weight is the easy part. Maintaining your results over a long period of time is often the most challenging aspect. And this maintenance is what most diet plans leave out. They show you how to drop weight fast, but they leave you hanging on how to prevent gaining the weight back.

Don't worry. I won't do that to you. I provide you with many tools and tips to help you become a huge success at weight maintenance for the rest of your life (after you first achieve your weight loss goals, of course!). In fact, I devote Chapter 18 to understanding weight maintenance, including meal plans.

Committing yourself to change

Because you're reading this book, you're obviously already motivated to lose weight, shrink your belly, and take control of your health. And that's great! Now you just have to commit yourself to making the required lifestyle changes. Doing so is easier said than done, but don't stress out — it's bad for your belly! (Check out the later section "Managing Stress for a Flatter Belly" for details.) In the following sections, I show you some of the easiest ways to start committing yourself to making the changes necessary to start fighting belly fat and keeping it off for good!

Write down your reasons to lose weight

I have a trick I like to recommend to my clients who struggle with motivation or temptation. Take out a piece of paper, grab a pen, and ask yourself why you want to lose weight. And don't just say to look better. Of course that's part of it, but really think about this question. What are *all* the reasons you want to lose weight? Is it to have more energy? To lower your blood pressure? To prevent heart disease or diabetes? To fit into an outfit you love? To help you keep up with your kids or grandkids? Or maybe to look and feel younger? Whatever your reasons, no matter how small or how ridiculous they may seem, write them all down!

After you have compiled your reasons for change, put this piece of paper somewhere you'll almost always have it with you. You can store it in your wallet or purse, or you can even text it to your cellphone if that's easier for you. Whatever you do, just make sure you have these reasons on hand at all times so you can take a look at them when you're struggling to stick with your lifestyle choices.

Think about the last time you tried to lose weight and were in a tempting situation. Maybe you went to a party and all of your favorite foods were out on display. What happened? Did you dive right in and then later regret it? Don't feel bad if you did. This reaction is normal. It happens to everyone at times, including me. Now think about being in the same situation with that list of every single reason you could think of for wanting to lose weight in front of you. Do you think you would have still overindulged? Or do you think you would have had just a few of the less healthy foods and looked for some better options as well?

Chances are, when you take the time to reflect on the reasons you're motivated to lose weight, you will almost always make the better choice. Looking at this list may not work 100 percent of the time, but even if it helps you prevent temptation 80 percent of the time, you're still better off.

Visualize success

In addition to keeping your reasons for change foremost in your mind, I want you to work on visualization as well. This amazing tool can help you stay motivated and resist temptations that come along.

Here's what to do: Think about how you want to look and feel at your goal weight. Picture yourself in an outfit you would love to be able to wear. Imagine yourself full of energy and vigor. Close your eyes and picture this image in as much detail as you can. Use as many senses as you can when creating this image. How do your new clothes feel on your skin? Is it a great feeling to put on pants that don't feel snug around the waistline? Can you run up the stairs without feeling winded? Are your skin and hair glowing due to your healthy diet? Are your muscles more defined from your new exercise routine? After you have a vivid image in your mind, open your eyes.

At least once a day, spend a few minutes calling on this image in your mind. When you're faced with a tempting situation or a stressful situation that may throw you off track, close your eyes for just a few seconds and remember this image. Remember that this image is your goal and is everything you're working so hard to attain. By constantly reminding yourself of what you're working toward and truly seeing the end result of all your efforts, you're more apt to stay motivated and on track.

Take stock of your habits

Some of your behaviors and habits can be damaging to your belly, so I want you to identify the biggest areas of your current diet and daily routine that need some work. No matter how healthfully you currently eat, you can always improve something.

The biggest contributors to belly fat are consuming refined carbohydrates, unhealthy saturated and trans fats, simple sugars, and excessive sodium. In addition, lifestyle factors like inadequate sleep, excessive stress, and limited physical activity can also pack on the pounds and expand your waistline.

It's vital to your Belly Fat Diet success to realize what current lifestyle behaviors are contributing to your belly fat and weight gain. If you don't know what's causing it, how are you going to fix it? So, for one full day, record your food intake as well as your other lifestyle behaviors. Here's what to write down:

✔ Everything you eat and drink, including any salt you may add to your food

✔ How long you slept, noting whether it was interrupted sleep and whether you felt rested when you awoke

✔ Your daily stress level, on a scale from 1 to 10, with 10 being the highest amount of stress

✔ Your level of physical activity and whether you performed any structured exercise, including how much and how often

After compiling it, examine the record that you kept. Are you consuming a large amount of fruits and vegetables? Out of the grains you're eating, are they mostly whole grain or are many refined? What type of fats are you consuming? Are they the healthy plant-based fats or the unhealthy saturated and trans fats? Are you inactive? Is your stress level high? After you start realizing your bad habits, you can begin trying to change them.

Transitioning to whole foods

Whole grains are bread products and starches that contain all parts of the grain: the bran, endosperm, and germ. These parts of the grain contain fiber and protein, which help to slow down digestion. Refined carbohydrates, on the other hand, have had the bran and germ removed, leaving only the endosperm. Because refined carbohydrates contain less fiber and protein, they're digested much more rapidly. This rapid digestion triggers a rise in blood sugar and insulin levels, which can cause you to begin storing more belly fat.

Transitioning away from refined carbohydrate sources and eating mainly whole grains is essential if you want to flatten your stomach once and for all. The increased insulin response caused by refined carbohydrates and simple sugars increases fat storage in your abdomen and makes your body more resistant to burning this fat. (You can read about the impact insulin has on belly fat in detail in Chapter 2.) To get your body on board with your plans to shed belly fat, you have to decrease this insulin response by consuming whole grains.

As you begin the Belly Fat Diet, start by going through your cabinets and pantry and look at the breads and grains you typically eat. For any refined grain you have, think of a healthier, belly-friendly option you can replace it with. For instance, if you have crackers made with white flour, switch them with 100 percent stone-ground wheat or brown rice crackers. If you have a loaf of white bread, replace it with 100 percent whole-wheat or oat bread. Check out Chapter 6 for more information on identifying whether a product is a whole grain or a refined grain.

Whole grains not only contain more fiber and nutrition, but they actually contain a lot more flavor as well. So these switches won't only be great for your waistline, but also for your taste buds!

Getting adequate sleep

The last thing you may think about when trying to lose weight is sleep, but it's actually a huge piece of the weight loss puzzle! Many studies have linked the amount and quality of sleep with appetite regulation and metabolism. Ghrelin and leptin are two hormones that regulate appetite in your body. *Ghrelin* is produced in the intestinal tract and helps stimulate appetite. *Leptin,* which is produced in your fat cells, tells your brain when you've eaten enough and are satisfied.

Lack of sleep leads to a decrease in leptin production, leaving you feeling less satisfied after eating. Even worse, too little sleep can trigger a rise in ghrelin, making you want to eat more. This combination is a recipe for weight gain. In fact, this sleep connection is so powerful, one study out of Stanford found a direct correlation with body weight and sleep. This study showed that those who slept the least weighed the most.

Being tired from lack of sleep can also cause you to seek out high-carbohydrate, high-sugar foods and snacks. Why? Perhaps because your body is looking for a quick burst of energy. Unfortunately, however, these simple sugars digest rapidly, giving you a quick burst of energy followed by a rapid decline in energy. If you continue to eat simple sugars over and over for energy, not only will your blood sugar become erratic, but so will your insulin levels, making it easier to store belly fat.

Sleep alone isn't the miracle cure to weight loss, but a lack of sleep can make it much harder to stay on track with a healthy eating plan. Increased hunger and cravings from fatigue can also increase the temptation to eat the foods that sabotage your belly-fighting efforts. So if you sleep six hours or less per night, work on increasing your amount of shut-eye. The ideal is to sleep seven to eight hours per night, but any amount more than what you're currently getting may be helpful, so work on increasing your sleep over time.

Managing Stress for a Flatter Belly

If you want to fight belly fat, you also have to fight stress. When you're constantly under stress, your body reacts. And, unfortunately, one of the ways in which your body reacts is to store fat right where you want it the least: in your belly!

Although you may not always notice it, your day can be filled with stressors. Think of the jerk who cut you off on the way to work or the person in front of you in the checkout line at the grocery store who had to count out hundreds of pennies to pay. Even if you don't think you're stressed, when you're in a hurry, these little annoyances can become stressful to your body. When your body is under stress, it releases stress hormones like cortisol and adrenaline.

And these hormones, when released into your body on a regular basis, can begin to increase fat storage in your midsection. (In Chapter 2, you can read about how these stress hormones can trigger belly fat storage.)

The stress response is your body's way of protecting you and helping you rise to address and fight off challenges. A certain level of stress can be healthy. However, at a certain point, stress levels can become too great and begin to impact your health, mood, and belly.

In the following sections, I show you how to determine the stressors in your life, explain how to know when your stress level is too high, and provide a few simple ways to start decreasing stress in your daily life. All these actions should help to reduce your belly fat (and make your life more enjoyable).

Identifying common stressors

Think about your day-to-day routine. What part of it brings on the most stress for you? Is it sitting in traffic? Is it running late to a meeting or having to drive the kids to multiple activities? Think about some of the stressful situations you run into on a regular basis. How do you react to these situations? Understanding the stress in your life and how you handle it is important to staying calm (and losing that gut!).

People handle stress in one of three main ways:

✓ **They become agitated.** These folks get angry and keyed up when stressed. They may yell, shout, or be unable to sit still.

✓ **They become quiet or withdrawn.** These people tend to shut down with stress. They may space out or just withdraw from the situation. A stressful situation may make them feel more depressed than agitated.

✓ **They freeze.** These individuals, on the surface, seem to freeze during a stressful situation. However, on the inside, they feel extremely agitated. They tend to hold everything in instead of expressing emotion.

There isn't necessarily a right way to react to stress, but you need to know how you respond to stress so you can recognize when you're under it. Recognizing when you're under stress is important so you can see how often you're stressed, what brings about this level of stress, and how you can manage it to decrease your overall stress levels.

Both external and internal causes can bring about stress. The most common external factors of stress include

✓ Family and children

✓ Financial stress

- ✔ Job-related stressors
- ✔ Major life changes
- ✔ Relationship difficulties

Internal causes of stress include

- ✔ Being too much of a perfectionist
- ✔ Engaging in negative self-talk
- ✔ Not being assertive enough
- ✔ Having a pessimistic attitude
- ✔ Setting unrealistic expectations for yourself

Make an effort to determine which of these factors brings on the majority of stress in your life and begin to work on reducing that stress load. The later section "Bringing your stress level down" can show you how.

Recognizing when stress is too high

Some stress can actually be good for you. It may help you to perform under pressure or give you added motivation to meet a deadline. But at a certain point, stress crosses from being healthy to being detrimental. Everyone has a different stress threshold, and your tolerance to stress depends on many things. You may be able to handle a larger amount of stress

- ✔ If you have a strong support system around you
- ✔ If you have a positive outlook on life
- ✔ If you know a stressful situation will present itself and you've prepared for it
- ✔ If you know how to calm yourself and self-soothe

You need to be on the lookout for stress overload, or the point at which stress can become both mentally and physically damaging. Figure 5-1 shows some common symptoms caused by stress overload. The more symptoms you display from the figure, the closer you may be to experiencing stress overload.

Mental and Emotional Symptoms	Physical Symptoms	Behavioral Changes
Decreased concentration	Muscle aches and pains	Eating too much or too little
Forgetfulness	Rapid heartbeat	Insomnia
Negative thinking	Gastrointestinal changes, such as constipation or diarrhea	Sleeping too much
Constant racing thoughts and worry		Isolating self from others
Moodiness		Using substances such as alcohol or cigarettes to relax
Agitation		
Feeling overwhelmed		

Figure 5-1:
Identifying symptoms of stress overload.

Bringing your stress level down

Learning strategies to reduce and manage stress is important for preventing the health effects that I discuss in the preceding section. Managing your stress is all about taking charge. If you start to take control of your emotions as well as your environment, schedules, and any other factors that may bring on stress, you can start to manage stress in a healthy way.

Be proactive. If you can change a stressful situation before it happens or while it's happening, do it. (However, if you can't change it, make sure to focus on yourself and those things you can control.) Also, make time every day to relax, rest, and unwind from the stressors of the day. Even if the stress in your life seems out of control, you can control the way you respond to it, which can make all the difference. With practice, you'll be able to better identify stressors in your life, be able to better handle them, and be able to better control the situation causing them. Doing so gives you more confidence that you can face these stressors and challenges, which in itself can help to reduce the overall stress you feel inside. As your levels of stress and anxiety decrease, the stress hormones your body releases also start to decline, helping you to shed excess weight around the middle.

In the following sections, I show you three techniques you can use to reduce stress and relax your body.

Breathing deeply

One of the easiest and best ways to reduce stress in the body is through deep breathing. It's simple to do and is a great way to cut stress almost immediately. The way you breathe affects your entire body, so when you breathe in deeply and slowly, it sends a message to your brain to relax and calm down. This message automatically helps to decrease your stress and put you in a more relaxed state.

To help reduce stress no matter what the situation and no matter where you are, start practicing *belly breathing*. You can master this simple technique quickly with just a little practice. To practice belly breathing, refer to Figure 5-2 and follow these steps:

1. **Sit or lay in a comfortable position.**

   You can sit in a comfy chair, on the floor, or even lay down on a couch, bed, or fitness mat. Remember that this exercise can be done anywhere, so even if you're sitting at your desk at work, in the car, on the train, or even a park bench, you can still practice this exercise.

2. **Place one hand on your chest and the other just below your ribs on your belly and take a deep breath through your nose.**

   Breathe in deep enough that it forces your belly to push your hand out. Your chest shouldn't be moving as you do this.

3. **Exhale through pursed lips (like when you're trying to whistle).**

   As you breathe out, focus on feeling the hand on your belly go in with your stomach.

4. **Repeat Steps 1 through 3 five to ten times, breathing in slowly and deeply.**

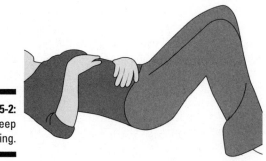

Figure 5-2:
Deep
breathing.

Illustration by Wiley, Composition Services Graphics

Progressive muscle relaxation

Progressive muscle relaxation, a stress-relieving technique, sounds complicated, but it's actually very simple. It involves focusing on each muscle group and slowly tensing and relaxing each muscle to help you calm and decompress. This technique forces you to focus on the difference between the tense muscle and the relaxed muscle, helping you become more aware of physical sensations and thus able to relax and release tension.

Here's how you do it:

1. **Tense the muscles in your toes, hold the tension for 5 to 10 seconds, and then relax the muscles for 30 seconds.**

2. **Move on to your legs, following the tension and relaxation directions in Step 1 for your calves, quadriceps, and even glutes. Slowly work your way up your body.**

   Practice tensing and relaxing your muscles all the way to your shoulders, neck, and even your face until you reach the top of your head.

Figure 5-3 illustrates another way of doing progressive muscle relaxation: in reverse order.

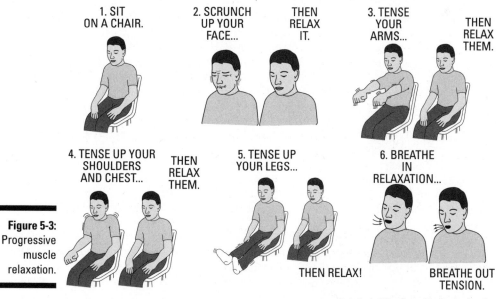

Figure 5-3: Progressive muscle relaxation.

1. SIT ON A CHAIR.
2. SCRUNCH UP YOUR FACE... THEN RELAX IT.
3. TENSE YOUR ARMS... THEN RELAX THEM.
4. TENSE UP YOUR SHOULDERS AND CHEST... THEN RELAX THEM.
5. TENSE UP YOUR LEGS... THEN RELAX!
6. BREATHE IN RELAXATION... BREATHE OUT TENSION.

Illustration by Wiley, Composition Services Graphics

Exercising

One of the best ways to reduce stress (and, of course, shrink your belly!) is through exercise. Here's why exercise is so important:

✔ **It improves the flow of blood to your brain.** This increased blood flow brings oxygen and energy (in the form of sugar) to your brain.

✔ **It fosters clear thinking.** When you're concentrating intensely, the neurons in your brain start working even harder than normal. These neurons then produce increased amounts of waste products, which, if built up, can cause you to suffer from foggy thinking. By exercising, however, you speed the flow of blood through your brain, moving these waste products faster and allowing your brain to function at its peak.

✔ **It releases endorphins into your bloodstream.** This release gives you a feeling of happiness, positively affects your overall sense of well-being, and helps reduce overall stress.

So what's the best exercise for stress reduction? A study out of the University of Missouri-Columbia found that high-intensity exercise was the best way to reduce overall stress and anxiety levels. This includes exercises like interval training. Here's the good news: The belly-blasting workout routines in Chapter 10 include this type of training, so they're perfect for your belly and your stress level!

Reducing stress with food

You may find this surprising, but your diet can actually impact your stress levels. The food you eat, how you eat it, and when you eat it can positively or negatively affect your overall stress levels. And as you know, if your stress level increases, so can your waistline. So in the same way that it's important to practice breathing exercises and get regular physical activity to manage stress, it's also just as important to focus on eating the right foods (at the right times) to help manage stress.

Specific nutrients can impact stress levels, but so can the timing of your meals and snacks. When you go long periods of time without eating, your blood sugar can drop. When your blood sugar drops, your energy level can decrease, your mental focus can decline, and you can become irritable. These feelings can all bring on and increase stress throughout the day. For this reason, along with the benefit to metabolism and weight loss, it's important to eat small meals and snacks frequently throughout the day.

Consuming adequate carbohydrates during the day is also helpful for managing stress (and therefore slimming your belly). When you eat carbohydrates, your body releases the hormone *serotonin,* which is a "feel good" chemical in the brain. Serotonin not only helps you feel good, but it also helps to reduce stress.

However, you can't just choose any carbohydrate. You need to consume only whole-grain carbohydrates. The fiber in these carbohydrates helps control appetite, decrease insulin response, and prevent midday dips in your energy level. You can read about whole grains and how to identify them in Chapter 6.

The following sections show you the specific nutrients and types of foods that can help decrease stress and belly fat.

Reach for vitamin C if you're stressed

The next time you're stressed, you may want to grab an orange. Why? A German study found a direct connection between vitamin C and stress hormones. This study showed that a diet rich in vitamin C can help reduce stress levels and return blood pressure and the stress hormone cortisol to normal levels after a stressful situation. So after a stressful situation, stress hormones will circulate in your body for shorter amounts of time, helping to fight against belly fat storage.

Don't worry if you don't love oranges. You can choose from plenty of great sources of vitamin C. Some of the best include

✔ Bell peppers

✔ Broccoli

✔ Grapefruit

✔ Kale

✔ Kiwi

✔ Oranges

✔ Papaya

✔ Strawberries

Although high in vitamin C, fruit juice contains limited amounts of fiber and large amounts of natural sugar, which can increase insulin response and increase belly fat storage. If you do reach for juice, choose only 100 percent fruit juice and limit the amount to 4 ounces per day.

Adding Belly-Slimming Foods to Your Diet

Believe it or not, you can reduce belly fat by eating! The catch is that you have to eat the right foods. The following sections cover the fats, beverages, and low-glycemic foods that need to be a part of your diet.

The best fats for your belly

Heart-healthy omega-3 fatty acids and monounsaturated fats have been found in research to help shrink belly fat. They also can help cut stress levels and reduce stress hormones, further reducing belly fat. I explain each of these good fats in the following sections.

Omega-3 fatty acids

Omega-3 fatty acids are a powerful fat with many anti-inflammatory properties. They not only promote health, but they also have been shown to impact belly fat in a positive way. In addition, studies have shown that eating a diet rich in omega-3 fatty acids can actually keep the stress hormones (cortisol and adrenaline) from peaking.

Imagine, for example, that you're faced with a stressful situation. Your boss comes to you at 2 p.m. with a major project that needs to be completed and turned in before the end of the day. Realizing that this task is next to impossible, you start feeling stressed. The more stressed you feel, the more your body releases stress hormones. These same hormones love filling up the fat cells in your belly. However, if your diet is rich in omega-3s, these stress hormones will be released, but they won't peak as high as they would otherwise. As a result, you have fewer stress hormones circulating in your body and, therefore, fewer stress hormones to store belly fat.

Monounsaturated fats

Monounsaturated fats are the fats found in many plant-based foods, such as olive oil, peanuts, and avocado. Although you may hear the word "fat" and think it's something damaging to your weight loss efforts, nothing is further from the truth. Actually, monounsaturated fats are powerful belly fat fighters.

A Spanish study published in *Diabetes Care,* an American Diabetes Association journal, found a very real connection between monounsaturated fats and a reduction in belly fat. The study looked at individuals with excessive belly fat and placed them on three different types of calorie-reduced diets: a diet high in saturated fat, a diet rich in monounsaturated fats, and a diet rich in carbohydrates. Only the individuals in the group consuming a diet rich in monounsaturated fats were found to have a reduction in belly fat accumulation. And the best part was they were found to lose both subcutaneous and visceral belly fat!

Drinking your way to a flatter belly

Did you know that what you drink can significantly impact your belly? For instance, you probably know that sugary drinks like soda and lemonade can spike insulin and cause your body to store belly fat. However, did you know that drinks with excessive amounts of caffeine can increase belly fat as well? And did you know that other drinks can actually help burn belly fat?

Caffeine can provide your body with a slight metabolism boost. So you may think you should consume lots of it to burn more calories and more fat. This thinking is true to a point, but it doesn't tell the whole story.

A general rule is to keep your caffeine intake to no more than 300 milligrams per day. That's equal to about 2 to 3 cups of coffee. Beyond this amount is where caffeine may have more of a negative impact than a positive one. Very high levels of caffeine in the body can start to impact you in a few unhealthy ways. You can start to feel more agitated, have trouble concentrating, and even suffer from a disrupted sleep cycle. These symptoms can all raise stress hormone production and slow metabolism.

If you need to cut back on your caffeine intake to stay within the suggested limits, try swapping your typical morning cup of coffee or your afternoon soda for decaffeinated green tea. This tea is loaded with stress-fighting antioxidants, which can help prevent cell damage and oxidation. Because green tea is one of the least processed teas, it also contains a high level of a catechin called *epigallocatechin-3-gallate* (EGCG). Promising studies have indicated that EGCG may help to reduce overall body fat, but especially belly fat. So drink up!

Eating foods with a low glycemic index

Throughout this book, I stress that you need to consume more whole grains and fewer refined carbohydrates. I suggest this change because refined carbohydrates have a high glycemic index (GI). The *glycemic index* is a scale that ranks foods based on how fast and how high they can raise your blood sugar. The lower a food ranks on the GI scale, the less of a rise in blood sugar it creates. A food ranking high on the GI scale causes a rapid spike in blood sugar.

When your blood sugar rises quickly, you experience an increased release of insulin into the bloodstream. And because insulin can store more abdominal fat, this news is bad for your belly. So choosing carbohydrates that rank lower on the GI scale helps to limit the blood sugar and insulin response, therefore giving you an added boost in the fight against belly fat.

In the following sections, I explain the glycemic index further and suggest low-GI foods to stock up on.

How the GI of a food is calculated

Carbohydrates are found in vegetables, fruits, starches, and dairy products like milk and yogurt. Any food that contains a source of carbohydrate can have a GI associated with it. In general, refined carbohydrates (processed starches, such as white bread, and foods high in added sugar, such as candy) tend to have a higher GI.

The most recent way devised to determine a food's GI has been to use white bread as a standard for comparison. White bread was given a GI value of 100. The GI of other foods is then calculated based on how quickly blood sugar rises after consumption of the food in comparison to the white bread standard. Foods with a GI greater than 100 raise blood sugar faster and higher than white bread, whereas foods with a GI less than 100 raise blood sugar slower and lower than this bread.

A GI value greater than 70 is considered to be a relatively high GI and may elevate insulin levels, working against your efforts to lose belly fat. But I want you to think of GI as a tool and not a rule. Even though consuming high-GI foods may make it more difficult to achieve your flat belly, you have to remember that GI is affected by more than just food itself. It can be elevated or lowered by what that food is eaten with and how much of the food is consumed. So if you do choose to have a high-GI food, try eating it at a meal that also contains lean protein, healthy fats, and high-fiber, low-GI foods. Doing so can minimize the high-GI food's impact on blood sugar and insulin.

Looking for low-GI foods

Table 5-1 lists the GI index categories of many common foods. The categories are as follows:

- ✔ GI ranking of 55 or less = Low-GI food
- ✔ GI ranking of 56–69 = Medium-GI food
- ✔ GI ranking of 70 or more = High-GI food

Proteins and fats aren't listed in the table, because these are all low-GI foods (unless additional ingredients like breading have been added).

Table 5-1   **The GI Index Category of Various Foods**

Food	GI Index Category	Food	GI Index Category
Apples	Low	Milk, fat-free or low-fat	Low
Asparagus	Low	Oatmeal	Medium
Baked russet potatoes	High	Pasta, white	Medium
Bananas	Low	Pasta, whole-grain	Low
Barley	Low	Peas	Low
Black beans	Low	Peppers, all	Low
Bran flake cereal	Medium	Pizza, white flour dough	High
Broccoli	Low	Popcorn	Medium
Brown rice	Low	Pretzels, white flour	High
Carrots	Low	Raisins	Medium
Cherries	Low	Rice cakes, white rice	High
Chickpeas	Low	Sweet potatoes	Medium
Corn	Medium	Tomatoes	Low
Corn flake cereal	High	Waffle, white flour	High
Cucumbers	Low	Watermelon	High
Donuts	High	White flour bread	High
Grapefruit	Low	White rice	Medium
Grapes	Low	Whole-wheat bread	Low
Kidney beans	Low	Yogurt	Low
Lettuce, all varieties	Low		

Chapter 6

The Key Nutritional Components for a Flat Belly

In This Chapter

▶ Understanding diet must-haves to achieve your flat belly

▶ Examining true portion sizes of everyday foods

▶ Increasing your metabolism with a few quick fixes

To be as successful as possible with your Belly Fat Diet plan, you need to understand the impact each food group has on your belly and know which foods are best and which may have a negative impact on your weight loss efforts. One of the easiest ways to get off track with your weight loss is to be unprepared.

So in this chapter, I show you what foods you need to have on hand at all times. I take a close look at each of the food groups in the Belly Fat Diet. I also explain why these foods are necessary. After all, knowing why you should eat something versus just being told to do it is much more beneficial in helping you achieve and maintain your weight loss goals.

I also help you identify and understand one of the biggest culprits of weight gain: portion distortion. Over the past 30 years, American portions have grown larger and larger. And now you probably have become accustomed to these huge portions without even realizing it. If you continue to eat these monster-sized portions, you'll take in far more calories than your body needs. And these excess calories are stored as fat right in your belly. In this chapter, I help you identify a true portion so you can combat portion distortion and achieve a slim waistline permanently!

Diet Basics that Lead to a Flatter Belly

Before I discuss each of the food groups, I want to give you a general overview of the key actions to take when beginning the Belly Fat Diet. To achieve the flat belly of your dreams, you must stick with the following habits:

✔ **Include at least one belly-burning food at each meal.**

✔ **Eat consistently throughout the day.** Don't wait too long in between meals and don't skip meals or snacks. Doing so can lead to overeating and can even slow your metabolism.

✔ **Avoid as many belly-bloating foods as possible on a regular basis.** Head to Chapter 19 for a list of foods to avoid.

✔ **Eat food you enjoy!** If you don't treat yourself to the foods you like to eat, you won't stick with your plan.

✔ **Incorporate variety in your meal plan.** You can eat the same things day in and day out, but doing so will likely lead to boredom. And with boredom comes cravings for less-than-healthy foods. Switching up your meals can help keep your meal plan interesting, thus helping you to stay on track.

The Power of Protein

Protein is essential to your body for many reasons. In fact, proteins are involved in almost all cellular function in your body! They help build and strengthen muscle tissue, build and repair cells, and process chemical reactions. Some even work as antibodies to ward off diseases and infections. Without an adequate amount of protein in your body, you would be in trouble.

Protein plays a critical role in weight loss and maintenance as well. By preserving and building lean muscle tissue and increasing the number of calories you burn during digestion, protein can help increase the amount of energy (in calories) you expend each day, promoting weight loss. It also helps to fight off hunger. Weight loss can be more difficult with an inadequate amount of protein.

Protein is found in the diet in two forms:

✔ **Animal proteins:** Protein in the form of beef, poultry, fish, game meats, eggs, and cheese

✔ **Plant-based proteins:** Protein from non-animal sources, such as tofu and other soy products, beans, and lentils

Before you get too wrapped up in eating all the protein you can get your hands on, remember the three types of protein: lean protein, medium-fat protein, and high-fat protein. Protein that contains a higher amount of fat also contains a higher number of calories per ounce. And because most high-fat protein also comes from animal sources, it's usually in the form of unhealthy, saturated fats. As you begin to add proteins to your meal plan, make sure to select lean proteins over the high-fat ones. Here's the skinny on the differences:

✓ **Lean protein:** Approximately 30–40 calories per ounce and 3 grams of fat or less per ounce

✓ **Medium-fat protein:** Approximately 45–55 calories per ounce and 5 grams of fat per ounce

✓ **High-fat protein:** Approximately 80–100 calories per ounce and 8 grams of fat per ounce

Because medium- and high-fat proteins contain a higher number of calories per ounce, consuming these types of proteins too often can slow your weight loss efforts. And, if they come from a source with an increased amount of saturated or trans fats, these proteins can increase inflammation, which may cause you to pack on more belly fat. So choosing lean proteins on a regular basis is essential to your success. The later section "Realizing true portion sizes" provides tables that show you which proteins are categorized as lean, medium-fat, and high-fat proteins.

In the following sections, I show you how protein impacts body weight so you can use this macronutrient to your advantage.

Protein: The hunger fighter

One of the main reasons you need to consume an adequate amount of protein when trying to lose or maintain a healthy body weight is that protein helps fight hunger. Unlike carbohydrates, which digest quickly, protein takes much longer to process. This slow digestion helps you feel satisfied for a longer period of time. And if you aren't feeling hungry, you're probably not suffering from food cravings or eating too quickly, which are behaviors that can contribute to weight gain.

Visualize yourself eating a big bowl of enriched white flour pasta with nothing but tomato sauce on top. How long do you think this meal will keep you full? One hour? Two? Now picture yourself sitting down to eat out of the exact same bowl, but this time you fill it with pieces of grilled chicken instead. You may not even be able to finish eating it, and, if you do, you'll feel uncomfortably full for four hours or more.

I don't want you to go and stuff yourself with huge bowls of chicken. The moral of the story is this: For the same number of calories, protein keeps you feeling much more satisfied for a longer period of time. And this benefit prevents you from eating too-large portions of other foods, which can pack on the pounds. So I recommend including a source of lean protein at each meal to avoid becoming too hungry in between meals and snacks.

Don't worry if you're a vegetarian or vegan. Plant-based proteins work perfectly at helping to control appetite. So if you don't consume any form of animal protein, adding a food like soy beans, lentils, or even tofu to your plate at each meal is important.

Protein: The metabolism booster

The most exciting benefit of eating protein is that it can help you burn more calories, therefore boosting your metabolism. Protein contains a high thermic effect. A *thermic effect* is the amount of energy (in calories) your body needs to burn in order to break down, digest, and metabolize a food. Because protein contains a higher thermic effect than other macronutrients, it causes your body to burn more calories to digest it than if you ate a carbohydrate or fat.

Its high thermic effect isn't the only way protein helps to boost metabolism. Your muscle tissue, which is made up largely of protein, is the most metabolically active tissue in your body. As a result, it burns many more calories than fat cells or other tissues.

When you start to lose weight, you can lose not just fat mass but muscle mass as well. If you lose too much muscle mass, your metabolism slows. Because muscle burns such a large number of calories, losing muscle means you burn fewer calories overall during the day, slowing your metabolism. As a result, further weight loss and even weight maintenance may become difficult. Protein, however, contains an amino acid called *leucine,* which helps protect you against muscle losses while you're losing weight. So be sure to consume an adequate amount of protein as you shed pounds.

Eating Fat to Reduce Belly Fat

Many folks think that they have to cut out fat entirely when they're trying to lose weight and belly fat. Believe it or not, though, certain dietary fats can actually help to burn belly fat. In fact, research has shown that diets rich in healthy fats promote increased fat loss, especially from the midsection. The main fat fighters are monounsaturated fats and omega-3 fatty acids. Here's how they work:

- ✔ **They help to fight off inflammation.** Inflammation can be damaging to your overall health and trigger your body to store more belly fat. By decreasing chronic inflammation in your body, these fats can help decrease internal stressors that pack on the pounds. To see how inflammation can increase belly fat, flip to Chapter 4.

- ✔ **They take longer to digest.** This extended digestion helps you feel full longer, preventing cravings and overeating. Do you remember the fat-free diet fad from the '90s? It didn't work because when you eat meals with little fat (and mostly carbohydrates), you have a limited feeling of satiety. As a result, you consume more food, and therefore more calories, throughout the day.

✔ **Omega-3 fatty acids help reduce stress hormones in your body.** Having increased belly fat can be a telltale sign of having too much stress in your life. This increased level of stress causes an increase in the production of stress hormones like cortisol. This increase in stress hormone production promotes an increase in the storage of belly fat. However, having more omega-3s in your meal plan helps cut stress hormones, and therefore, cut down on the amount of belly fat they can store. For more on how stress hormones promote the storage of belly fat, head to Chapter 5.

Some dietary fats can be quite negative to your health and can increase belly fat. These are the fats you want to limit:

✔ **Saturated fats:** These fats are mainly found in animal proteins, so a diet rich in high-fat dairy, red meat, and processed meat is high in saturated fat. These fats have been linked with an increased risk for heart disease, elevated cholesterol levels, and inflammation in the body.

A small amount of saturated fat each day is alright, but you want to make sure that less than 10 percent of your total daily calories comes from saturated fat. So on the Belly Fat Diet plan, you're allotted 14–18 grams of saturated fat per day.

✔ **Trans fats:** These fats are found mostly in processed foods, such as fried foods, pastries and other baked goods, biscuits, muffins, crackers, and even some brands of microwave popcorn. These fats can lower your good cholesterol, raise your bad cholesterol, and trigger inflammation. In fact, research has shown that even just 2 grams of trans fats per day can have a negative impact on your health. Because these fats can pack inches onto your waistline, you need to eliminate them from your diet to successfully reach your flat-belly goals. To identify trans fats in your foods, check out Chapter 11.

Although healthy fats can be essential for getting rid of belly fat, balance is key. Too much of a good thing can be bad, especially when it comes to fats. Healthy fats have powerful health and weight loss benefits, but they're also high in calories. So it's important that you consume just enough of these healthy fats to reap their belly-flattening benefits without consuming so much that you cancel out their effects.

Great sources of monounsaturated fats include

✔ Almonds

✔ Avocado

✔ Cashews

- ✔ Natural peanut or almond butter
- ✔ Olives
- ✔ Olive oil
- ✔ Peanuts
- ✔ Peanut oil
- ✔ Sesame oil

Terrific sources of omega-3 fatty acids include

- ✔ Chia seeds
- ✔ Cod
- ✔ Flaxseed
- ✔ Halibut
- ✔ Omega-3 eggs
- ✔ Salmon
- ✔ Sardines
- ✔ Scallops
- ✔ Seaweed
- ✔ Soybeans
- ✔ Tofu
- ✔ Walnuts

In Chapter 7, I outline the number of servings of these healthy fats you should have per day based on your individual meal plan. This balance provides you with all the health benefits of these healthy fats and none of the negative impacts of eating too many or too few.

Carbohydrates: Belly Shrinkers and Belly Bloaters

Carbohydrates play a critical role in belly fat in two ways: by increasing it or decreasing it. To successfully achieve your weight loss and belly-flattening goals, you must know the carbohydrate sources that can shrink belly fat as well as the ones that can actually increase it.

Describing the sources is pretty simple: Whole-grain carbohydrates help fight belly fat, and refined carbohydrates increase it. So the key is to identify which carbs are whole grain and which are refined. After you can distinguish one from another, you're on your way to selecting only belly-friendly carbohydrates that will have you burning up belly fat and slimming down!

The following sections give you the lowdown on both whole and refined carbohydrates.

Identifying whole grains

A grain is made of the following three elements:

- ✔ **Bran:** This is the outer layer of the grain. It's rich in B vitamins, antioxidants, minerals, and fiber.
- ✔ **Endosperm:** This is the middle starchy layer of the grain. It's where complex carbohydrates and some proteins are found.
- ✔ **Germ:** This innermost layer of the grain is rich in B vitamins, vitamin E, minerals, antioxidants, and even essential fatty acids.

A whole grain, which is basically in its original form, contains all three of these important elements, making it rich in essential vitamins, minerals, antioxidants, complex carbohydrates, and fiber.

When trying to find whole-grain products, you need to look closely at the packaging. Look for the words "100%" followed by a grain on the product packaging. If your product says "100% whole wheat," for example, you're getting all parts of the grain, or a whole-grain product. You can also look at the ingredients. The first ingredient is what makes up the majority of the food. The first ingredient should be a "whole" product like whole-wheat flour or whole-rye flour. If the second ingredient lists a "whole" ingredient (and the first one doesn't) you can't be sure of the proportion of whole grain in the product, so it may not be your best choice.

Avoiding refined carbohydrates

Refined carbohydrates are processed, or refined, to remove layers of the original grain (see the preceding section for details on the layers). Typically, when grains are refined both the inner layer (germ) and outer layer (bran) are removed, leaving just the middle starchy layer (endosperm). This processing leaves behind all the energy (calories) but little to no fiber, vitamins, minerals, and antioxidants. About 25 percent of the protein in the grain is removed during refining as well.

Some processers replace some vitamins and minerals to their products. These products are known as *enriched grains*. However, these enriched grains don't contain the original amount of antioxidants, fiber, or protein of the whole grain.

When trying to identify a refined grain, look for any of the following terms as the first ingredient listed on the product packaging:

- ✔ Bran flour (without the word "whole")
- ✔ Cornmeal
- ✔ Durum wheat
- ✔ Enriched flour
- ✔ Mixed grain
- ✔ Multigrain
- ✔ Semolina
- ✔ Unbleached flour
- ✔ Wheat flour (without the word "whole")

You want to see the word "whole" before any grain; otherwise, some parts of the grain may be missing and won't provide all the nutrients and nutrient benefits.

Comparing the impact of whole grains and refined carbohydrates on belly fat

When you eat a refined grain, you're consuming mostly carbohydrates with very little fiber or protein to help slow down the absorption of the food. Because digestion happens rapidly, your body quickly converts the carbohydrates into glucose (sugar). After glucose enters your bloodstream, your body releases insulin to bring the sugar into your cells for energy. But here's where the problem arises: When your blood sugar increases quickly (which is what happens when a food is digested rapidly), your body releases that much more insulin to quickly bring your blood sugar back down by transporting it into your cells.

Insulin is one of the main culprits of belly fat (see Chapter 2 to understand why). The more insulin that's introduced into your bloodstream, the more your body stores fat, specifically belly fat.

All foods create an insulin response. However, certain foods, specifically refined carbohydrates and simple sugars, cause the largest spike in insulin, which is why you want to avoid them. These foods not only lack nutrients, but because of the insulin response, they also store belly fat — even if you keep your overall calories reduced!

Whole grains trigger an insulin response, but because of the fiber and protein in the whole grain, this response is reduced. As a result, you have less insulin circulating throughout your body, and therefore less belly fat is being stored.

Just because all grains, even whole grains, cause an insulin response doesn't mean that you should avoid them all together. Carbohydrates are essential to your body in many ways, with the main reason being energy. If you reduce your intake of grains too much, you may notice a dip in energy levels. In fact, you may even have trouble thinking clearly (because sugar is the main source of energy for your brain).

You need whole grains daily. Besides helping you achieve and maintain a healthy body weight, these grains have quite a few health benefits, including the following:

✔ Reduced risk of heart disease and stroke

✔ Reduced risk of type 2 diabetes and help promoting the maintenance of blood sugar levels

✔ Reduction in cancers related to the digestive system

✔ Help in lowering cholesterol

✔ Help in maintaining digestive system regularity

Reviewing the whole grain and hunger connection

In addition to limiting the insulin response, whole grains help promote weight loss and a reduction in belly fat in another way: They help control your appetite. Because whole grains are digested more slowly than their refined counterparts, they help provide an increased feeling of satiety after eating. However, when you eat a refined carbohydrate and promote an increase in insulin, not only does the insulin store fat, but it also increases your appetite. So after eating a refined carbohydrate, you may feel hungrier sooner and even experience cravings for more simple sugars. As a result, you end up in a cycle of eating too many refined carbohydrates over and over, which just causes you to continue to pack on belly fat.

By decreasing hunger and preventing cravings, whole grains can help you stay on track with your Belly Fat Diet plan, helping you to achieve your weight loss goals even faster.

Fruit: It's Essential, but Watch the Sugar

Fruit is an essential component of a healthy meal plan. It's not only essential for good health, but it's also needed for sustainable weight loss. Fruit provides you with a large amount of antioxidants, fiber, phytochemicals, and carbohydrates. And the best benefit of fruit is that it provides you with a sweet satisfaction, which can help reduce cravings for less-than-belly-friendly sweets like candy.

Studies have shown that people who eat a large amount of fruit lose more weight than people who eat a large amount of vegetables (but not as much fruit). What a great incentive to start eating more fruit!

Even though fruit has many powerful health benefits and can promote weight loss, you still need to watch your intake of it. Fruit is rich in vitamins and minerals, but it's also rich in natural sugars. These sugars are fine to eat, but if you consume more natural sugars than your body truly needs, you may find that the increased intake slows or even stops your weight loss efforts.

In this section, I show you the best fruits to consume and tell you which ones to limit. In the later section "Realizing true portion sizes," I explain what a portion of fruit actually is. In Chapter 7, I show you how many portions of fruit per day are recommended (based on your individual meal plan) so you gain all the benefits from fruit without any of the negative effects.

The best fruits for your belly

All fruits contain health benefits, such as providing you with large amounts of disease- and inflammation-fighting antioxidants, but some fruits play a more powerful role in shrinking belly fat than others. The following sections uncover some of the most powerful belly-fighting fruits and why you want to eat them.

Blueberries

Blueberries may be small, but they're powerhouses! These tasty berries have many health and weight loss benefits. Consider the following:

- ✔ They're powerful inflammation fighters thanks to their super-high antioxidant content.
- ✔ They're potent belly shrinkers. A study at the University of Michigan Cardiovascular Center found that when rats consumed just 2 percent of their calories from blueberries over a 90-day period, they significantly reduced their percentage of belly fat.

- ✔ According to a study by the University of Michigan, they can reduce triglyceride levels and increase insulin sensitivity, perhaps cutting the risk for cardiovascular disease and diabetes.

- ✔ They have been shown to help reduce food cravings.

Pomegranate

Pomegranates with their red, juicy seeds are a potent tool to include in your weight loss arsenal. Here are the main benefits:

- ✔ They have some of the highest levels of antioxidants when compared to many fruits.

- ✔ They contain high levels of the polyphenol *catechin.* This powerful chemical has been shown to increase your body's fat-burning potential and may even help to boost metabolism, making it a strong belly-fat fighter. To further promote weight loss, catechins may also decrease appetite, helping to prevent overeating.

- ✔ They may help decrease fat buildup in the arteries, making them as healthy for the heart as they are for your waistline.

Tart cherries

Tart cherries are rich in the plant chemical *anthocyanin.* Not only does this chemical give the cherries their bright color, but it also helps you burn belly fat.

A study conducted by the University of Michigan found that when mice were given food that contained added tart cherry powder, their body fat reduced by 9 percent more than mice fed the same diet without the additional cherry powder. Even better, most of the weight loss came from fat stores in the abdominal area. The mice fed the cherry powder also showed significant decreases in cholesterol levels as well as a decline in inflammatory markers.

Tart cherries are different from the sweet cherries you may often eat raw. They're not usually found in the fresh produce aisle. Instead, you can usually find them frozen or dried. Just be sure you buy an unsweetened variety.

Grapefruit

Grapefruit is a super fat burner. It also has diuretic properties, which help you shed any unwanted water retention, leaving you looking and feeling slimmer, especially in the midsection. This refreshing citrus fruit has long been linked with many promising studies touting its weight loss benefits. Here are a couple to chew on:

- ✔ A 2011 study in *Nutrition & Metabolism* by researchers at Vanderbilt University found that when obese adults consumed half a grapefruit or 4 ounces of 100 percent grapefruit juice before three main meals, they experienced a significant decrease in both body weight and waist circumference. Why? Perhaps the high water content and volume of the grapefruit prior to meals helped make them feel fuller sooner, allowing them to eat smaller portions at the next meals.

✔ A 2009 study in the *Journal of Nutrition* found that eating a low-glycemic-index food, such as grapefruit, for breakfast before exercising helps you burn 50 percent more fat. (Check out Chapter 5 for more information on glycemic index.)

 If you're taking medications, make sure to check with your doctor or pharmacist before eating grapefruit or drinking grapefruit juice. Grapefruit products can have potentially adverse interactions with some medications.

More fruits to enjoy

No fruit is bad for your belly as long as you consume the right portions per day (I provide guidelines based on your individual meal plan in Chapter 7). In the preceding sections, I list some of the best fruits for your belly, but you have many, many more great options, including

✔ Apples

✔ Blackberries

✔ Grapes

✔ Mango

✔ Nectarines

✔ Oranges

✔ Peaches

✔ Pears

✔ Plums

✔ Raspberries

✔ Strawberries

The fruits to limit

Fruit is great for you, but you do have to keep in mind the glycemic index (GI) of the type you choose. Choosing foods with a lower GI can help promote the loss of belly fat (see Chapter 5 for details). Most fruits are in the low range on the GI scale, but a few are higher, most specifically watermelon. Because it has an elevated GI, watermelon may cause spikes in both blood sugar and insulin levels, which can trigger storage of belly fat.

Watermelon isn't all bad, however. Out of almost all fruits and vegetables, it contains the highest content of *lycopene,* which is a phytochemical that has been shown to protect the heart by decreasing the buildup of plaque in the arteries. Some studies have also shown a positive correlation between increased lycopene intake and a decreased risk of certain cancers, such as prostate cancer. Watermelon is also rich in the amino acid *arginine,* which has been shown to promote fat loss and increase muscle mass.

You don't need to avoid watermelon, just watch how often you eat it and how much you eat at one sitting. For the best belly-flattening results, keep your watermelon intake to about 1 cup per day. This way you get all the great benefits of watermelon without too much impact on your insulin levels.

Other fruits that can contain a high GI include

- ✔ **Dried fruits with added sugar:** When choosing dried fruit, buy brands that only contain fruit. Dried fruits that list sugar, cane juice, or corn syrup in the ingredients are loaded with added sweeteners that can raise your GI and promote increased belly fat storage.

- ✔ **Fruits that have been canned in heavy syrup:** If you enjoy canned fruits, choose varieties canned in 100 percent fruit juice rather than those packed in syrups.

- ✔ **Fruit juices, specifically juices that aren't 100 percent juice:** Because juices contain limited amounts of fiber, they aren't as filling as eating a piece of fruit. They also may potentially raise blood sugar and insulin levels higher than a piece of fruit would. If you do have juice, drink it in moderation (approximately ½ to 1 cup per day). Also be sure to select a brand that contains only 100 percent fruit juice. If you love juice in larger quantities, try this trick: Dilute 4 ounces of juice with 8 ounces of water for a delicious and refreshing beverage with less sugar.

To identify and avoid these high-GI fruits, make sure you read labels. You can find out more about reading labels in Chapter 11.

Vegetables: You Gotta Have 'Em

Vegetables can help to shrink belly fat and promote weight loss in so many great ways! One of the greatest benefits of vegetables when you're trying to lose weight is that they provide you with a great amount of volume and satiety with few calories.

Think about it this way: If you were hungry and ate six plain crackers, would you feel full? Probably not. What if you ate 6 cups of raw, sliced cucumbers? I bet you would feel a lot more satisfied. And what if I told you that 6 cups of cucumbers contains the same number of calories as those six crackers? Amazing! That's one of the benefits of vegetables: You can eat plates full of them without taking in many calories. If you ate plates full of other foods, on the other hand, you'd gain weight. But when you eat large amounts of vegetables, you feel satisfied and eat less of other food groups, helping you to shed weight quickly without feeling hungry or deprived!

Most vegetables on your Belly Fat Diet plan are unlimited. In fact, I want you to eat lots of them. I want you to strive to take in at least the minimum recommended amount of vegetables each day (see Chapter 7 for your individual meal plan guidelines). If you don't eat enough vegetables, chances are you'll feel hungrier and eat more of another food group, which will contain additional calories that can make it more difficult to lose weight.

I provide all the info you need on adding veggies to your diet in the following sections.

Getting your antioxidants

In addition to helping you feel full with few calories, vegetables also help promote weight loss by being rich in many powerful antioxidants, vitamins, minerals, and phyotochemicals. Some of these nutrients, such as catechins and anthocyanins, by themselves can help increase your body's ability to burn fat. But as a whole, antioxidants help to decrease oxidative stress in your body.

Your body needs oxygen to live and to perform many essential functions. However, high concentrations of oxygen in your body can actually cause damage. The way you obtain energy to live and perform day-to-day functions is by taking the fuel you put in your body (food) and combining it with the air you breathe (oxygen). This metabolic process provides your body with energy, but it also creates byproducts, such as free radicals, that can be damaging to your body's cells.

Oxidative stress is essentially the stress placed on your body from the free radicals produced during digestion and metabolism as well as the environmental toxins your body is exposed to, such as pollutants in the air, cigarette smoke, and so on. Poor dietary habits, such as diets high in simple sugars and trans fats and low in antioxidants, can increase the oxidative damage to your cells as well.

Increased oxidative stress can increase inflammation in the body. And, as I describe in Chapter 4, inflammation can trigger increased fat storage, especially in the belly. The good news is that antioxidants are warriors that fight off the free radicals that can attack and damage your body's cells. Because vegetables contain incredibly high amounts of antioxidants, the more you eat, the more you increase your defense mechanisms against these attackers, cutting down on cell damage as well as inflammation. And when inflammation decreases, so does belly fat!

Filling your plate with color

Have you ever heard the rule to eat a rainbow on your plate? Maybe in school? Well even though this guideline may sound a bit childish, adults need to eat the colors of the rainbow as much as little ones. Every color vegetable contains a different type and amount of antioxidants. If you only eat one or two colors, you may be missing out on some potent belly fat and disease fighters. In the following sections, I give you the lowdown on some of the best colors of fresh vegetables.

Orange and yellow vegetables

The orange and yellow group is terrific for your skin, eyes, and heart. Some research also suggests this group may fight off some cancers. Beta carotene is plentiful in this group. This compound has been shown to promote eye health and protect skin from sun damage, and it may even delay cognitive aging. Beta carotene is also a precursor for vitamin A, meaning it's a vitamin that can help neutralize the damage of free radicals in the body, helping to fight off oxidative stress and inflammation. This group of veggies is also rich in vitamin C, which can help decrease stress hormones in the body, helping to prevent storage of belly fat.

Examples of orange and yellow vegetables include

- Carrots
- Corn
- Pumpkin
- Summer squash
- Sweet potatoes
- Yellow and orange peppers
- Yellow tomatoes

Green vegetables

The green vegetable group contains high levels of vitamins A and C, which, just like in orange and yellow vegetables, can help decrease oxidative stress and cut down on the stress hormones in the body that can store belly fat. In addition, green leafy vegetables are a fantastic source of folic acid, which plays a critical role in protein digestion and metabolism. Because adequate folic acid helps ensure that protein is metabolized properly, it may also help your body's insulin levels remain stable. Spiking or rapidly fluctuating insulin levels can trigger fat storage, especially in the belly. So consuming foods rich in folic acid may help to better stabilize insulin levels, decreasing the storage of belly fat.

Examples of green vegetables include

- ✔ Asparagus
- ✔ Broccoli
- ✔ Brussels sprouts
- ✔ Cabbage
- ✔ Cucumbers
- ✔ Green beans
- ✔ Kale
- ✔ Lettuce
- ✔ Spinach
- ✔ Zucchini

White vegetables

The white group is colored by pigments called *anthoxanthins,* which contain disease-fighting chemicals like allicin. This chemical may help reduce overall cholesterol and blood pressure levels as well as fight off inflammation in the body.

Examples of the white vegetables include

- ✔ Cauliflower
- ✔ Mushrooms
- ✔ Onions
- ✔ Parsnips
- ✔ Potatoes
- ✔ Turnips

Red and purple vegetables

The red coloring of these vegetables is an indication they're high in the phytochemical lycopene. This nutrient is a potent antioxidant that has been shown to protect your heart (by decreasing the buildup of plaque in your arteries) and may even protect against cancers like prostate cancer.

Examples of red and purple vegetables include

- ✔ Beets
- ✔ Eggplant
- ✔ Red cabbage

> ✔ Red onions
> ✔ Red peppers
> ✔ Tomatoes

Starchy vegetables: Good for you in limited quantities

As I mention earlier, many vegetables are essentially unlimited because they provide so many health benefits and so much volume with so few calories. A few vegetables are the exception to this rule, however. These are known as *starchy vegetables*. These vegetables are still loaded with healthy and belly-shrinking benefits, but they're higher in carbohydrates and calories, so they can't be consumed in unlimited quantities.

Eating too many of these starchy vegetables may slow down your weight loss progress. So for your Belly Fat Diet plan, these particular vegetables fall into the starch category, which is the same food group that contains breads, cereal, and pasta. (The starchy veggies have an equivalent amount of carbohydrates per serving as these bread products.) In Chapter 7, I show you just how many servings of starch you can have per day based on your individual meal plan. The vegetables that fall into the starch category are

> ✔ Beans and lentils
> ✔ Corn
> ✔ Peas
> ✔ Plantains
> ✔ Potatoes
> ✔ Sweet potatoes
> ✔ Winter squash (acorn, butternut, spaghetti, pumpkin)
> ✔ Yams

Dairy Done Right

Consuming an adequate amount of dairy products, such as milk and yogurt, is important to your success with your Belly Fat Diet plan. Dairy products are packed with whey, a protein that helps promote the formation of lean body mass (which in turn helps you burn more calories). Because dairy contains a high level of protein, it helps keep you feeling full and satisfied. As a result, you reduce your portions and, therefore, promote weight loss.

Some research has found that a diet rich in dairy may also directly promote weight loss. A study published in *Obesity Research* showed that obese individuals who ate a diet rich in dairy lost significantly more body fat and weight than other individuals eating the same number of calories but following a low-dairy diet. In fact, the dairy-rich group lost almost double the amount of fat and weight. The best part was that a majority of the fat lost came from the midsection. So increasing your intake of dairy may help you flatten your belly faster than just cutting calories alone.

These findings may be in part due to calcium's crucial role in regulating how fat is stored and broken down by the body. Researchers think that the more calcium a fat cell has, the more fat it will burn. Dairy products are also rich in the amino acid arginine, which has been shown to help promote fat loss and increase muscle mass. Other studies have shown that an increased intake of dietary calcium may also increase fat excretion in stool. So a diet high in calcium may slightly decrease calorie absorption from dietary fat intake, which may help promote weight loss as well.

For the Belly Fat Diet, the dairy group consists of milk and yogurt. Cheese falls into the protein food group. Here's why: Milk and yogurt contain high levels of both protein and carbohydrates as well as fat depending on the variety you choose, and cheese contains just protein and fat.

In the following sections, I give you the skinny on blasting belly fat by increasing your dairy intake.

CLA and belly fat

Dairy products may help to promote weight loss because of a fatty acid called *conjugated linoleic acid* (CLA). This acid is found mainly in dairy and beef products and has recently been gaining attention for its potential to aid in weight loss. In fact, if you look in any supplement store, you can find many products containing CLA promoted for weight and fat loss. One reason CLA may help promote weight loss is that it's thought to help trigger fat cells to shrink and die off.

Some promising research shows that these claims may be true. Animal studies show that mice consuming a diet high in CLA had significant reductions in body fat. However, more research is needed in the human population. The few studies that have been done show that the results of an increased intake of CLA weren't as significant in humans as they were in mice. And one other caution: In animal studies, a high CLA intake actually caused fatty liver disease in some test samples.

All is not lost, however. CLA has also shown some potential to improve insulin resistance, decrease blood sugar levels, and fight off some cancers. Human studies seem to indicate that 3.2 grams of CLA daily may help reduce body fat and promote health benefits. Foods don't list the CLA content on nutrition labels, but consuming the correct portions of dairy and protein on your Belly Fat Diet plan can help you to take in adequate CLA.

Due to the findings in some studies that high supplemental levels of CLA can potentially increase the risk of fatty liver disease, I recommend increasing your intake of CLA through food. If you wish to consume CLA as a supplement, make sure to speak to your physician first to make sure doing so is appropriate for you.

Choosing the right milk and yogurt

Dairy can play a huge role in helping to reduce belly fat, but it's important to make sure you're choosing the right forms of dairy. A stroll down the milk aisle in your grocery store shows that the options are vast. Should you buy low-fat, full-fat, organic, nondairy? The decision can feel overwhelming. That's why I give you some simple guidelines here to help you select the best milk and yogurt for your belly without spending half your day examining the cartons.

Milking it

You want to choose low-fat milk. Full-fat and 2 percent milk is rich in saturated fat, which can clog arteries and trigger an increase in inflammation. Aim to choose either 0 percent fat (skim) or 1 percent fat milk as your milk of choice.

Also, select dairy that comes from grass-fed cows whenever possible. Cows that feed on grass and grains have a much more favorable milk composition, such as a higher CLA content. In fact, it's believed that milk from grass-fed cows contains almost five times more CLA than grain-fed cows. Cows fed a diet composed of mostly grains, blood meal, or bone meal contain higher levels of unhealthy fats and little to no CLA. Some organic milk contains milk from grass-fed cows, but not all. So check the labels to be sure.

Some individuals can't tolerate dairy or prefer to remove it from their diets. No problem. Suitable substitutes include soy, almond, and coconut milk. Rice milk isn't recommended (unless you have allergies to the other milk substitutes) because it contains a higher percentage of carbohydrates and a lower percentage of protein than other milk alternatives. When choosing nondairy milk substitutes, unsweetened varieties are the best choice. If you do select a sweetened variety, pick a brand with 10 grams of sugar or less per cup, and try to avoid brands that contain high fructose corn syrup in the ingredients.

Picking yogurt

Do you find the sea of never-ending yogurt options in the grocery store a bit overwhelming? You're not alone! Between light yogurt, plain, flavored, Greek, and everything in between, it can feel like an impossible decision to choose the best yogurt for your belly and health. No need to feel defeated. Just use these simple guidelines:

✔ **Choose low-fat or fat-free yogurt (0 percent or 1 percent) over the higher fat varieties.** You can go for plain or Greek yogurt. Greek yogurt is strained, providing it with a thicker consistency and a higher protein content, which can fill you up.

✔ **Watch out for flavored yogurts.** These varieties often contain large amounts of added sugars. All yogurt contains some naturally occurring sugar, so no need to choose a sugar-free yogurt, but do look at the labels. Aim for a yogurt with no more than 15 grams of sugar per 8-ounce serving.

Portion Distortion: When Enough Just Isn't Enough Anymore

Portion distortion is the phenomenon that occurs when you start to view excessively large portions as the normal servings you should eat. When eating in a restaurant, you can see that portions have been slowly increasing in size. Over the past 20 to 30 years, portions on average have increased dramatically. Check out the portion increase statistics in Table 6-1.

Table 6-1	Portion Increases in Restaurant Foods	
Food	*20 years ago*	*Today*
Bagel	3-inch diameter, 140 calories	6-inch diameter, 350 calories
Cheeseburger	4 ounces, 330 calories	8 ounces, 590 calories
Spaghetti	1 cup with 3 small meatballs, 500 calories	2 cups with 3 large meatballs, 1,025 calories
French Fries	2.4 ounces, 210 calories	6.9 ounces, 610 calories
Soda	6.5 ounces, 80 calories	20 ounces, 250 calories

Source: USDA

Even if you have been ordering the same foods at restaurants over the years, you can be gaining weight simply because the portions continue to enlarge. What's worse is that you may view these super-sized portions as normal. As a result, you're now conditioned to recognize these portions as standard and you may fill your plate with more food than your body really needs — whether you're eating out or at home.

So what's the solution? I don't want you to shrink your portions overnight. If you go cold turkey on your portion sizes, you'll find yourself hungry and feeling deprived. And deprivation can lead to everything from cravings to binge eating, which isn't the solution to weight loss. The solution to permanent weight loss is to eat filling foods that are low in calories. That way you can continue to fill your plate but actually take in fewer calories overall without feeling hungry or deprived.

For example, check out the food comparisons in Figure 6-1. Consider which options help you feel more satisfied for a longer period of time.

I show you the true portion sizes of some of the most common foods in the following sections. I also show you how to trick yourself into thinking you're eating more.

Realizing true portion sizes

In order to be successful with your weight loss and belly-flattening efforts, you need to be able to identify a true portion of food. Being able to do so helps you recognize portion distortion, which can cause you to overeat without even realizing it.

The following sections outline the true portion sizes in each food group of your Belly Fat Diet plan. These portion sizes are based on the American Diabetes Association (ADA) Diabetic Exchange List.

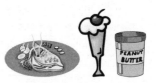

Deli bagel with 2 tablespoons
cream cheese

VS.

Egg-white omlet with lowfat cheese
and
Nonfat yogurt parfait with 1 cup berries
and 1/2 c cereal
and
1 slice whole-wheat toast with
2 teaspoons of peanut butter

Total Calories: 600   **Total Calories: 600**

Figure 6-1:
High-calorie
foods
versus high-
volume,
low-calorie
foods.

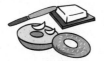

16-ounce soft drink

VS.

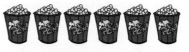

6 cups of air-popped popcorn

Total Calories: 200   **Total Calories: 200**

Illustration by Wiley, Composition Services Graphics

To find out how alcohol fits into your Belly Fat Diet plan, including the portions allowed, head to Chapter 17.

Fruits and vegetables

In Chapter 7, I outline exactly how many servings of fruits and vegetables you need each day to stay on track with your Belly Fat Diet plan and achieve your weight loss goals. But what exactly is a serving? In Table 6-2, I show you just how much of a certain vegetable or certain fruit is considered one serving. This information can help you see whether you're eating too little, too much, or just enough.

Table 6-2	Portion Sizes of Fruits and Vegetables
Food	**Size of a Serving**
Cooked vegetables	½ cup
Raw vegetables	1 cup
100% vegetable juice	6 ounces
Whole fruit (apples, oranges, pears, peaches, and so on)	1 medium piece (size of a baseball)
Bananas	Half of a medium banana
Berries, melons, grapes	1 cup
Canned fruit in juice	½ cup
No-sugar-added dried fruit	¼ cup
100% fruit juice	½ cup

Dairy

For the Belly Fat Diet plan, the dairy group contains milk and yogurt. Cheese and eggs are included in the protein group. Consuming adequate dairy during the day is essential to making sure you're taking in adequate amounts of CLA, calcium, vitamin D, and protein. Table 6-3 outlines what a serving of dairy is equal to. In Chapter 7, you can see how many servings of dairy you need each day on your individualized meal plan.

Table 6-3	Portion Sizes of Dairy Products
Food or Drink	**Size of a Serving**
Fat-free or 1% milk	1 cup
Soy or almond milk (with less than 10 grams of sugar per cup)	1 cup

Food or Drink	Size of a Serving
2% or whole milk (equals 1 dairy + 1 fat serving)	1 cup
Fat-free or lowfat plain yogurt	1 cup
Fat-free or lowfat flavored yogurt (15 grams of sugar or less per serving)	1 cup
2% or full-fat yogurt (equals 1 dairy + 1 fat serving)	1 cup
Fat-free or 1% Greek yogurt (equals 1 dairy + 1 protein)	1 cup
Fat-free or lowfat pudding	½ cup

Starches

The starch group incorporates everything from breads to cereal to snack foods and even starchy vegetables. The trickiest part with starches is to know how many servings you should eat each day and what a serving size truly is. In Chapter 7, I provide you with individualized meal plan goals for daily starch servings. In Table 6-4, I list what portion is equal to one serving. Limit your intake of refined starches as much as possible.

Table 6-4	Portion Sizes of Starches
Food	**Size of a Serving**
Breads and Sides	
100% whole-grain bread	1 slice
100% whole-grain cereal	½ cup
Cooked steel-cut oatmeal	½ cup
Cooked whole-grain pasta	½ cup
Cooked brown or wild rice	⅓ cup
Cooked whole-grain couscous	⅓ cup
Cooked quinoa	½ cup
Whole-grain tortillas	One 6-inch tortilla
Whole-grain English muffin	Half of a muffin
Whole-grain pita	Half of a 6-inch pita
Whole-grain bagel	A quarter of a large, deli-size bagel
Whole-grain flour	3 tablespoons

(continued)

Table 6-4 *(continued)*

Food	Size of a Serving
Snack Foods	
Air-popped popcorn	3 cups
Whole-grain pretzels	¾ cup
Whole-grain crackers	6 crackers (or 1 ounce)
Whole-grain baked chips	15 chips
Graham crackers	3 squares
Dark chocolate (equals 1 starch + 1 fat serving)	1 ounce
Starchy Vegetables	
Cooked corn	½ cup
Corn on the cob	1 medium ear
Cooked beans and lentils	½ cup
Cooked peas	½ cup
Plantains	½ cup
Baked russet potato	3 ounces
Baked sweet potato	3 ounces
Cooked winter squash	1 cup
Refined Starches	
White or Italian bread	1 slice
White rice	⅓ cup
White rice cakes	2 large cakes
Cookies (1 starch + 2 fats)	One 2¼-inch cookie
Ice cream (lowfat) or frozen yogurt (1 starch + 1 fat)	½ cup
White flour	3 tablespoons
Sugar, syrup, jelly, or honey	1 tablespoon

Proteins

Protein is essential to your belly-blasting plan because it helps to keep you full and prevents muscle loss while losing fat mass. However, you need to take in the right amount of protein each day. Taking in too much or too little can sabotage your weight loss efforts. In Chapter 7, I show you how many servings of protein you need each day on your Belly Fat Diet plan. In Tables 6-5 and 6-6, I categorize the protein into two groups: lean protein and medium/high-fat protein. Except where noted, one serving size of each of the foods in the following tables equals 1 ounce of protein.

Table 6-5   Portion Sizes of Lean Protein Choices

Food	Size of a Serving
Fish	
All fish, including salmon, flounder, halibut, trout, cod, tilapia, herring, grouper, swordfish, and so on	1 ounce
Canned tuna in water	¼ cup
Canned sardines in water	2 sardines
Shellfish (clams, shrimp, crab, lobster, scallops, oysters, and so on)	1 ounce
Imitation shellfish	1 ounce
Poultry	
Chicken breast, white meat, skinless	1 ounce
Turkey breast, white meat, skinless	1 ounce
Cornish hen, skinless	1 ounce
Ground turkey, 100% breast meat	1 ounce
Ground chicken, 100% breast meat	1 ounce
Pork	
Tenderloin	1 ounce
Center chop loin	1 ounce
Fresh ham	1 ounce
Boiled ham	1 ounce
Canadian bacon	1 ounce
Beef *(for all cuts, choose USDA Select and Choice cuts and trim all visible fat)*	
Flank steak	1 ounce
Round	1 ounce
Tenderloin	1 ounce
Eye of round roast or steak	1 ounce
Sirloin tip side steak	1 ounce
Top round roast and steak	1 ounce
Bottom round roast and steak	1 ounce
Top sirloin steak	1 ounce

(continued)

Table 6-5 *(continued)*

Food	Size of a Serving
Game	
Buffalo (bison)	1 ounce
Venison	1 ounce
Ostrich	1 ounce
Goose (cooked without skin)	1 ounce
Lamb	
Leg of lamb	1 ounce
Loin chops	1 ounce
Loin shoulder	1 ounce
Cheese	
Fat-free or part-skim varieties with 3 grams of fat or less per ounce	1 ounce
Fat-free or part-skim cottage cheese	¼ cup
Fat-free or part-skim ricotta cheese	¼ cup
Parmesan cheese	2 tablespoons
Other	
Legumes/lentils (equals 1 protein and 1 starch serving)	½ cup
Eggs	1 egg
Egg whites	2 egg whites or ¼ cup liquid egg substitute
Tofu	½ cup
Edamame	¼ cup
Vegetable burger	1 burger (equals 2 ounces protein)
Deli meat (choose varieties with 3 grams of fat or less per serving)	1 ounce

Table 6-6　Portion Sizes of Medium- and High-Fat Protein Choices

Food	Size of a Serving
Fish	
Fried fish	1 ounce
Fried shellfish	1 ounce
Sautéed fish or shellfish in oil/butter	1 ounce

Food	Size of a Serving
Fish	
Tuna canned in oil	¼ cup
Poultry	
Chicken, dark meat	1 ounce
Chicken, with skin	1 ounce
Turkey, dark meat	1 ounce
Turkey, with skin	1 ounce
Fried chicken or turkey	1 ounce
Ground chicken/turkey, dark meat	¼ cup
Pork	
Top loin	1 ounce
Chop	1 ounce
Cutlet	1 ounce
Boston butt	1 ounce
Taylor ham	1 ounce
Spare ribs	1 ounce
Ground pork	1 ounce
Pork sausage	1 ounce
Bacon	3 slices
Hot dog	1 ounce
Beef *(any USDA Prime grade of meat counts as a medium/high-fat protein)*	
Ground beef	¼ cup
Corned beef	1 ounce
Filet mignon	1 ounce
Porterhouse steak	1 ounce
New York strip steak	1 ounce
T-bone	1 ounce
Rib-eye	1 ounce
Prime rib	1 ounce
Short rib	1 ounce
Lamb	
Rib roast	1 ounce
Ground lamb	1 ounce

(continued)

Table 6-6 *(continued)*

Food	Size of a Serving
Cheese	
Part-skim or full-fat cheese with more than 3 grams of fat per ounce	1 ounce
Other	
Sandwich meats with more than 3 grams of fat per ounce	1 ounce

Fats

Fats play a critical role in your Belly Fat Diet plan. In fact, some fats even help to burn belly fat. I've divided the fats in Table 6-7 into two groups so you can easily identify which fats are best for your belly and which fats can pack on the fat. In Chapter 7, I show you how many servings of fat you should have each day. And in the following table, I explain what portion is equal to one serving of fat.

Table 6-7	Portion Sizes of Fats
Food	Size of a Serving
Belly-Friendly Fats	
Oil (olive, canola, peanut, grapeseed)	1 teaspoon
Nut butter, natural	2 teaspoons
Hummus	2 tablespoons
Tahini paste	2 teaspoons
Avocado	Quarter of an avocado
Olives	8 large
Almonds	6 nuts
Cashews	6 nuts
Peanuts	10 nuts
Pistachios	10 nuts
Pecans	4 halves
Walnuts	4 halves or 1 tablespoon crushed
Seeds (flax, chia, sesame, pumpkin, sunflower)	1 tablespoon
Salad dressing, olive oil-based, trans-fat-free	1 tablespoon

Food	Size of a Serving
Belly-Friendly Fats	
Salad dressing, reduced fat	2 tablespoons
Spreads, olive oil- or canola oil-based	1 teaspoon
Less-than-Belly-Friendly Fats	
Butter, stick	1 teaspoon
Butter, whipped	1 teaspoon
Shortening	1 teaspoon
Lard	1 teaspoon
Creamer	2 tablespoons
Sour cream	2 tablespoons
Cream cheese	1 tablespoon

Condiments and seasonings

Condiments and seasonings are a great way to add flavor and variety to your meals. Many seasonings and spices can be used in unlimited amounts. However, a few condiments do contain some calories or even small amounts of sugar. These condiments are allowed on your Belly Fat Diet plan, but you do need to monitor the portions. In Table 6-8, I show you what seasonings and condiments are unlimited and which ones you need to measure.

Table 6-8   Portion Sizes of Belly-Friendly Condiments and Seasonings

Food	Size of a Serving
All dry seasonings and spices	Unlimited
Barbeque sauce	1 tablespoon per day
Garlic	Unlimited
Horseradish	½ cup per day
Ketchup (choose no-sugar-added varieties)	2 tablespoons per day
Lemon and lime juice (in cooking)	¼ cup per day
Mustard	¼ cup per day
Nonstick cooking sprays	Unlimited
Pickle relish	1 tablespoon per day
Pickles (avoid brands with added sugars)	3 pickles per day
Salsa (choose fresh varieties)	Unlimited

(continued)

Table 6-8 *(continued)*

Food	Size of a Serving
Soy sauce (choose low-sodium varieties)	2 teaspoons per day
Taco seasoning	1 tablespoon per day
Teriyaki sauce (choose low-sodium varieties)	2 teaspoons per day
Vinegar	Unlimited
Worcestershire sauce	2 tablespoons per day

Trimming your portions to trim your waistline

To help you balance your food intake and stay within the recommended portions per day without feeling hungry or deprived, you have a few strategies to use:

- **Try using smaller plates.** Many times you can eat with your eyes rather than your stomach. When using a large plate, you may fill your plate so it looks visually appealing, even if that amount is more food than you truly need. Using a smaller plate, such as a salad plate rather than a dinner plate, is a great way to trick yourself into thinking that your plate is full even though you're filling it with smaller amounts of food.

- **Visualize your plate divided into four equal sections.** Fill two of these sections with nonstarchy vegetables, one section with lean protein, and the last section with a whole-grain starch. By doing so, you have filled your plate. But half of your plate is filled with low-calorie, but quite filling, vegetables, helping you keep your portions of protein and starch in check.

Revving Up Your Metabolism

Metabolism is the process by which the body makes and uses energy (calories) for everything from the cellular absorption of nutrients to running a marathon. Efficiently metabolizing calories can lead to a healthier body weight and a reduction in belly fat. In other words, the better your metabolism, the more calories you burn throughout the day. Because weight loss and body fat loss are dependent on creating a calorie deficit, increasing your metabolism makes losing weight and keeping it off easier.

Metabolism can decline for many reasons, including the following:

- ✔ **Aging:** As you age, your metabolism begins to slow. This slowing is due in part to a decline in muscle mass. However, if you start to build muscle back (using the belly-blasting workouts in Chapter 10), you can begin to increase your metabolism.

- ✔ **Lifestyle behaviors:** Behaviors, such as being sedentary, being under large amounts of stress, skipping meals, and not getting adequate sleep, can negatively impact your metabolism.

The good news is that a decline in metabolism doesn't have to be permanent. You can increase it and, therefore, the number of calories you burn each day. I show you how in the following sections.

Noshing on foods that fire up your metabolism

Some foods, seasonings, and spices directly boost your metabolism (and therefore promote fat loss and weight reduction). Here are some great belly-burners to aim to eat on a regular basis:

- ✔ **Apples:** This fruit is rich in the flavonoid quercetin, which has been shown to block baby fat cells from maturing. It's also a powerful inflammation fighter.

- ✔ **Cinnamon:** This spice has been found in studies to make fat cells more responsive to insulin, helping to better regulate blood sugar levels.

- ✔ **Ginger:** This spice has been found to have a thermogenic effect and to aid in digestion.

- ✔ **Green tea:** The main polyphenol, EGCG, in green tea has been shown to have thermogenic properties and to increase fat oxidation.

- ✔ **Hot peppers:** Rich in capsaicin, these peppers have a thermogenic effect on the body, boosting metabolism and calorie burn. These can be used fresh or in ground and flaked forms.

- ✔ **Red and purple grapes:** These fruits are rich in resveratrol. Studies have shown that this polyphenol helps increase metabolism and suppress estrogen production, which may help decrease body fat and increase muscle mass.

- ✔ **Soup:** Research has found that individuals who eat soup rather than solid foods consumed fewer overall calories throughout the day. Soup's high fluid volume may be the reason for this decreased consumption of calories. But watch out for the sodium content of canned soups. Homemade soup is best whenever possible. If you do choose a canned soup, make sure to select a low-sodium variety. And also watch your choice in soup; cream-based soups can be rich in saturated fat and high in calories. Choose mostly broth-based options, and if you do opt for a cream-based soup, make sure to select a lowfat option.

Eating your way to a better metabolism

By making some simple changes to your eating habits and behaviors, you can boost your metabolism (and, therefore, burn more calories every day). Here are a few easy changes you can make:

- ✔ **Eat!** Sounds easy enough, right? Who doesn't want to eat more? Studies have shown that eating smaller meals every three to four hours speeds up both metabolism and weight loss progress. When you wait too long between meals to eat, your body begins to wonder when the next meal is coming. So your body goes into a starvation mode of sorts; it stores fat in the rare chance that another meal never comes. This protective mechanism is useful in times of famine but not dieting.

  Because of this fat-storing mechanism, those who drastically restrict their caloric intake generally don't lose much weight. So not only is it important to eat regularly, but you never want to cut your portions too dramatically (under 1,000–1,200 calories per day depending on age and height). Otherwise, you sabotage your weight loss efforts.

- ✔ **Ditch the simple sugars.** When you eat large amounts of sugar, your body produces more insulin. And the more insulin that's constantly being produced, the more fat your body stores. Consuming low-glycemic-index foods and avoiding refined carbohydrates helps to prevent an excessive production of insulin and, therefore, results in less fat storage.

- ✔ **Don't discount breakfast.** When you skip breakfast, you sabotage the rest of your day as well as your weight loss efforts. Studies show that people who eat a healthy breakfast weigh less than people who don't. When you eat breakfast, you're doing two things: jump-starting your metabolism and preventing excessive hunger later in the day. Your body doesn't begin to burn calories as effectively until you eat something. And remember that excessive hunger leads to cravings, which leads to overeating.

- ✔ **Drink plenty of water.** A German study found that drinking water can actually raise your metabolism. Increased fluid volume in the body may actually help to break down fat. And not drinking enough water can lead to dehydration, which can lower your metabolic rate. And at times, your brain can confuse thirst for hunger. So slight dehydration may increase your appetite and make it harder to resist the temptation to overeat. So on your Belly Fat Diet plan, drink at least 8 to 10 cups of water daily. If you can, drink your water chilled. Cold water may give your metabolism a small boost because some energy is required to heat the body.

Chapter 7

Jumping into Your Meal Plan

· ·

In This Chapter

▶ Preparing for meal plan success

▶ Determining which meal plan is right for you

▶ Knowing what to expect from your meal plan

· ·

*1*f you've been reading this book from the start, you know the foods that are best for your belly and the appropriate serving size of each of these foods. (If you need a refresher, check out Chapter 6.) Now you need to know just how many portions per day of each food group you need to achieve your weight loss and health goals. Luckily, you've come to the right place. This chapter shows you just that.

Because no two people are exactly alike, weight loss plans shouldn't be a one-size-fits-all approach either. The same approach may not work in the same way for two different people. So throughout this chapter, I outline three different weight loss plans, noting who each plan is most appropriate for. Male and female metabolisms also differ. So I outline meal plans geared toward women and men. With all this specialized info, you can follow a plan targeted toward your individual needs and be as successful as possible.

Gathering What You Need

Planning ahead is the key to being successful with your weight loss goals. You probably know the saying "Failing to plan is planning to fail." I don't want you to fail at your weight loss effort, and I'm sure you don't want to fail either. So in this section, I show you exactly how to prepare so you can maximize your results.

Planning your meals ahead of time

When trying to lose weight, eating on a whim can throw you off track. So I suggest planning out your meals and snacks in advance. This preparation not only helps keep you focused on making the right food choices, but it also helps you to know what foods you need to have on hand. Planning out your meals in advance is a great way to create your shopping list for the week as well.

Think about it this way: It's almost lunch time, and you decide you want to have a salad topped with grilled chicken. It fits right in with your weight loss plan, and it's a meal you love. But when you go to the refrigerator, you're out of lettuce and tomatoes, and the chicken isn't cooked. Now what do you do? You're hungry and have limited options on hand, so you pick up the phone and call in a takeout order, which may be loaded with sodium, fat, and calories. See how a lack of planning can throw you off track? Instead, if you plan your lunches in advance, you can have everything you need for the whole week (and have it prepared for a quick and easy meal).

In Chapter 8, I provide you with two weeks of meal plans that you can follow as you get started with your Belly Fat Diet plan. Keep in mind, however, that these meal plans are just to give you ideas. You don't need to follow them to the letter (or even use them at all). If you prefer, you can make your own meal plans by using the belly-friendly food options listed in Chapter 6 and by following the meal planning portion guidelines in this chapter.

Regardless of which meal plans you choose to follow, creating meal plans in advance and sticking to them is one of the best ways to be successful with your weight loss efforts.

Keeping the correct supplies on hand

In addition to creating and following a meal plan, you want to keep a few items on hand to help you be successful with your belly-flattening efforts. Make sure you stock up on the following supplies:

- **Measuring cups and spoons:** These tools are essential for helping you recognize a portion and for knowing how many servings you're truly having. For instance, a serving of oil is 1 teaspoon. This small amount is hard to portion correctly by just eyeballing it. Because excessive intake of portions from any food group can stall your weight loss efforts, you need to measure your servings, especially in the beginning, to make sure you're on track with your meal plan and staying within the guidelines.

✔ **Food scale:** Because proteins come in all shapes and sizes, trying to visualize the serving size can be challenging. A food scale is a great way to determine exactly how many ounces of protein you're really getting.

Always weigh animal proteins after cooking, not before. Doing so gives you an accurate measurement of how many ounces of protein you're truly consuming.

✔ **Smaller plates:** How big are your dinner plates at home? In the 1950s, the average dinner plate was about 9 inches. By the 1980s, it grew to 11 inches. Today many dinner plates are as large as 13 inches in diameter! Overeating isn't always caused just by how hungry you are. Many environmental factors can play a role too. One of these factors is the size of your plate.

By shaving inches off your plate, you can also shave inches off your waistline. Why? Because often you eat with your eyes, not just your stomach. Putting smaller portions on a large plate can make you feel cheated and cause you to crave additional servings. Seeing a full plate in front of you can help you feel more satisfied. So eat on a salad plate rather than on a dinner plate.

Maintaining a food journal

Do you want to double the amount of weight you lose? Keeping a food journal is a simple way to do it. Studies have shown that keeping a record of what you eat throughout the day can actually help you lose twice as much weight as someone who doesn't. There's a good reason for this success: It's easy to lose track of what you're actually eating in a day, including the actual portions and the small snacks you grab on the run. So writing everything down keeps your intake in the forefront of your mind.

Research indicates that most folks underestimate their caloric intake by as much as 25 to 40 percent. This inaccuracy can have a dramatic effect on your waistline.

A food journal helps you really see what and how much you're truly eating. It's also a terrific way to make sure what you're eating is balanced. It's important that you're eating the foods that help shrink belly fat on a regular basis (see Chapter 6 for the list). And how are you going to make sure you're doing that? With a food journal, of course!

Keeping a food journal is easy and requires little time. You can keep a food journal in a number of ways. I like keeping a small bound notebook with me. But people use all sorts of methods, including computers, text messages, and cellphone applications. You can keep track whatever way works best for you as long as you make sure to follow a few simple rules. When keeping a food journal, always include each of the following items:

- ✔ Time of the meal or snack eaten.

- ✔ How hungry you were before eating and how full you were after. (Try using a rating scale from 1 to 10, with 1 being not hungry at all and 10 being famished.)

- ✔ The location of where you ate, such as at home, at work, in the car, at a restaurant, and so on.

- ✔ Any emotions you were experiencing before you ate, such as stress, frustration, and so on.

- ✔ Everything you ate and drank as well as the portion of each food or beverage. (For example, don't just write olive oil. Make sure you write 1 teaspoon of olive oil.)

Keeping track of your food intake helps you see whether you may be consuming too much or too little of a particular food group, whether you're experiencing any sort of emotional eating, and whether you're waiting too long and letting yourself get too hungry before eating.

In Figure 7-1, I include an example of the food journal I use with my weight loss clients. This food journal is my favorite because it allows you to track the time and location of your meal, your hunger and emotions, the portion size, and the food group your food or beverage falls into. You can copy it and easily keep it with you wherever you go.

Date: _____

Time	Hunger / Fullness	Location / Emotions	Food Eaten (Include Portions)	Vegetables	Starchy Vegetables	Fruit	Milk	Starch	Protein	Fat
			Totals							

Figure 7-1:
A sample food journal.

Figure 7-2 shows an example of a completed journal so you can see how it works. After you complete your food journal, add up your totals to see whether you met your meal plan goals for the day or whether you need to work on certain areas so you can be more in line with your daily goals.

Date: _____

Time	Hunger / Fullness	Location / Emotions	Food Eaten (Include Portions)	Vegetables	Starchy Vegetables	Fruit	Milk	Starch	Protein	Fat
7 a.m.	Hunger – 4 Fullness – 6	home relaxed	1 cup yogurt 1 cup berries			1	1			
10 a.m.	Hunger – 5 Fullness – 7	work slight stress	12 almonds							2
1 p.m.	Hunger – 8	work	2 slices whole-wheat bread					2		
	Fullness – 8	high stress	3 ounces turkey breast 1 teaspoon mayo 2 cups salad 1 tablespoon olive oil	2					3	1 1
4 p.m.	Hunger – 4 Fullness – 5	car relaxed	1 small apple 1 ounce lowfat string cheese			1			1	
7 p.m.	Hunger – 6 Fullness – 8	home relaxed	6 ounces chicken breast 1 cup steamed mixed vegetables 1 small sweet potato 1 teaspoon olive oil spread	2	1				6	1
			Totals	4	1	2	1	2	10	5

Figure 7-2: A completed food journal for one day.

Choosing the Most Appropriate Plan for You

Because every individual dieter has different needs, the Belly Fat Diet includes three unique weight loss plans: the Turbo-Charged plan, the Moderation plan, and the Gradual-Change plan. In the following sections, I outline each of the three plans, the philosophy behind each, and who the plan is best for.

The Turbo-Charged plan for quick results

Are you impatient about weight loss? Do you want to see results on the scale overnight? Have you tried many other weight loss programs with no results? Are you someone who feels your metabolism is practically nonexistent? If you answered yes to any of these questions, the Turbo-Charged plan may be the best option for you.

This weight loss plan is the strictest of the three I introduce in this chapter, and it's not for everyone. I developed this plan to help the resistant dieter. This person struggles to lose even 1 or 2 pounds and feels she gains weight just by looking at food. This plan is also for the person who wants to see progress and see it quickly.

This plan requires the most dedication, especially in Level 1 (the first two weeks of the plan). Depending on your age, activity level, and weight loss progress, you may choose to stay in Level 2 of your Turbo-Charged plan until you reach your weight loss goals.

If you exercise for more than 60 minutes per day or are losing weight too quickly (more than 2 pounds per week after the first few weeks of your plan), I recommend transitioning to Level 2 of the Moderation plan. This plan helps you continue to safely reach your weight loss goals and keep the weight off for good.

The basics of the Turbo-Charged plan

The Turbo-Charged plan includes two levels to work through to achieve your weight loss goals:

- **Level 1:** This level, which comprises the first two weeks of the Turbo-Charged plan, focuses on reducing your intake of carbohydrates while increasing your intake of lean protein. This isn't a low-carb diet, though. Level 1 simply reduces the amount of carbohydrates while still providing you with a healthy level for energy. By slightly reducing carbohydrates and increasing lean protein, you gain a slight metabolism boost. This slight decrease in carbs also helps your body to quickly shed any excess water weight you may be carrying, helping to deflate your belly and provide you with an energy boost.

- **Level 2:** Level 2 of the Turbo-Charged plan increases your intake of healthy carbohydrates to ensure adequate energy throughout your weight loss efforts. The added carbs also increase your food options to encourage variety with your meal plan and prevent boredom. As healthy carbohydrates are reintroduced, protein and fat intake decrease slightly.

Follow these main guidelines when following the Turbo-Charged plan:

✓ **Pay attention to your plan levels.** Level 1 is designed to last for only two weeks. At the end of these two weeks, you want to move into Level 2. You can stay in Level 2 of the Turbo-Charged plan until you meet your weight loss goals. However, if you find the Turbo-Charged plan to be too restrictive or you feel that your energy levels have declined, you can move into Level 2 of the Moderation plan, which continues to promote a healthy rate of weight loss until you reach your long-term weight loss goals.

✓ **Eat your nonstarchy veggies.** Nonstarchy vegetables are unlimited in both Level 1 and Level 2. It's important to consume at least four servings of nonstarchy veggies per day.

✓ **Take notice of the differing starchy vegetable requirements in Levels 1 and 2.** They're considered a separate category in Level 1 to ensure you're taking in enough nutrients, fiber, and healthy carbohydrates. In Level 2, starchy vegetables are included in the starch group and are optional.

✓ **Select your proteins judiciously.** When choosing protein options, make sure to select mainly lean proteins. If you select medium/high-fat proteins, each ounce that you eat counts as one protein and one fat serving. See Chapter 6 for a full list of protein options.

✓ **Get the right kinds of fat.** Aim to choose your daily fat servings from belly-blasting choices like monounsaturated fats and omega-3 fatty acids. Chapter 6 can help you choose wisely.

✓ **Stay hydrated.** Make sure to drink at least 64 ounces of water daily to stay hydrated and decrease belly bloat.

Who should opt for the Turbo-Charged plan?

The Turbo-Charged plan is most appropriate for the following people:

✓ Inactive individuals

✓ Individuals of short stature

✓ Individuals over the age of 40

✓ Individuals who feel their metabolism has slowed with age

✓ Individuals who have had little to no success with previous weight loss programs

✓ Individuals who want to see quick results to keep them motivated

✓ Pre- and postmenopausal women

The Turbo-Charged plan is not appropriate for

- ✔ Individuals with diabetes (the reduced carbohydrate level may lead to dangerous drops in blood sugar)
- ✔ Women who have just given birth and are breastfeeding
- ✔ Very active individuals (90 minutes of intense exercise or more per day)

The Moderation plan for steady changes

The Moderation plan provides a steady and significant rate of weight loss. This plan focuses on making realistic, healthy changes to your dietary habits that you can stick with for life. The Moderation plan provides a balance of healthy carbohydrates, lean proteins, and belly-fighting fats that keep you feeling full and satisfied while losing pounds and trimming off body fat.

The basics of the Moderation plan

The Moderation plan contains two levels:

- ✔ **Level 1:** This level is designed to last for two weeks. It helps to banish belly-fat-storing foods from your meal plan while helping you introduce foods that increase metabolism and promote fat loss in the abdomen.
- ✔ **Level 2:** After completing your first two weeks of Level 1, you transition to Level 2. At this level, your servings of healthy carbohydrates increase slightly, helping you to maintain your energy level and increase variety in your meal plan. These additional healthy carbohydrates also provide you with an increased amount of filling fiber. As your fiber intake gradually increases, your portions of lean protein decrease just slightly.

Here are a few guidelines to keep in mind when following the Moderation plan:

- ✔ **Pay attention to your plan levels.** Level 1 is designed to last for only two weeks. At the end of these two weeks, you move into Level 2. You can stay in Level 2 of the Moderation plan until you meet your weight loss goals.
- ✔ **Eat your nonstarchy veggies.** Nonstarchy vegetables are unlimited in both Level 1 and Level 2; however, you need to consume at least four servings per day.
- ✔ **Take notice of the differing starchy vegetable requirements in Levels 1 and 2.** Starchy vegetables are considered a separate category in Level 1 to ensure you're taking in enough nutrients, fiber, and healthy carbohydrates. In Level 2, starchy vegetables are included in the starch group and are optional.

✔ **Select your proteins judiciously.** When choosing protein options, make sure to select mainly lean proteins. If you select medium/high-fat proteins, each ounce that you eat counts as one protein and one fat serving. See Chapter 6 for a full list of protein options.

✔ **Get the right kind of fats.** Aim to choose your daily fat servings from belly-blasting choices like monounsaturated fats and omega-3 fatty acids. Check out Chapter 6 for details.

✔ **Stay hydrated.** Make sure to drink at least 64 ounces of water daily to stay hydrated and decrease belly bloat.

Who should opt for the Moderation plan?

The Moderation plan is perfect for almost everyone. This plan provides a great balance of healthy nutrients that help you feel satisfied while shedding those unwanted pounds. This plan is designed to promote a slow, steady rate of weight loss, which not only helps you get the weight (and belly!) off, but also keep it off for good.

This plan is perfect for

✔ Individuals looking for steady weight loss results.

✔ Individuals with moderate to high levels of physical activity.

✔ Individuals with moderate to tall stature. (Individuals of short stature may have faster results with the earlier Turbo-Charged plan.)

Individuals with medical conditions, including diabetes, should consult their personal physician or dietitian to determine whether the Moderation plan is appropriate for them. Individuals with inconsistent blood sugar readings may be best suited for the upcoming Gradual-Change plan.

The Gradual-Change plan for leisurely results

The Gradual-Change plan is very much like it sounds: It allows you to make small changes over time that lead to big results. Not everyone is ready to jump in with both feet when starting a weight loss program. And there's nothing wrong with that! Slowly making changes over time is a great way to make permanent lifestyle changes that help you keep the weight off for good.

Although the results of the Gradual-Change plan are a bit slower than the other two weight loss plans in this chapter, it's still an effective weight loss program that helps you blast belly fat, improve health, and yield long-lasting results.

The basics of the Gradual-Change plan

The Gradual-Change plan shows you how to gradually improve your eating habits to make them more healthy and belly friendly. The focus of this plan is on consuming the proper portions from each food group each day, particularly fruits and vegetables. The plan comprises the following two levels:

- ✔ **Level 1:** This level, which lasts two weeks, starts out by encouraging you to increase your intake of fruits and vegetables, which are low in calories, rich in nutrients, and quite filling. To help prevent you from feeling overwhelmed with the dietary change, Level 1 starts out by recommending you consume fewer vegetables than Level 1 in the Turbo-Charged and Moderation plans, but helps you build up gradually over time.

- ✔ **Level 2:** As you become more accustomed to adding vegetables and fruits into your diet, you'll begin to increase your daily amount in this level. This increase allows you to take in more fiber and belly-burning antioxidants to help you shed excess body weight and improve overall health. Your intake of whole grains and healthy fats also slightly increases in this level, which provides you with increased variety and satiety.

Consider these key principles of the Gradual-Change plan:

- ✔ **Pay attention to your plan levels.** Level 1 is designed to last for only two weeks. At the end of these two weeks, you move into Level 2. You can stay in Level 2 of the Gradual-Change plan until you meet your weight loss goals. If your weight loss slows or stalls in the Gradual-Change plan, you may move into Level 2 of the Moderation plan to continue to promote weight loss until you reach your long-term goals.

- ✔ **Eat your nonstarchy veggies.** Nonstarchy vegetables are unlimited in both Level 1 and Level 2, but you need to consume at least three servings per day.

- ✔ **Take notice of the differing starchy vegetable requirements in Levels 1 and 2.** Starchy vegetables are considered a separate category in Level 1 to ensure you're taking in enough nutrients, fiber, and healthy carbohydrates. In Level 2, starchy vegetables are included in the starch group and are optional.

- ✔ **Select your proteins judiciously.** When choosing protein options, make sure to select mainly lean proteins. If you select medium/high-fat proteins, each ounce that you eat counts as one protein and one fat serving. Head to Chapter 6 for a full list of protein options.

✔ **Get the right kinds of fats.** Aim to choose your daily fat servings from belly-blasting choices like monounsaturated fats and omega-3 fatty acids.

✔ **Stay hydrated.** Make sure to drink at least 64 ounces of water daily to stay hydrated and decrease belly bloat.

Who should opt for the Gradual-Change plan?

The Gradual-Change plan is the perfect plan if you're looking to lose some weight, improve your health, and flatten your belly. This plan promotes all the principles of the Belly Fat Diet plan while showing you how to slowly transition your dietary habits to become more belly friendly. This plan is best for

✔ Individuals with less than 10 pounds to lose and who want to shrink their waistlines

✔ Individuals who are very active and have high energy demands

✔ Individuals who get burned out when following crash diets and who instead want to make gradual changes

✔ New mothers who would like to lose weight but are also breastfeeding

✔ Individuals already at or near their weight loss goals but who want to improve their health and further reduce their belly fat

Women who are breastfeeding should wait six to eight weeks after birth before beginning a weight loss plan. To prevent a decrease in milk supply, don't lose more than ½ pound per week when breastfeeding. Also, if you're a new mom, be sure to check with your physician before starting any weight loss plan.

Setting Your Expectations

Each of the three Belly Fat Diet plans I introduce earlier in the chapter help you to shrink your waistline, improve your energy level, and lose weight. The results and expectations of each plan vary slightly and depend on some personal factors. I explain what you can generally expect in the following sections.

Because results vary from person to person and plan to plan, it's important that you're aware of the expected results and are monitoring your progress. This way you know when you're on track and when you may need to make some changes to your meal plan.

What you can expect from Level 1

During the first two weeks of your Belly Fat Diet plan, you'll notice some significant changes. First, you should start to feel an improvement in your energy level. Also, you'll likely begin to shed unwanted water weight, allowing you to notice that your belly is visually smaller and your clothes are looser. During the first two weeks, you can expect to lose 2–10 pounds and ½–3 inches from your waistline.

But keep in mind that because everyone is different, your results can vary and are dependent on a few factors. Here are some of the main factors that affect your results during the first two weeks:

- **Age:** Younger individuals tend to lose weight faster than older individuals because their metabolisms are functioning at their peak.

- **Gender:** Although it seems unfair, men naturally have faster metabolisms than women because they contain a larger amount of lean body mass. For this reason, men often can lose weight at a faster rate.

- **Height:** The taller you are, the higher your metabolism. If you're 6 feet tall, you'll most likely lose weight quicker than a person who's only 5 feet tall.

- **Water weight changes:** Diets high in sodium, refined carbohydrates, simple sugars, and processed foods tend to pack on the water weight. So when you begin any weight loss plan, some of the first weight you lose is water weight. Although it isn't recommended to lose more than 2 pounds per week, during the first few weeks of a weight loss plan, your weight may decrease at a faster rate because you're losing both body fat and water weight.

Some individuals will appear to lose more weight during the first few weeks of the Belly Fat Diet plan because they're holding onto larger amounts of water weight. If you already avoid many of the foods that promote this water weight, you may have less to lose. So don't panic if your weight loss isn't rapid during this time. If you don't have much water weight to lose, the weight you're losing is mostly fat mass!

- **Your activity level:** If you stay on track with the exercise guidelines and routines outlined in Chapter 10, you'll see results faster than an inactive individual.

- **Your starting weight:** Individuals with a large amount of weight to lose tend to lose weight quicker than individuals near their ideal weight.

The only progress that matters is your progress. Don't try to compare yourself to others. Just focus on making healthy dietary changes and increasing your level of physical activity, and you'll see great results over time!

What you can expect from Level 2 and beyond

After you've completed your first two weeks on Level 1, you'll transition to Level 2. This level continues to encourage the healthy meal plan guidelines of the Belly Fat Diet while promoting a healthy, steady rate of weight loss. When you reach Level 2, most of your water weight has been lost, so what you'll be seeing on the scale will be mostly body fat losses.

You must take in adequate amounts of lean protein daily and increase your physical activity to help prevent loss of muscle mass as you lose weight. Muscle mass is what makes up the majority of your metabolism, so losing this mass may slow your weight loss efforts. Aim to meet your meal plan protein goals every day, and follow one of the exercise routines in Chapter 10. (Always consult your physician before starting or changing an exercise routine.)

In Level 2, you can expect to lose anywhere from ½ pound to 2 pounds per week. If you're losing weight at a rate slower than this, you may want to adjust your meal plan. Consider the following adjustments:

- ✔ If you're following the Gradual-Change plan, switch to Level 2 of the Moderation plan for a boost in your weight loss.

- ✔ If you're in Level 2 of the Moderation plan, you can move to Level 2 of the Turbo-Charged plan.

- ✔ If you're in the Turbo-Charged plan and not losing at least ½ pound per week, aim to increase your level of physical activity and make sure you're keeping accurate food records and measuring your food intake.

As tempting as it may be, after your first two weeks on your Belly Fat Diet plan, don't skip back to Level 1. This level is meant to help jumpstart your weight loss efforts, helping to shed both belly fat and water weight. However, staying in Level 1 for extended periods of time or jumping back and forth between levels can start to impact your metabolism, making continued weight loss more challenging. Also, because Level 1 is a more restrictive plan, extending it for too long can cause you to become burned out with your weight loss efforts and make it challenging to stay on track.

Track your waist measurement throughout your plan so you can monitor your changes in belly fat. Measure your waistline once a week and write down your measurements. Doing so allows you to track your body and belly fat losses and see the fantastic progress you're making! Chapter 3 outlines how to take an accurate waist measurement.

Getting an Overview of the Meal Plans

As I note throughout this chapter, sticking with an effective meal plan is the most important aspect of the Belly Fat Diet. In Tables 7-1 through 7-4, I show both women's and men's meal plans for each of the levels of the plans I describe earlier in the chapter. These tables show how many servings of each food group you should eat daily. You can get an idea of portions for each of the groups in Chapter 6.

Table 7-1		Level 1 Meal Plans for Women					
Plan	*Vegetables*	*Starchy Vegetables*	*Fruit*	*Milk/ Yogurt*	*Starch*	*Protein*	*Fat*
Turbo-Charged	4+	1	1	1	0	12 ounces	6
Moderation	4+	1	2	1	2	10 ounces	5
Gradual-Change	3+	1	2	2	4	8 ounces	5

Table 7-2		Level 1 Meal Plans for Men					
Plan	*Vegetables*	*Starchy Vegetables*	*Fruit*	*Milk/ Yogurt*	*Starch*	*Protein*	*Fat*
Turbo-Charged	4+	1	1	2	0	14 ounces	8
Moderation	4+	1	2	2	3	12 ounces	7
Gradual-Change	3+	1	3	2	4	12 ounces	6

Table 7-3   **Level 2 Meal Plans for Women**

Plan	Vegetables	Fruit	Milk/Yogurt	Starch	Protein	Fat
Turbo-Charged	4+	2	2	2	10 ounces	5
Moderation	4+	3	2	3	8 ounces	5
Gradual-Change	4+	3	2	5	8 ounces	6

Table 7-4   **Level 2 Meal Plans for Men**

Plan	Vegetables	Fruit	Milk/Yogurt	Starch	Protein	Fat
Turbo-Charged	4+	2	2	4	12 ounces	7
Moderation	4+	3	2	5	10 ounces	6
Gradual-Change	4+	3	2	6	12 ounces	7

Chapter 8

Meal Plans

• •

In This Chapter

▶ Creating meal plans based on your individual Belly Fat Diet plan

▶ Identifying belly-flattening foods to incorporate daily at each meal

• •

*I*n this chapter, I provide you with a detailed meal plan for both Level 1 and Level 2 of your Belly Fat Diet plan. (What do I mean by Level 1 and Level 2? See Chapter 7 for all the details.) These meal plans are meant to help give you meal planning ideas and show you how to correctly space out your meals and snacks. I encourage you to create your own customized meal plans using the meal plan guidelines provided in Chapter 7.

Here are a few things to keep in mind as you're looking through the meal plans:

✔ You can substitute lowfat plain Greek yogurt for the regular lowfat plain yogurt. If you do opt for the Greek-style yogurt, however, just be sure to remember that it adds an additional ounce of protein.

✔ I don't always provide a drink choice for the meals and snacks in this chapter, so when I don't, you can choose whatever zero-calorie drink you want. Water is best, but unsweetened green tea is a solid choice as well. Diet soda isn't ideal, because the carbonation can cause bloating.

The Turbocharged Plan, Level 1: Sample Week Meal Plan for Men

Day 1

Breakfast
Breadless Breakfast Quiche, 2 servings (Chapter 12)
Equals 2 vegetables, 4 ounces protein, 2 fats

Snack
1 cup lowfat plain yogurt topped with 1 cup blackberries
Equals 1 milk, 1 fruit

Lunch
Tuna and Salsa Stuffed Pepper, 2 servings (Chapter 13)
Equals 2 vegetables, 4 ounces protein

Snack
18 almonds
Equals 3 fats

Dinner
6 ounces chicken breast, grilled
10 asparagus spears (5 inches long), steamed and drizzled with 1 teaspoon olive oil
1 small sweet potato topped with 2 teaspoons olive oil-based spread
1 cup lowfat or fat-free milk
Equals 2 vegetables, 1 starchy vegetable, 1 milk, 6 ounces protein, 3 fats

Day 2

Breakfast
2 eggs, scrambled
½ cup diced potatoes, sautéed in 1 teaspoon olive oil
1 cup lowfat plain yogurt
Equals 1 starchy vegetable, 2 ounces protein, 1 fat

Snack
Belly-Blasting Berry Smoothie (Chapter 12)
Equals 1 fruit, 1 milk, 1 fat

Lunch
Grilled Chicken Salad (Chapter 13)
Equals 1.5 vegetables, 4 ounces protein, 2.5 fats

Snack
1 cup raw celery sticks topped with 5 teaspoons natural peanut butter
Equals 1 vegetable, 2.5 fats

Dinner
8 ounces flank steak, grilled or broiled
1 cup green beans, sautéed in 1 teaspoon olive oil
Equals 2 vegetables, 8 ounces protein, 1 fat

Day 3

Breakfast
Tropical Yogurt Parfait (Chapter 12)
Equals 1 fruit, 1 milk, 4 fats

Snack
½ cup edamame (fresh or dry roasted)
Equals 2 ounces protein

Lunch
4 ounces turkey breast, baked
1 medium ear of corn coated with 2 teaspoons olive oil-based spread
1 cup steamed broccoli
1 cup lowfat or fat-free milk or yogurt
Equals 2 vegetables, 1 starchy vegetable, 1 milk, 4 ounces protein, 2 fats

Snack
1 cup raw carrot sticks topped with 4 tablespoons hummus
Equals 1 vegetable, 2 fats

Dinner
Belly-Friendly Chicken Marsala, 2 servings (Chapter 14)
1 cup cauliflower, sautéed in 2 teaspoons olive oil
Equals 4 vegetables, 8 ounces protein, 2 fats

Day 4

Breakfast
1 medium apple, sliced and topped with
6 teaspoons natural almond butter
Equals 1 fruit, 3 fats

Snack
2 cups lowfat plain yogurt topped with 2
tablespoons chopped walnuts and
1 tablespoon cinnamon
Equals 2 milk, 2 fats

Lunch
Turkey Burger with Sweet Potato Fries
(Chapter 13) *(replace hamburger bun with
a bed of lettuce or spinach leaves)*
*Equals 1 vegetable, 1 starchy vegetable,
4 ounces protein, 1 fat*

Snack
1 cup raw bell pepper slices
2 ounces lowfat cheese
Equals 1 vegetable, 2 ounces protein

Dinner
Herb-Roasted Salmon, 2 servings
(Chapter 14)
1 cup summer squash slices, steamed
*Equals 2 vegetables, 8 ounces protein,
2 fats*

Day 5

Breakfast
Veggie-Egg Muffin (Chapter 12)
Half a grapefruit
1 cup lowfat plain yogurt topped with
6 almonds
*Equals ½ vegetable, 1 fruit, 1 milk,
2 ounces protein, 1 fat*

Snack
30 pistachio nuts
Equals 3 fats

Lunch
Chicken Cordon Bleu, 2 servings (Chapter 14)
1½ cups zucchini slices, sautéed in
2 teaspoons olive oil
*Equals 3 vegetables, 8 ounces protein,
2 fats*

Snack
1 cup lowfat plain yogurt topped with
2 tablespoons chopped walnuts
Equals 1 milk, 2 fats

Dinner
Roasted Pork Tenderloin with Vegetables
(Chapter 14)
*Equals 1 vegetable, 1 starchy vegetable,
4 ounces protein*

Day 6

Breakfast
Omelet made with 1 cup egg substitute (or
8 egg whites), 1 ounce lowfat cheese, and
½ cup chopped onions and bell peppers
that were sautéed in 1 teaspoon olive oil
Equals 1 vegetable, 5 ounces protein, 1 fat

Snack
Half a pomegranate
1 cup lowfat plain yogurt topped with
6 almonds
Equals 1 fruit, 1 milk, 1 fat

Lunch
Portobello Mushroom Salad (Chapter 14)
1 cup fat-free or lowfat milk
Equals 2.5 vegetables, 1 milk, 1.5 fats

Snack
Half an avocado
Equals 2 fats

Dinner
9 ounces salmon, grilled or broiled and
drizzled with ½ teaspoon olive oil
½ cup peas, steamed
1 cup bell pepper slices, sautéed in 2 teaspoons olive oil
*Equals 2 vegetables, 1 starchy vegetable,
9 ounces protein, 2.5 fats*

Day 7

Breakfast
1 cup lowfat yogurt topped with ¼ cup
dried tart cherries and 2 tablespoons
chopped almonds
Equals 1 fruit, 1 milk, 2 fats

Snack
2 hard-boiled eggs
Equals 2 ounces protein

Lunch
Belly-Beating Bean Burrito (Chapter 13)
*(wrap burrito in lettuce leaves instead of
a tortilla)*
*Equals 2 vegetables, 1 starchy vegetable,
1 ounce protein, 1 fat*

Snack
1 medium tomato, sliced
3 ounces fresh mozzarella, sliced
Equals 1 vegetable, 3 ounces protein, 3 fats

Dinner
Walnut-Encrusted Flounder, 2 servings
(Chapter 14)
1 cup carrots, steamed
1 cup fat-free or lowfat milk
*Equals 2 vegetables, 1 milk, 8 ounces
protein, 2 fats*

The Turbocharged Plan, Level 1: Sample Week Meal Plan for Women

Day 1

Breakfast
Breadless Breakfast Quiche (Chapter 12)
Equals 1 vegetable, 2 ounces protein, 1 fat

Snack
1 cup lowfat plain yogurt topped with
1 cup blackberries
Equals 1 milk, 1 fruit

Lunch
Tuna and Salsa Stuffed Pepper, 2 servings
(Chapter 13)
Equals 2 vegetables, 4 ounces protein

Snack
18 almonds
Equals 3 fats

Dinner
6 ounces chicken breast, grilled
10 asparagus spears (5 inches long),
steamed and drizzled with 1 teaspoon
olive oil
1 small sweet potato topped with
1 teaspoon olive oil-based spread
*Equals 2 vegetables, 1 starchy vegetable,
6 ounces protein, 2 fats*

Day 2

Breakfast
2 eggs, scrambled
½ cup diced potatoes, sautéed in 1 teaspoon olive oil
*Equals 1 starchy vegetable, 2 ounces
protein, 1 fat*

Snack
Belly-Blasting Berry Smoothie (Chapter 12)
Equals 1 fruit, 1 milk, 1 fat

Lunch
Grilled Chicken Salad (Chapter 13)
*Equals 1.5 vegetables, 4 ounces protein,
2.5 fats*

Snack
1 cup raw celery sticks topped with
3 teaspoons natural peanut butter
Equals 1 vegetable, 1.5 fats

Dinner
6 ounces flank steak, grilled or broiled
1 cup green beans, steamed
Equals 2 vegetables, 6 ounces protein

Day 3

Breakfast
Tropical Yogurt Parfait (Chapter 12)
Equals 1 fruit, 1 milk, 4 fats

Snack
½ cup edamame (fresh or dry roasted)
Equals 2 ounces protein

Lunch
6 ounces turkey breast, baked
1 medium ear of corn coated with
1 teaspoon olive oil-based spread
1 cup steamed broccoli
*Equals 2 vegetables, 1 starchy vegetable,
6 ounces protein, 1 fat*

Snack
1 cup raw carrot sticks topped with
2 tablespoons hummus
Equals 1 vegetable, 1 fat

Dinner
Belly-Friendly Chicken Marsala
(Chapter 14)
1 cup cauliflower, sautéed in 2 teaspoons
olive oil
*Equals 3 vegetables, 4 ounces protein,
2 fats*

Day 4

Breakfast
1 medium apple, sliced and topped with
4 teaspoons natural almond butter
Equals 1 fruit, 2 fats

Snack
1 cup lowfat plain yogurt topped with
1 tablespoon chopped walnuts and
1 tablespoon cinnamon
Equals 1 milk, 1 fat

Lunch
Turkey Burger with Sweet Potato Fries
(Chapter 13) *(replace hamburger bun with
a bed of lettuce or spinach leaves)*
*Equals 1 vegetable, 1 starchy vegetable,
4 ounces protein, 1 fat*

Snack
1 cup raw bell pepper slices
Equals 1 vegetable

Dinner
Herb-Roasted Salmon, 2 servings
(Chapter 14)
1 cup summer squash slices, steamed
*Equals 2 vegetables, 8 ounces protein,
2 fats*

Day 5

Breakfast
90-Second Omelet (Chapter 12)
Half a grapefruit
*Equals 1 vegetable, 1 fruit, 1 milk,
3 ounces protein, 2 fats*

Snack
30 pistachio nuts
1 stick lowfat string cheese
Equals 1 ounce protein, 3 fats

Lunch
Chicken Cordon Bleu (Chapter 14)
1 cup zucchini slices, steamed
Equals 2 vegetables, 4 ounces protein

Snack
1 cup lowfat plain yogurt
1 tablespoon chopped walnuts
Equals 1 milk, 1 fat

Dinner
Roasted Pork Tenderloin with Vegetables
(Chapter 14)
*Equals 1 vegetable, 1 starchy vegetable,
4 ounces protein*

Day 6

Breakfast
Veggie-Egg Muffins, 2 servings (Chapter 12)
Equals 1 vegetable, 4 ounces protein

Snack
Half a pomegranate
Equals 1 fruit

Lunch
Portobello Mushroom Salad (Chapter 14)
1 cup fat-free or lowfat milk
Equals 2.5 vegetables, 1 milk, 1.5 fats

Snack
Half an avocado
Equals 2 fats

Dinner
8 ounces salmon, grilled or broiled and
drizzled with ½ teaspoon olive oil
½ cup peas, steamed
1 cup bell pepper slices, sautéed in
2 teaspoons olive oil
*Equals 2 vegetables, 1 starchy vegetable,
8 ounces protein, 2.5 fats*

Day 7

Breakfast
1 cup lowfat yogurt topped with ¼ cup
dried tart cherries and 1 tablespoon
chopped almonds
Equals 1 fruit, 1 milk, 1 fat

Snack
1 hard-boiled egg
Equals 1 ounce protein

Lunch
Belly-Beating Bean Burrito (Chapter 13)
*(wrap burrito in lettuce leaves instead of
tortilla)*
*Equals 2 vegetables, 1 starchy vegetable,
1 ounce protein, 1 fat*

Snack
1 medium tomato, sliced
2 ounces fresh mozzarella, sliced
*Equals 1 vegetable, 2 ounces protein,
2 fats*

Dinner
Walnut-Encrusted Flounder, 2 servings
(Chapter 14)
1 cup carrots, steamed
*Equals 2 vegetables, 8 ounces protein,
2 fats*

Turbocharged Plan, Level 2: Sample Week Meal Plan for Men

Day 1

Breakfast
Banana-Almond Breakfast Toast
(Chapter 12)
1 cup fat-free or lowfat milk
Equals 1 fruit, 1 milk, 1 starch, 1 ounce protein, 1 fat

Snack
Baked Apple (Chapter 15)
1 cup lowfat plain yogurt
Equals 1 fruit, 1 milk

Lunch
6 ounces flounder, grilled or broiled
1 cup frozen spinach, thawed and sautéed in 2 teaspoons olive oil
1 cup cooked whole-grain pasta
Equals 2 vegetables, 2 starches, 6 ounces protein, 2 fats

Snack
1 cup raw celery sticks topped with
4 teaspoons natural peanut butter
Equals 1 vegetable, 2 fats

Dinner
Low-Calorie Chicken Parmesan
(Chapter 14)
1 cup Brussels sprouts, sautéed in
2 teaspoons olive oil
Equals 2 vegetables, 0.5 starch, 5 ounces protein, 2 fats

Snack
1½ cups air-popped popcorn
Equals 0.5 starch

Day 2

Breakfast
Waistline-Slimming Omelet (Chapter 12)
½ cup mandarin oranges
1 slice 100% whole-grain bread topped
with 1 teaspoon olive oil-based spread
Equals 1 vegetable, 0.5 fruit, 1 starch, 3 ounces protein, 2 fats

Snack
Belly-Blasting Trail Mix (Chapter 15)
Equals 0.5 fruit, 1 starch, 2 fats

Lunch
Shockingly Healthy (and Easy!) Calzone
(Chapter 13)
Equals 1 vegetable, 1 starch, 2 ounces protein

Snack
Smoothie made with 1 cup lowfat yogurt,
1 cup mixed berries, and 1 tablespoon
flaxseed
Equals 1 milk, 1 fruit, 1 fat

Dinner
7 ounces pork tenderloin, grilled or broiled
½ cup carrots, sautéed in 1 teaspoon
olive oil
½ cup zucchini slices, sautéed in
1 teaspoon olive oil
½ cup cooked quinoa
1 cup fat-free or lowfat milk
Equals 2 vegetables, 1 milk, 1 starch, 7 ounces protein, 2 fats

Day 3

Breakfast
Quick and Belly-Friendly Cold Cereal with
Fruit (Chapter 12)
Equals 1 fruit, 1 milk, 2 starches

Snack
1 cup raw carrot sticks
4 tablespoons hummus spread on
6 whole-grain crackers
Equals 1 vegetable, 1 starch, 2 fats

Lunch
Spicy Shrimp Kabobs (Chapter 14)
2 cups salad tossed with 3 tablespoons
vinaigrette dressing
Equals 3 vegetables, 4 ounces protein, 3 fats

Snack
1 cup lowfat plain yogurt topped with
1 cup raspberries
Equals 1 milk, 1 fruit

Dinner
8 ounces flounder, sautéed in 1 teaspoon
olive oil
1 cup frozen kale, thawed and sautéed in
1 teaspoon olive oil
½ cup corn, steamed
Equals 2 vegetables, 1 starch, 8 ounces protein, 2 fats

Day 4

Breakfast
Bean, Ham, and Cheese Breakfast Burrito
(Chapter 12)
Equals 2 starches, 4 ounces protein, 1 fat

Snack
1 cup diced papaya
12 almonds
Equals 1 fruit, 2 fats

Lunch
4 ounces chicken breast, grilled or broiled
1 cup chopped vegetables (onions, bell
peppers, and mushrooms), stir-fried in
2 teaspoons olive oil
⅔ cup brown rice, cooked
*Equals 2 vegetables, 2 starches, 4 ounces
protein, 2 fats*

Snack
1 cup lowfat plain yogurt
1 cup grapes
Equals 1 milk, 1 fruit

Dinner
4 ounces London broil, grilled or broiled
1 cup green beans, sautéed in
2 teaspoons olive oil
1 cup fat-free or lowfat milk
*Equals 2 vegetables, 1 milk, 4 ounces
protein, 2 fats*

Day 5

Breakfast
1 cup blackberries
½ cup lowfat cottage cheese
1 tablespoon chopped walnuts
Equals 1 fruit, 2 ounces protein, 1 fat

Snack
1 small banana
¼ cup edamame (fresh or dry roasted)
Equals 1 fruit, 1 ounce protein

Lunch
Hummus and Avocado Sandwich
(Chapter 13)
1 cup lowfat plain yogurt
Equals 1 vegetable, 1 milk, 2 starches, 3 fats

Snack
1 cup raw carrot sticks
1 hard-boiled egg
Equals 1 vegetable, 1 ounce protein

Dinner
Pepper Steak with Fresh Vegetables,
2 servings (Chapter 14)
1 large sweet potato topped with
1 teaspoon olive oil-based spread
1 cup fat-free or lowfat milk
*Equals 4 vegetables, 1 milk, 2 starches,
8 ounces protein, 3 fats*

Day 6

Breakfast
Veggie-Egg Muffins, 2 servings
(Chapter 12)
1 cup lowfat plain yogurt
18 almonds
*Equals 1 vegetable, 1 milk, 4 ounces
protein, 3 fats*

Snack
Chocolate-Drizzled Strawberries
(Chapter 15)
Equals 1 fruit, 0.5 starch

Lunch
Hot and Spicy Vegetarian Chili (Chapter 13)
*Equals 1.5 vegetables, 1.5 starches,
2 ounces protein, 1 fat*

Snack
½ cup lowfat cottage cheese
½ cup pineapple
Equals 1 fruit, 2 ounces protein

Dinner
4 ounces chicken breast, grilled or broiled
1 cup chopped bell peppers, ½ cup
chopped mushrooms, ½ cup chopped
onions, stir-fried in 1 tablespoon soy
sauce and 1 tablespoon olive oil
⅔ cup cooked wild rice
1 cup fat-free or lowfat milk
*Equals 2 vegetables, 1 milk, 2 starches,
4 ounces protein, 3 fats*

Day 7

Breakfast
1 cup liquid egg substitute (or 8 egg
whites), scrambled
Yogurt parfait made with 1 cup lowfat
yogurt, 1 cup mixed berries, and 1 tablespoon chopped walnuts
*Equals 1 fruit, 1 milk, 4 ounces protein,
1 fat*

Snack
1 medium plum
1 stick lowfat string cheese
Equals 1 fruit, 1 ounce protein

Lunch
Herb-Roasted Salmon (Chapter 14)
1 cup frozen spinach, thawed and sautéed
in 1 teaspoon olive oil
*Equals 2 vegetables, 4 ounces protein,
2 fats*

Snack
1 cup lowfat plain yogurt
¼ cup soy nuts
Equals 1 milk, 1 ounce protein

Dinner
Whole-Grain Bruschetta Pizza, 2 servings
(Chapter 14)
2 cups salad tossed with 2 tablespoons
balsamic vinegar and 2 teaspoons olive oil
*Equals 4 vegetables, 4 starches, 2 ounces
protein, 4 fats*

Turbocharged Plan, Level 2: Sample Week Meal Plan for Women

Day 1

Breakfast
Banana-Almond Breakfast Toast
(Chapter 12)
1 cup fat-free or lowfat milk
Equals 1 fruit, 1 milk, 1 starch, 1 ounce protein, 1 fat

Snack
Baked Apple (Chapter 15)
1 cup lowfat plain yogurt
Equals 1 fruit, 1 milk

Lunch
4 ounces flounder, grilled or broiled
1 cup frozen spinach, thawed and sautéed
in 2 teaspoons olive oil
Equals 2 vegetables, 6 ounces protein, 2 fats

Snack
1 cup raw celery sticks topped with
4 teaspoons natural peanut butter
Equals 1 vegetable, 2 fats

Dinner
Low-Calorie Chicken Parmesan
(Chapter 14)
1 cup Brussels sprouts, steamed
Equals 2 vegetables, 0.5 starch, 5 ounces protein

Snack
1½ cups air-popped popcorn
Equals 0.5 starch

Day 2

Breakfast
Waistline-Slimming Omelet (Chapter 12)
½ cup mandarin oranges
Equals 1 vegetable, 0.5 fruit, 3 ounces protein, 1 fat

Snack
Belly-Blasting Trail Mix (Chapter 15)
Equals 0.5 fruit, 1 starch, 2 fats

Lunch
Shockingly Healthy (and Easy!) Calzone
(Chapter 13)
Equals 1 vegetable, 1 starch, 2 ounces protein

Snack
Smoothie made with 1 cup lowfat yogurt,
1 cup mixed berries, and 1 tablespoon
flaxseed
Equals 1 milk, 1 fruit, 1 fat

Dinner
5 ounces pork tenderloin, grilled or broiled
½ cup carrots, steamed and topped with
1 teaspoon olive oil-based spread
½ cup zucchini slices, steamed
1 cup fat-free or lowfat milk
Equals 2 vegetables, 1 milk, 5 ounces protein, 1 fat

Day 3

Breakfast
Quick and Belly-Friendly Cold Cereal
(Chapter 12)
Equals 1 fruit, 1 milk, 2 starches

Snack
1 cup raw carrot sticks topped with
2 tablespoons hummus
Equals 1 vegetable, 1 fat

Lunch
Spicy Shrimp Kabobs (Chapter 14)
2 cups salad tossed with 2 tablespoons
vinaigrette dressing
Equals 3 vegetables, 4 ounces protein, 2 fats

Snack
1 cup lowfat plain yogurt topped with
1 cup raspberries
Equals 1 milk, 1 fruit

Dinner
6 ounces flounder, sautéed in 1 teaspoon
olive oil
1 cup frozen kale, thawed and sautéed
in 1 teaspoon olive oil
Equals 2 vegetables, 6 ounces protein, 2 fats

Day 4

Breakfast
Bean, Ham, and Cheese Breakfast Burrito
(Chapter 12)
Equals 2 starches, 4 ounces protein, 1 fat

Snack
1 cup diced papaya
12 almonds
Equals 1 fruit, 2 fats

Lunch
3 ounces chicken breast, grilled or broiled
1 cup chopped vegetables (onions,
peppers, and mushrooms), stir-fried in
1 teaspoon olive oil
*Equals 2 vegetables, 3 ounces protein,
1 fat*

Snack
1 cup lowfat plain yogurt
1 cup grapes
Equals 1 milk, 1 fruit

Dinner
3 ounces London broil, grilled or broiled
1 cup green beans, sautéed in 1 teaspoon
olive oil
1 cup fat-free or lowfat milk
*Equals 2 vegetables, 1 milk, 3 ounces
protein, 1 fat*

Day 5

Breakfast
1 cup lowfat plain yogurt topped with 1
cup blackberries
Equals 1 fruit, 1 milk

Snack
1 small banana
¼ cup edamame (fresh or dry roasted)
Equals 1 fruit, 1 ounce protein

Lunch
Hummus and Avocado Sandwich
(Chapter 13)
1 cup lowfat plain yogurt
*Equals 1 vegetable, 1 milk, 2 starches,
3 fats*

Snack
1 cup raw carrot sticks
1 hard-boiled egg
Equals 1 vegetable, 1 ounce protein

Dinner
Pepper Steak with Fresh Vegetables,
2 servings (Chapter 14)
*Equals 4 vegetables, 8 ounces protein,
2 fats*

Day 6

Breakfast
Veggie-Egg Muffin (Chapter 12)
1 cup lowfat plain yogurt
6 almonds
*Equals 0.5 vegetable, 1 milk, 2 ounces
protein, 1 fat*

Snack
Chocolate-Drizzled Strawberries
(Chapter 15)
Equals 1 fruit, 0.5 starch

Lunch
Hot and Spicy Vegetarian Chili (Chapter 13)
*Equals 1.5 vegetables, 1.5 starches, 2
ounces protein, 1 fat*

Snack
½ cup lowfat cottage cheese
½ cup pineapple
Equals 1 fruit, 2 ounces protein

Dinner
4 ounces chicken breast, grilled or broiled
1 cup chopped bell peppers, ½ cup
chopped mushrooms, ½ cup chopped
onions, stir-fried in 1 tablespoon soy
sauce and 1 tablespoon olive oil
1 cup fat-free or lowfat milk
*Equals 2 vegetables, 1 milk, 4 ounces
protein, 3 fats*

Day 7

Breakfast
1 cup liquid egg substitute (or 8 egg
whites), scrambled
Yogurt parfait made with 1 cup lowfat
yogurt, 1 cup mixed berries, and 1 tablespoon chopped walnuts
*Equals 1 fruit, 1 milk, 4 ounces protein,
1 fat*

Snack
1 medium plum
1 stick lowfat string cheese
Equals 1 fruit, 1 ounce protein

Lunch
Herb-Roasted Salmon (Chapter 14)
1 cup frozen spinach, thawed and sautéed
in 1 teaspoon olive oil
*Equals 2 vegetables, 4 ounces protein,
2 fats*

Snack
1 cup lowfat plain yogurt
Equals 1 milk

Dinner
Whole-Grain Bruschetta Pizza, 1 serving
(Chapter 14)
2 cups salad tossed with 2 tablespoons
balsamic vinegar and 1 teaspoon olive oil
*Equals 3 vegetables, 2 starches, 1 ounce
protein, 2 fats*

Moderation Plan, Level 1: Sample Week Meal Plan for Men

Day 1

Breakfast
Breadless Breakfast Quiche (Chapter 12)
2 slices 100% whole-grain toast topped with 2 teaspoons olive oil-based spread
Equals 1 vegetable, 2 starches, 2 ounces protein, 3 fats

Snack
1 cup lowfat plain yogurt topped with 1 cup blackberries and 1 tablespoon chopped walnuts
Equals 1 milk, 1 fruit, 1 fat

Lunch
Tuna and Salsa Stuffed Pepper (Chapter 13)
1 medium pear
Equals 1 vegetable, 1 fruit, 2 ounces protein

Snack
6 whole-grain crackers topped with 4 teaspoons natural almond butter
Equals 1 starch, 2 fats

Dinner
8 ounces chicken breast, grilled
10 asparagus spears (5 inches long), steamed
1 small sweet potato topped with 1 teaspoon olive oil-based spread
1 cup lowfat or fat-free milk
Equals 2 vegetables, 1 starchy vegetable, 1 milk, 8 ounces protein, 1 fat

Day 2

Breakfast
2 eggs, scrambled
½ cup diced potatoes, sautéed in nonstick cooking spray
1 cup blueberries
Equals 1 starchy vegetable, 2 ounces protein, 1 fruit

Snack
Belly-Blasting Berry Smoothie (Chapter 12)
Equals 1 fruit, 1 milk, 1 fat

Lunch
Grilled Chicken Salad (Chapter 13)
Equals 1.5 vegetables, 4 ounces protein, 2.5 fats

Snack
1 cup raw celery sticks topped with 5 teaspoons natural peanut butter
Equals 1 vegetable, 2.5 fats

Dinner
6 ounces flank steak, grilled or broiled
1 cup green beans, sautéed in 1 teaspoon olive oil
1 cup cooked brown rice
1 cup fat-free or lowfat milk
Equals 2 vegetables, 1 milk, 3 starches, 6 ounces protein, 1 fat

Day 3

Breakfast
Tropical Yogurt Parfait (Chapter 12)
Equals 1 fruit, 1 milk, 4 fats

Snack
½ cup edamame (fresh or dry roasted)
1 cup fruit salad
1 cup lowfat yogurt
Equals 1 fruit, 1 milk, 2 ounces protein

Lunch
6 ounces turkey breast, baked
1 medium ear of corn coated with 2 teaspoons olive oil-based spread
1 cup broccoli, steamed
Equals 2 vegetables, 1 starchy vegetable, 6 ounces protein, 2 fats

Snack
1 cup raw carrot sticks topped with 4 tablespoons hummus
Equals 1 vegetable, 2 fats

Dinner
Belly-Friendly Chicken Marsala (Chapter 14)
1 cup cauliflower, sautéed in 1 teaspoon olive oil
1½ cups cooked whole-grain pasta
Equals 3 vegetables, 3 starches, 4 ounces protein, 1 fat

Day 4

Breakfast
1 medium apple, sliced and topped with
4 teaspoons natural almond butter
Equals 1 fruit, 2 fats

Snack
1 cup lowfat plain yogurt topped with
1 tablespoon chopped walnuts, ¼ cup
dried tart cherries, and 1 tablespoon
cinnamon
Equals 1 milk, 1 fruit, 1 fat

Lunch
Turkey Burger with Sweet Potato Fries
(Chapter 13)
1 cup fat-free or lowfat milk
*Equals 1 starchy vegetable, 1 milk,
2 starches, 4 ounces protein, 1 fat*

Snack
1 cup raw bell pepper slices topped with
2 tablespoons hummus
Equals 1 vegetable, 1 fat

Dinner
Herb-Roasted Salmon, 2 servings
(Chapter 14)
1½ cups string beans, steamed
½ cup cooked quinoa
*Equals 3 vegetables, 1 starch, 8 ounces
protein, 2 fats*

Day 5

Breakfast
1 cup lowfat cottage cheese
½ cup pineapple
Equals 1 fruit, 4 ounces protein

Snack
30 pistachio nuts
1 medium orange
Equals 1 fruit, 3 fats

Lunch
Chicken Cordon Bleu (Chapter 14)
4 cups zucchini slices, sautéed in
2 teaspoons olive oil
½ cup cooked whole-grain pasta
*Equals 4 vegetables, 1 starch, 4 ounces
protein, 2 fats*

Snack
1 cup lowfat plain yogurt
2 tablespoons chopped walnuts
Equals 1 milk, 2 fats

Dinner
Roasted Pork Tenderloin with Vegetables
(Chapter 14)
⅔ cup cooked wild rice
1 cup fat-free or lowfat milk
*Equals 1 vegetable, 1 starchy vegetable,
1 milk, 2 starches, 4 ounces protein*

Day 6

Breakfast
On-the-Go Breakfast Sandwich
(Chapter 12)
1 cup fat-free or lowfat milk
Equals 1 milk, 2 starches, 3 ounces protein

Snack
¼ cup dried cranberries mixed with ½ cup
whole-grain cereal
Equals 1 fruit, 1 starch

Lunch
Portobello Mushroom Salad (Chapter 14)
topped with ½ cup fresh edamame
1 cup fat-free or lowfat milk
*Equals 2.5 vegetables, 1 milk, 2 ounces
protein, 1.5 fats*

Snack
Half an avocado
1 small banana
Equals 1 fruit, 2 fats

Dinner
7 ounces salmon, grilled or broiled and
drizzled with 1½ teaspoons olive oil
½ cup peas, steamed
1 cup bell pepper slices, sautéed in
2 teaspoons olive oil
*Equals 2 vegetables, 1 starchy vegetable,
7 ounces protein, 3.5 fats*

Day 7

Breakfast
1 cup lowfat ricotta cheese topped with ¼
cup dried blueberries and 2 tablespoons
chopped almonds
Equals 1 fruit, 4 ounces protein, 2 fats

Snack
1 hard-boiled egg
Half a grapefruit
Equals 1 fruit, 1 ounce protein

Lunch
Belly-Beating Bean Burrito (Chapter 13)
1 cup lowfat plain yogurt
*Equals 2 vegetables, 1 starchy vegetable,
1 milk, 1 starch, 1 ounce protein, 1 fat*

Snack
1 medium tomato, sliced
2 ounces fresh mozzarella, sliced
*Equals 1 vegetable, 2 ounces protein,
2 fats*

Dinner
Walnut-Encrusted Flounder (Chapter 14)
1 cup carrots, steamed and topped with
1 teaspoon olive oil-based spread
⅔ cup cooked whole-grain couscous
1 cup fat-free or lowfat milk
*Equals 2 vegetables, 1 milk, 2 starches,
4 ounces protein, 2 fats*

Moderation Plan, Level 1: Sample Week Meal Plan for Women

Day 1

Breakfast
Breadless Breakfast Quiche (Chapter 12)
1 slice 100% whole-grain toast topped
with 1 teaspoon olive oil-based spread
*Equals 1 vegetable, 1 starch, 2 ounces
protein, 2 fats*

Snack
1 cup lowfat plain yogurt topped with
1 cup blackberries
Equals 1 milk, 1 fruit

Lunch
Tuna and Salsa Stuffed Pepper
(Chapter 13)
1 medium pear
*Equals 1 vegetable, 1 fruit, 2 ounces
protein*

Snack
6 whole-grain crackers topped with
4 teaspoons natural almond butter
Equals 1 starch, 2 fats

Dinner
6 ounces chicken breast, grilled
10 asparagus spears (5 inches long),
steamed
1 small sweet potato topped with
1 teaspoon olive oil-based spread
*Equals 2 vegetables, 1 starchy vegetable,
6 ounces protein, 1 fat*

Day 2

Breakfast
2 eggs, scrambled
½ cup diced potatoes, sautéed in nonstick
cooking spray
1 cup blueberries
*Equals 1 starchy vegetable, 2 ounces
protein, 1 fruit*

Snack
Belly-Blasting Berry Smoothie (Chapter 12)
Equals 1 fruit, 1 milk, 1 fat

Lunch
Grilled Chicken Salad (Chapter 13)
*Equals 1.5 vegetables, 4 ounces protein,
2.5 fats*

Snack
1 cup raw celery sticks topped with
3 teaspoons natural peanut butter
Equals 1 vegetable, 1.5 fats

Dinner
4 ounces flank steak, grilled or broiled
1 cup green beans, steamed
⅔ cup cooked brown rice
*Equals 2 vegetables, 2 starches, 4 ounces
protein*

Day 3

Breakfast
Tropical Yogurt Parfait (Chapter 12)
Equals 1 fruit, 1 milk, 4 fats

Snack
½ cup edamame (fresh or dry roasted)
1 cup fruit salad
Equals 1 fruit, 2 ounces protein

Lunch
4 ounces turkey breast, baked
1 medium ear of corn coated with
1 teaspoon olive oil-based spread
1 cup steamed broccoli
*Equals 2 vegetables, 1 starchy vegetable,
4 ounces protein, 1 fat*

Snack
1 cup raw carrot sticks topped with 2
tablespoons hummus
Equals 1 vegetable, 1 fat

Dinner
Belly-Friendly Chicken Marsala
(Chapter 14)
1 cup cauliflower, sautéed in 1 teaspoon
olive oil
1 cup cooked whole-grain pasta
*Equals 3 vegetables, 2 starches, 4 ounces
protein, 1 fat*

Day 4

Breakfast
1 medium apple, sliced and topped with
4 teaspoons natural almond butter
Equals 1 fruit, 2 fats

Snack
1 cup lowfat plain yogurt topped with
1 tablespoon chopped walnuts, ¼ cup
dried tart cherries, and 1 tablespoon
cinnamon
Equals 1 milk, 1 fruit, 1 fat

Lunch
Turkey Burger with Sweet Potato Fries
(Chapter 13) *(replace hamburger bun with
a bed of lettuce or spinach leaves)*
*Equals 1 vegetable, 1 starchy vegetable,
4 ounces protein, 1 fat*

Snack
1 cup raw bell pepper slices
2 ounces lowfat cheese
Equals 1 vegetable, 2 ounces protein

Dinner
Herb-Roasted Salmon (Chapter 14)
1 cup string beans, steamed
1 cup cooked quinoa
*Equals 3 vegetables, 2 starches, 4 ounces
protein, 1 fat*

Day 5

Breakfast
½ cup lowfat cottage cheese
½ cup pineapple
Equals 1 fruit, 2 ounces protein

Snack
30 pistachio nuts
1 medium orange
Equals 1 fruit, 3 fats

Lunch
Chicken Cordon Bleu (Chapter 14)
4 cups zucchini slices, sautéed in
1 teaspoon olive oil
½ cup whole-grain pasta
*Equals 4 vegetables, 1 starch, 4 ounces
protein, 1 fat*

Snack
1 cup lowfat plain yogurt topped with
1 tablespoon chopped walnuts
Equals 1 milk, 1 fat

Dinner
Roasted Pork Tenderloin with Vegetables
(Chapter 14)
⅓ cup cooked wild rice
*Equals 1 vegetable, 1 starchy vegetable,
1 starch, 4 ounces protein*

Day 6

Breakfast
On-the-Go Breakfast Sandwich
(Chapter 12)
Equals 2 starches, 3 ounces protein

Snack
1 small pomegranate

Lunch
Portobello Mushroom Salad (Chapter 14)
1 cup fat-free or lowfat milk
Equals 2.5 vegetables, 1 milk, 1.5 fats

Snack
A quarter of an avocado
1 small banana
Equals 1 fruit, 1 fat

Dinner
7 ounces salmon, grilled or broiled and
drizzled with ½ teaspoon olive oil
½ cup peas, steamed
1 cup bell pepper slices, sautéed in 2 teaspoons olive oil
*Equals 2 vegetables, 1 starchy vegetable,
7 ounces protein, 2.5 fats*

Day 7

Breakfast
½ cup lowfat ricotta cheese topped with
¼ cup dried blueberries and 1 tablespoon
chopped almonds
Equals 1 fruit, 2 ounces protein, 1 fat

Snack
1 hard-boiled egg
Half a grapefruit
Equals 1 fruit, 1 ounce protein

Lunch
Belly-Beating Bean Burrito (Chapter 13)
*(wrap burrito in lettuce leaves instead of
tortilla)*
*Equals 2 vegetables, 1 starchy vegetable,
1 ounce protein, 1 fat*

Snack
1 medium tomato, sliced
2 ounces fresh mozzarella, sliced
Equals 1 vegetable, 2 ounces protein, 2 fats

Dinner
Walnut-Encrusted Flounder (Chapter 14)
1 cup carrots, steamed
⅔ cup cooked whole-grain couscous
1 cup fat-free or lowfat milk
*Equals 2 vegetables, 1 milk, 2 starches,
4 ounces protein, 1 fat*

Moderation Plan, Level 2: Sample Week Meal Plan for Men

Day 1

Breakfast
Banana-Almond Breakfast Toast
(Chapter 12)
1 cup fat-free or lowfat milk
Equals 1 fruit, 1 milk, 1 starch, 1 ounce protein, 1 fat

Snack
Baked Apple (Chapter 15)
1 cup lowfat plain yogurt
Equals 1 fruit, 1 milk

Lunch
4 ounces flounder, grilled or broiled
1 cup frozen spinach, thawed and sautéed in 2 teaspoons olive oil
1 cup cooked whole-grain pasta
1 cup fruit salad
Equals 2 vegetables, 1 fruit, 2 starches, 4 ounces protein, 2 fats

Snack
1 cup raw celery sticks topped with 4 teaspoons natural peanut butter
Equals 1 vegetable, 2 fats

Dinner
Low-Calorie Chicken Parmesan (Chapter 14)
1 cup Brussels sprouts, sautéed in 1 teaspoon olive oil
Equals 2 vegetables, 0.5 starch, 5 ounces protein, 1 fat

Snack
4½ cups air-popped popcorn
Equals 1.5 starch

Day 2

Breakfast
Waistline-Slimming Omelet (Chapter 12)
½ cup mandarin oranges
2 slices of 100% whole-grain toast topped with 1 teaspoon olive oil-based spread
Equals 1 vegetable, 0.5 fruit, 2 starches, 3 ounces protein, 2 fats

Snack
Belly-Blasting Trail Mix (Chapter 15)
Equals 0.5 fruit, 1 starch, 2 fats

Lunch
Shockingly Healthy (and Easy!) Calzone (Chapter 13)
1 medium apple
Equals 1 vegetable, 1 fruit, 1 starch, 2 ounces protein

Snack
Smoothie made with 1 cup lowfat yogurt, 1 cup mixed berries, and 1 tablespoon flaxseed
Equals 1 milk, 1 fruit, 1 fat

Dinner
5 ounces pork tenderloin, grilled or broiled
½ cup carrots, steamed and topped with 1 teaspoon olive oil-based spread
½ cup zucchini slices, steamed
1 cup fat-free or lowfat milk
½ cup cooked quinoa
Equals 2 vegetables, 1 milk, 1 starch, 5 ounces protein, 1 fat

Day 3

Breakfast
Quick and Belly-Friendly Cold Cereal with Fruit (Chapter 12)
Equals 1 fruit, 1 milk, 2 starches

Snack
1 cup raw carrot sticks topped with 4 tablespoons hummus
Equals 1 vegetable, 2 fats

Lunch
Spicy Shrimp Kabobs (Chapter 14)
2 cups salad tossed with 2 tablespoons vinaigrette dressing
1 cup fruit salad
Equals 3 vegetables, 1 fruit, 4 ounces protein, 2 fats

Snack
1 cup lowfat plain yogurt topped with 1 cup raspberries
Equals 1 milk, 1 fruit

Dinner
6 ounces flounder, sautéed in 1 teaspoon olive oil
1 cup frozen kale, thawed and sautéed in 1 teaspoon olive oil
1½ cups cooked whole-grain pasta
Equals 2 vegetables, 3 starches, 6 ounces protein, 2 fats

Day 4

Breakfast
Bean, Ham, and Cheese Breakfast Burrito (Chapter 12)
Equals 2 starches, 4 ounces protein, 1 fat

Snack
1 cup diced papaya
12 almonds
Equals 1 fruit, 2 fats

Lunch
3 ounces chicken breast, grilled or broiled
1 cup chopped vegetables (onions, peppers, and mushrooms), stir-fried in 2 teaspoons olive oil
1 medium peach
Equals 2 vegetables, 1 fruit, 3 ounces protein, 2 fats

Snack
1 cup lowfat plain yogurt
1 cup grapes
Equals 1 milk, 1 fruit

Dinner
3 ounces London broil, grilled or broiled
1 cup green beans, sautéed in 1 teaspoon olive oil
1 cup cooked wild rice
1 cup fat-free or lowfat milk
Equals 2 vegetables, 1 milk, 3 starches, 3 ounces protein, 1 fat

Day 5

Breakfast
1 cup blackberries
1¼ cups lowfat cottage cheese
1 cup cooked steel-cut oatmeal (prepared with water)
Equals 1 fruit, 2 starches, 5 ounces protein

Snack
1 small banana
1 cup lowfat plain yogurt
12 almonds
Equals 1 fruit, 1 milk, 2 fats

Lunch
Hummus and Avocado Sandwich (Chapter 13)
1 cup lowfat plain yogurt
Equals 1 vegetable, 1 milk, 2 starches, 3 fats

Snack
1 hard-boiled egg on 1 slice of 100% whole-grain toast
1 cup raw carrot sticks
Equals 1 vegetable, 1 starch, 1 ounce protein

Dinner
Pepper Steak with Fresh Vegetables (Chapter 14)
1 cup strawberries
Equals 2 vegetables, 1 fruit, 4 ounces protein, 1 fat

Day 6

Breakfast
Veggie-Egg Muffin (Chapter 12)
1 cup lowfat plain yogurt
12 almonds
Equals 0.5 vegetable, 1 milk, 2 ounces protein, 2 fats

Snack
Chocolate-Drizzled Strawberries (Chapter 15)
Equals 1 fruit, 0.5 starch

Lunch
Hot and Spicy Vegetarian Chili (Chapter 13)
1 cup blueberries
Equals 1.5 vegetables, 1 fruit, 1.5 starches, 2 ounces protein, 1 fat

Snack
½ cup lowfat cottage cheese
½ cup pineapple
6 rye crisps
Equals 1 fruit, 1 starch, 2 ounces protein

Dinner
4 ounces chicken breast, grilled or broiled
1 cup chopped bell peppers, ½ cup chopped mushrooms, ½ cup chopped onions, stir-fried in 1 tablespoon soy sauce and 1 tablespoon olive oil
⅔ cup cooked brown rice
1 cup fat-free or lowfat milk
Equals 2 vegetables, 1 milk, 2 starches, 4 ounces protein, 3 fats

Day 7

Breakfast
1 cup liquid egg substitute (or 8 egg whites), scrambled
Yogurt parfait made with 1 cup lowfat yogurt, 1 cup mixed berries, and 2 tablespoons chopped walnuts
Equals 1 fruit, 1 milk, 4 ounces protein, 2 fats

Snack
1 medium plum
1 stick lowfat string cheese
Equals 1 fruit, 1 ounce protein

Lunch
Herb-Roasted Salmon (Chapter 14)
1 cup frozen spinach, thawed and sautéed in 1 teaspoon olive oil
1 cup kidney beans, cooked
Half a grapefruit
Equals 2 vegetables, 1 fruit, 2 starches, 4 ounces protein, 2 fats

Snack
1 cup lowfat plain yogurt topped with ½ cup whole-grain cereal
Equals 1 milk, 1 starch

Dinner
Whole-Grain Bruschetta Pizza, 1 serving (Chapter 14)
2 cups salad tossed with 2 tablespoons balsamic vinegar and 1 teaspoon olive oil
Equals 3 vegetables, 2 starches, 1 ounce protein, 2 fats

Moderation Plan, Level 2:
Sample Week Meal Plan for Women

Day 1

Breakfast
Banana-Almond Breakfast Toast
(Chapter 12)
1 cup fat-free or lowfat milk
*Equals 1 fruit, 1 milk, 1 starch, 1 ounce
protein, 1 fat*

Snack
Baked Apple (Chapter 15)
1 cup lowfat plain yogurt
Equals 1 fruit, 1 milk

Lunch
2 ounces flounder, grilled or broiled
1 cup frozen spinach, thawed and sautéed
in 2 teaspoons olive oil
½ cup cooked whole-grain pasta
1 cup fruit salad
*Equals 2 vegetables, 1 fruit, 1 starch,
2 ounces protein, 2 fats*

Snack
1 cup raw celery sticks topped with
4 teaspoons natural peanut butter
Equals 1 vegetable, 2 fats

Dinner
Low-Calorie Chicken Parmesan
(Chapter 14)
1 cup Brussels sprouts, steamed
*Equals 2 vegetables, 0.5 starch, 5 ounces
protein*

Snack
1½ cups air-popped popcorn
Equals 0.5 starch

Day 2

Breakfast
Waistline-Slimming Omelet (Chapter 12)
½ cup mandarin oranges
*Equals 1 vegetable, 0.5 fruit, 3 ounces
protein, 1 fat*

Snack
Belly-Blasting Trail Mix (Chapter 15)
Equals 0.5 fruit, 1 starch, 2 fats

Lunch
Shockingly Healthy (and Easy!) Calzone
(Chapter 13)
1 medium apple
*Equals 1 vegetable, 1 fruit, 1 starch,
2 ounces protein*

Snack
Smoothie made with 1 cup lowfat yogurt,
1 cup mixed berries, and 1 tablespoon
flaxseed
Equals 1 milk, 1 fruit, 1 fat

Dinner
3 ounces pork tenderloin, grilled or broiled
½ cup carrots, steamed and topped with
1 teaspoon olive oil-based spread
½ cup zucchini slices, steamed
1 cup fat-free or lowfat milk
½ cup cooked quinoa
*Equals 2 vegetables, 1 milk, 1 starch,
3 ounces protein, 1 fat*

Day 3

Breakfast
Quick and Belly-Friendly Cold Cereal with
Fruit (Chapter 12)
Equals 1 fruit, 1 milk, 2 starches

Snack
1 cup raw carrot sticks topped with
2 tablespoons hummus
Equals 1 vegetable, 1 fat

Lunch
Spicy Shrimp Kabobs (Chapter 14)
2 cups salad tossed with 2 tablespoons
vinaigrette dressing
1 cup fruit salad
*Equals 3 vegetables, 1 fruit, 4 ounces
protein, 2 fats*

Snack
1 cup lowfat plain yogurt topped with
1 cup raspberries
Equals 1 milk, 1 fruit

Dinner
4 ounces flounder, sautéed in 1 teaspoon
olive oil
1 cup frozen kale, thawed and sautéed
in 1 teaspoon olive oil and 1 teaspoon
minced garlic
½ cup cooked whole-grain pasta
*Equals 2 vegetables, 1 starch, 4 ounces
protein, 2 fats*

Day 4

Breakfast
Bean, Ham, and Cheese Breakfast Burrito
(Chapter 12)
Equals 2 starches, 4 ounces protein, 1 fat

Snack
1 cup diced papaya
12 almonds
Equals 1 fruit, 2 fats

Lunch
2 ounces chicken breast, grilled or broiled
1 cup chopped vegetables (onions,
peppers, and mushrooms), stir-fried in
1 teaspoon olive oil
1 medium peach
*Equals 2 vegetables, 1 fruit, 2 ounces
protein, 1 fat*

Snack
1 cup lowfat plain yogurt
1 cup grapes
Equals 1 milk, 1 fruit

Dinner
2 ounces London broil, grilled or broiled
1 cup green beans, sautéed in 1 teaspoon
olive oil
1 cup fat-free or lowfat milk
⅓ cup cooked wild rice
*Equals 2 vegetables, 1 milk, 1 starch,
2 ounces protein, 1 fat*

Day 5

Breakfast
1 cup blackberries
¾ cup lowfat cottage cheese
½ cup cooked steel-cut oatmeal (prepared
with water)
Equals 1 fruit, 1 starch, 3 ounces protein

Snack
1 small banana
1 cup lowfat plain yogurt
6 almonds
Equals 1 fruit, 1 milk, 1 fat

Lunch
Hummus and Avocado Sandwich
(Chapter 13)
1 cup lowfat plain yogurt
*Equals 1 vegetable, 1 milk, 2 starches,
3 fats*

Snack
1 hard-boiled egg
1 cup raw carrot sticks
Equals 1 vegetable, 1 ounce protein

Dinner
Pepper Steak with Fresh Vegetables
(Chapter 14)
1 cup strawberries
*Equals 2 vegetables, 1 fruit, 4 ounces
protein, 1 fat*

Day 6

Breakfast
Veggie-Egg Muffin (Chapter 12)
1 cup lowfat plain yogurt
6 almonds
*Equals 0.5 vegetable, 1 milk, 2 ounces
protein, 1 fat*

Snack
Chocolate-Drizzled Strawberries
(Chapter 15)
Equals 1 fruit, 0.5 starch

Lunch
Hot and Spicy Vegetarian Chili (Chapter 13)
1 cup blueberries
*Equals 1.5 vegetables, 1 fruit, 1.5 starches,
2 ounces protein, 1 fat*

Snack
¼ cup lowfat cottage cheese
½ cup pineapple
6 rye crisps
Equals 1 fruit, 1 starch, 1 ounce protein

Dinner
3 ounces chicken breast, grilled or broiled
1 cup chopped bell peppers, ½ cup
chopped mushrooms, ½ cup chopped
onions, stir-fried in 1 tablespoon soy
sauce and 1 tablespoon olive oil
1 cup fat-free or lowfat milk
*Equals 2 vegetables, 1 milk, 3 ounces
protein, 3 fats*

Day 7

Breakfast
½ cup liquid egg substitute (or 4 egg
whites), scrambled
Yogurt parfait made with 1 cup lowfat
yogurt, 1 cup mixed berries, and 1 tablespoon chopped walnuts
Equals 1 fruit, 1 milk, 2 ounces protein, 1 fat

Snack
1 medium plum
1 stick lowfat string cheese
Equals 1 fruit, 1 ounce protein

Lunch
Herb-Roasted Salmon (Chapter 14)
1 cup frozen spinach, thawed and sautéed
in 1 teaspoon olive oil
Half a grapefruit
*Equals 2 vegetables, 1 fruit, 4 ounces
protein, 2 fats*

Snack
1 cup lowfat plain yogurt topped with ½
cup whole-grain cereal
Equals 1 milk, 1 starch

Dinner
Whole-Grain Bruschetta Pizza, 1 serving
(Chapter 14)
2 cups salad tossed with 2 tablespoons
balsamic vinegar and 1 teaspoon olive oil
*Equals 3 vegetables, 2 starches, 1 ounce
protein, 2 fats*

Gradual-Change Plan, Level 1: Sample Week Meal Plan for Men

Day 1

Breakfast
Breadless Breakfast Quiche (Chapter 12)
1 slice 100% whole-grain toast topped with 1 teaspoon olive oil-based spread
1 kiwi
Equals 1 vegetable, 1 fruit, 1 starch, 2 ounces protein, 2 fats

Snack
Yogurt parfait made with 1 cup lowfat plain yogurt, 1 cup blackberries, ½ cup whole-grain cereal, and 2 tablespoons chopped walnuts
Equals 1 milk, 1 fruit, 1 starch, 2 fats

Lunch
Tuna and Salsa Stuffed Pepper (Chapter 13)
1 medium pear
Equals 1 vegetable, 1 fruit, 2 ounces protein

Snack
12 whole-grain crackers topped with 2 tablespoons hummus
Equals 2 starches, 2 fats

Dinner
8 ounces chicken breast, grilled
5 asparagus spears (5 inches long), steamed
1 small sweet potato topped with 1 teaspoon olive oil-based spread
1 cup fat-free or lowfat milk
Equals 1 vegetable, 1 starchy vegetable, 1 milk, 8 ounces protein, 1 fat

Day 2

Breakfast
2 eggs, scrambled
½ cup diced potatoes, sautéed in nonstick cooking spray
1 slice 100% whole-grain toast topped with 1 teaspoon olive oil-based spread
1 cup blueberries
Equals 1 starchy vegetable, 1 starch, 2 ounces protein, 1 fruit, 1 fat

Snack
Belly-Blasting Berry Smoothie (Chapter 12)
Equals 1 fruit, 1 milk, 1 fat

Lunch
Grilled Chicken Salad (Chapter 13)
Equals 1.5 vegetables, 4 ounces protein, 2.5 fats

Snack
½ cup raw celery sticks topped with 3 teaspoons natural peanut butter
Equals 0.5 vegetable, 1.5 fats

Dinner
6 ounces flank steak, grilled or broiled
½ cup green beans, steamed
1 cup cooked brown rice
1 cup lowfat plain yogurt
1 cup honeydew melon
Equals 1 vegetable, 1 fruit, 3 starches, 1 milk, 6 ounces protein

Day 3

Breakfast
Tropical Yogurt Parfait (Chapter 12)
Equals 1 fruit, 1 milk, 4 fats

Snack
3 cups Homemade Spicy Microwave Popcorn (Chapter 15)
1 cup lowfat milk
Equals 1 milk, 2.5 starches

Lunch
8 ounces turkey breast, baked
1 medium ear of corn coated with 2 teaspoons olive oil-based spread
½ cup broccoli, steamed
Equals 1 vegetable, 1 starchy vegetable, 8 ounces protein, 2 fats

Snack
1 cup raw carrot sticks topped with 4 tablespoons hummus
Equals 1 vegetable, 2 fats

Dinner
Belly-Friendly Chicken Marsala (Chapter 14)
1½ cups cooked whole-grain pasta
1 cup fruit salad
Equals 1 vegetable, 1 fruit, 3 starches, 4 ounces protein

Day 4

Breakfast
1 medium apple, sliced and topped with 2 teaspoons natural almond butter
Equals 1 fruit, 1 fat

Snack
1 cup lowfat plain yogurt topped with 1 tablespoon chopped walnuts, ¼ cup dried tart cherries, and 1 tablespoon cinnamon
Equals 1 milk, 1 fruit, 1 fat

Lunch
Turkey Burger with Sweet Potato Fries (Chapter 13)
1 cup fat-free or lowfat milk
Equals 1 starchy vegetable, 1 milk, 2 starches, 4 ounces protein, 1 fat

Snack
1 cup raw bell pepper slices topped with 2 tablespoons hummus
Equals 1 vegetable, 1 fat

Dinner
Herb-Roasted Salmon, 2 servings (Chapter 14)
1 cup string beans, steamed
1 cup cooked quinoa
1 cup watermelon
Equals 2 vegetables, 1 fruit, 2 starches, 8 ounces protein, 2 fats

Day 5

Breakfast
Cinnamon Oatmeal with Almonds (Chapter 12)
1 small banana
Equals 1 starch, 1 fruit, 1 fat

Snack
20 pistachio nuts
1 medium orange
Equals 1 fruit, 2 fats

Lunch
Chicken Cordon Bleu, 2 servings (Chapter 14)
4 cups zucchini slices, sautéed in 1 teaspoon olive oil
½ cup cooked whole-grain pasta
Equals 2 vegetables, 1 starch, 8 ounces protein, 1 fat

Snack
1 cup lowfat plain yogurt topped with 2 tablespoons chopped walnuts and 1 cup blueberries
Equals 1 milk, 1 fruit, 2 fats

Dinner
Roasted Pork Tenderloin with Vegetables (Chapter 14)
⅔ cup cooked wild rice
1 cup fat-free or lowfat milk
Equals 1 vegetable, 1 starchy vegetable, 1 milk, 2 starches, 4 ounces protein

Day 6

Breakfast
On-the-Go Breakfast Sandwich (Chapter 12)
1 cup fat-free or lowfat milk
Equals 2 starches, 1 milk, 3 ounces protein

Snack
¼ cup dried cranberries mixed with ½ cup whole-grain cereal and 1 tablespoon chopped walnuts
Equals 1 fruit, 1 starch, 1 fat

Lunch
Portobello Mushroom Salad (Chapter 14)
6 whole-grain crackers
1 cup fat-free or lowfat milk
Equals 2.5 vegetables, 1 milk, 1 starch, 1.5 fats

Snack
Quarter of an avocado
1 small banana
Equals 1 fruit, 1 fat

Dinner
9 ounces salmon, grilled or broiled and drizzled with 1½ teaspoons olive oil
½ cup peas, steamed
½ cup bell pepper slices, sautéed in 1 teaspoon olive oil
Equals 1 vegetable, 1 starchy vegetable, 9 ounces protein, 2.5 fats

Day 7

Breakfast
1¼ cup lowfat ricotta cheese topped with ¼ cup dried tart cherries and 2 tablespoons chopped almonds
Equals 1 fruit, 5 ounces protein, 2 fats

Snack
2 hard-boiled eggs
Half a grapefruit
Equals 1 fruit, 2 ounces protein

Lunch
Belly-Beating Bean Burrito (Chapter 13)
1 cup lowfat plain yogurt
Equals 2 vegetables, 1 starchy vegetable, 1 milk, 1 starch, 1 ounce protein, 1 fat

Snack
Baked Apple (Chapter 15) topped with 1 tablespoon chopped almonds
Equals 1 starch, 1 fat

Dinner
Walnut-Encrusted Flounder (Chapter 14)
½ cup carrots, steamed and topped with 1 teaspoon olive oil-based spread
1 cup cooked whole-grain pasta
1 cup fat-free or lowfat milk
Equals 1 vegetable, 1 milk, 2 starches, 4 ounces protein, 2 fats

Gradual-Change Plan, Level 1:
Sample Week Meal Plan for Women

Day 1

Breakfast
Breadless Breakfast Quiche (Chapter 12)
1 slice 100% whole-grain toast topped
with 1 teaspoon olive oil-based spread
*Equals 1 vegetable, 1 starch, 2 ounces
protein, 2 fats*

Snack
Yogurt parfait made with 1 cup lowfat
plain yogurt, 1 cup blackberries, ½ cup
whole-grain cereal, and 1 tablespoon
chopped walnuts
Equals 1 milk, 1 fruit, 1 starch, 1 fat

Lunch
Tuna and Salsa Stuffed Pepper
(Chapter 13)
1 medium pear
*Equals 1 vegetable, 1 fruit, 2 ounces
protein*

Snack
12 whole-grain crackers topped with
2 tablespoons hummus
Equals 2 starches, 2 fats

Dinner
4 ounces chicken breast, grilled
10 asparagus spears (5 inches long),
steamed
1 small sweet potato topped with
1 teaspoon olive oil-based spread
1 cup fat-free or lowfat milk
*Equals 2 vegetables, 1 starchy vegetable,
1 milk, 4 ounces protein, 1 fat*

Day 2

Breakfast
1 egg, scrambled
½ cup diced potatoes, sautéed in nonstick
cooking spray
1 slice 100% whole-grain toast topped
with 1 teaspoon peanut butter
1 cup blueberries
*Equals 1 starchy vegetable, 1 starch,
1 ounce protein, 0.5 fat, 1 fruit*

Snack
Belly-Blasting Berry Smoothie (Chapter 12)
Equals 1 fruit, 1 milk, 1 fat

Lunch
Grilled Chicken Salad (Chapter 13)
*Equals 1.5 vegetables, 4 ounces protein,
2.5 fats*

Snack
1 cup raw celery sticks topped with
2 teaspoons natural peanut butter
Equals 1 vegetable, 1 fat

Dinner
3 ounces flank steak, grilled or broiled
½ cup green beans, steamed
1 cup cooked brown rice
1 cup lowfat plain yogurt
*Equals 1 vegetable, 3 starches, 1 milk,
3 ounces protein*

Day 3

Breakfast
Tropical Yogurt Parfait (Chapter 12)
Equals 1 fruit, 1 milk, 4 fats

Snack
3 cups Homemade Spicy Microwave
Popcorn (Chapter 15)
1 cup lowfat milk
Equals 1 milk, 2.5 starches

Lunch
4 ounces turkey breast, baked
1 medium ear of corn coated with
1 teaspoon olive oil-based spread
½ cup broccoli, steamed
*Equals 1 vegetable, 1 starchy vegetable,
4 ounces protein, 1 fat*

Snack
1 cup raw carrot sticks topped with
4 tablespoons hummus
Equals 1 vegetable, 2 fats

Dinner
Belly-Friendly Chicken Marsala
(Chapter 14)
1½ cups cooked whole-grain pasta
1 medium apple
*Equals 1 vegetable, 1 fruit, 3 starches,
4 ounces protein*

Day 4

Breakfast
1 medium apple, sliced and topped with
2 teaspoons natural almond butter
Equals 1 fruit, 1 fat

Snack
1 cup lowfat plain yogurt topped with
1 tablespoon chopped walnuts, ¼ cup
dried tart cherries, and 1 tablespoon
cinnamon
Equals 1 milk, 1 fruit, 1 fat

Lunch
Turkey Burger with Sweet Potato Fries
(Chapter 13)
1 cup fat-free or lowfat milk
*Equals 1 starchy vegetable, 1 milk,
2 starches, 4 ounces protein, 1 fat*

Snack
1 cup raw bell pepper slices topped with
2 tablespoons hummus
Equals 1 vegetable, 1 fat

Dinner
Herb-Roasted Salmon (Chapter 14)
1 cup string beans, steamed
1 cup cooked quinoa
*Equals 2 vegetables, 2 starches, 4 ounces
protein, 1 fat*

Day 5

Breakfast
Cinnamon Oatmeal with Almonds
(Chapter 12)
Equals 1 starch, 1 fat

Snack
20 pistachio nuts
1 medium orange
Equals 1 fruit, 2 fats

Lunch
Chicken Cordon Bleu (Chapter 14)
4 cups zucchini slices, sautéed in
1 teaspoon olive oil
½ cup cooked whole-grain pasta
*Equals 2 vegetables, 1 starch, 4 ounces
protein, 1 fat*

Snack
1 cup lowfat plain yogurt topped with
1 tablespoon chopped walnuts and
1 cup blueberries
Equals 1 milk, 1 fruit, 1 fat

Dinner
Roasted Pork Tenderloin with Vegetables
(Chapter 14)
⅔ cup cooked wild rice
1 cup fat-free or lowfat milk
*Equals 1 vegetable, 1 starchy vegetable,
1 milk, 2 starches, 4 ounces protein*

Day 6

Breakfast
On-the-Go Breakfast Sandwich
(Chapter 12)
1 cup fat-free or lowfat milk
Equals 2 starches, 1 milk, 3 ounces protein

Snack
¼ cup dried cranberries mixed with ½ cup
whole-grain cereal
Equals 1 fruit, 1 starch

Lunch
Portobello Mushroom Salad (Chapter 14)
1 cup fat-free or lowfat milk
6 whole-grain crackers
*Equals 2.5 vegetables, 1 milk, 1 starch,
1.5 fats*

Snack
Quarter of an avocado
1 small banana
Equals 1 fruit, 1 fat

Dinner
5 ounces salmon, grilled or broiled and
drizzled with 1½ teaspoons olive oil
½ cup peas, steamed
½ cup bell pepper slices, sautéed in
1 teaspoon olive oil
*Equals 1 vegetable, 1 starchy vegetable,
5 ounces protein, 2.5 fats*

Day 7

Breakfast
½ cup lowfat ricotta cheese topped with ¼
cup dried tart cherries and 2 tablespoons
chopped almonds
Equals 1 fruit, 2 ounces protein, 2 fats

Snack
1 hard-boiled egg
Half a grapefruit
Equals 1 fruit, 1 ounce protein

Lunch
Belly-Beating Bean Burrito (Chapter 13)
1 cup lowfat plain yogurt
*Equals 2 vegetables, 1 starchy vegetable,
1 milk, 1 starch, 1 ounce protein, 1 fat*

Snack
Mock Ice Cream Sandwich (Chapter 15)
Equals 1 starch

Dinner
Walnut-Encrusted Flounder (Chapter 14)
½ cup carrots, steamed and topped with
1 teaspoon olive oil-based spread
⅔ cup cooked whole-grain couscous
1 cup fat-free or lowfat milk
*Equals 1 vegetable, 1 milk, 2 starches,
4 ounces protein, 2 fats*

Gradual-Change Plan, Level 2: Sample Week Meal Plan for Men

Day 1

Breakfast
Banana-Almond Breakfast Toast
(Chapter 12)
1 cup fat-free or lowfat milk
Equals 1 fruit, 1 milk, 1 starch, 1 ounce protein, 1 fat

Snack
Baked Apple (Chapter 15)
1 cup lowfat plain yogurt
Equals 1 fruit, 1 milk

Lunch
6 ounces flounder, grilled or broiled
1 cup frozen spinach, thawed and sautéed in 2 teaspoons olive oil
1 cup cooked whole-grain pasta
1 cup fruit salad
Equals 2 vegetables, 1 fruit, 2 starches, 6 ounces protein, 2 fats

Snack
1 cup celery sticks topped with
4 teaspoons natural peanut butter
Equals 1 vegetable, 2 fats

Dinner
Low-Calorie Chicken Parmesan
(Chapter 14)
1 cup Brussels sprouts, sautéed in
2 teaspoons olive oil
1 medium ear of corn
Equals 2 vegetables, 1.5 starches, 5 ounces protein, 2 fats

Snack
4½ cups air-popped popcorn
Equals 1.5 starches

Day 2

Breakfast
Waistline-Slimming Omelet (Chapter 12)
½ cup mandarin oranges
2 slices 100% whole-grain toast topped with 2 teaspoons olive oil-based spread
Equals 1 vegetable, 0.5 fruit, 2 starches, 3 ounces protein, 3 fats

Snack
Belly-Blasting Trail Mix (Chapter 15)
Equals 0.5 fruit, 1 starch, 2 fats

Lunch
Shockingly Healthy (and Easy!) Calzone
(Chapter 13)
1 medium apple
Equals 1 vegetable, 1 fruit, 1 starch, 2 ounces protein

Snack
Smoothie made with 1 cup lowfat yogurt, 1 cup mixed berries, and 1 tablespoon flaxseed
Equals 1 milk, 1 fruit, 1 fat

Dinner
7 ounces pork tenderloin, grilled or broiled
½ cups carrots, steamed and topped with
1 teaspoon olive oil-based spread
½ cups zucchini, steamed
1 cup fat-free or lowfat milk
1 cup cooked quinoa
Equals 2 vegetables, 1 milk, 2 starches, 7 ounces protein, 1 fat

Day 3

Breakfast
Quick and Belly-Friendly Cold Cereal with Fruit (Chapter 12)
Equals 1 fruit, 1 milk, 2 starches

Snack
1 cup raw carrot sticks topped with
4 tablespoons hummus
Equals 1 vegetable, 2 fats

Lunch
Spicy Shrimp Kabobs (Chapter 14)
2 cups salad tossed with 3 tablespoons vinaigrette dressing
1 cup fruit salad
Equals 3 vegetables, 1 fruit, 4 ounces protein, 3 fats

Snack
1 cup lowfat plain yogurt topped with
½ cup whole-grain cereal
1 cup raspberries
Equals 1 milk, 1 starch, 1 fruit

Dinner
8 ounces flounder, sautéed in 1 teaspoon olive oil
1 cup frozen kale, thawed and sautéed in 1 teaspoon olive oil and 1 teaspoon minced garlic
1½ cups cooked whole-grain pasta
Equals 2 vegetables, 3 starches, 8 ounces protein, 2 fats

Day 4

Breakfast
Bean, Ham, and Cheese Breakfast Burrito
(Chapter 12)
Equals 2 starches, 4 ounces protein, 1 fat

Snack
1 cup diced papaya
12 almonds
Equals 1 fruit, 2 fats

Lunch
4 ounces chicken breast, grilled or broiled
1 cup chopped vegetables (onions,
peppers, and mushrooms), stir-fried in
2 teaspoons olive oil and served over
½ cup cooked barley
1 medium peach
*Equals 2 vegetables, 1 fruit, 1 starch,
4 ounces protein, 2 fats*

Snack
1 cup lowfat plain yogurt
1 cup grapes
Equals 1 milk, 1 fruit

Dinner
4 ounces London broil, grilled or broiled
1 cup green beans, sautéed in
2 teaspoons olive oil
1 cup fat-free or lowfat milk
1 cup cooked wild rice
*Equals 2 vegetables, 1 milk, 3 starches,
4 ounces protein, 2 fats*

Day 5

Breakfast
1 cup blackberries
¾ cup lowfat cottage cheese
1 cup cooked steel-cut oatmeal (prepared
with water)
Equals 1 fruit, 2 starches, 3 ounces protein

Snack
1 small banana
1 cup lowfat plain yogurt or 1 cup lowfat milk
6 almonds
Equals 1 fruit, 1 milk, 1 fat

Lunch
Hummus and Avocado Sandwich
(Chapter 13)
1 cup lowfat plain yogurt
*Equals 1 vegetable, 1 milk, 2 starches,
3 fats*

Snack
1 hard-boiled egg
1 slice 100% whole-grain toast topped
with 2 teaspoons almond butter
Equals 1 starch, 1 fat, 1 ounce protein

Dinner
Pepper Steak with Fresh Vegetables,
2 servings (Chapter 14)
1 cup strawberries
½ cup butternut squash, steamed
½ cup steamed cabbage
*Equals 4 vegetables, 1 fruit, 1 starch,
8 ounces protein, 2 fats*

Day 6

Breakfast
Veggie-Egg Muffins, 2 servings (Chapter 12)
Half a small whole-grain bagel topped
with 1 teaspoon olive oil-based spread
1 cup lowfat plain yogurt
12 almonds
*Equals 1 vegetable, 1 milk, 1 starch,
4 ounces protein, 3 fats*

Snack
Chocolate-Drizzled Strawberries (Chapter 15)
Equals 1 fruit, 0.5 starch

Lunch
Hot and Spicy Vegetarian Chili (Chapter 13)
1 cup blueberries
*Equals 1½ vegetables, 1 fruit, 1.5 starches,
2 ounces protein, 1 fat*

Snack
½ cup lowfat cottage cheese
½ cup pineapple
6 rye crisps
Equals 1 fruit, 1 starch, 2 ounces protein

Dinner
4 ounces chicken breast, grilled or broiled
1 cup chopped bell peppers, ½ cup
chopped mushrooms, ½ cup chopped
onions, stir-fried in 1 tablespoon soy
sauce and 1 tablespoon olive oil
⅔ cup cooked brown rice
1 cup fat-free or lowfat milk
*Equals 2 vegetables, 1 milk, 2 starches,
4 ounces protein, 3 fats*

Day 7

Breakfast
1¼ cups liquid egg substitute (or 8 egg
whites), scrambled
Yogurt parfait made with 1 cup lowfat
yogurt, 1 cup mixed berries, and 2 tablespoons chopped walnuts
Equals 1 fruit, 1 milk, 5 ounces protein, 2 fats

Snack
1 medium plum
1 stick lowfat string cheese
Equals 1 fruit, 1 ounce protein

Lunch
Herb-Roasted Salmon (Chapter 14)
1 cup frozen spinach, thawed and sautéed
in 1 teaspoon olive oil
1 cup cooked kidney beans
Half a grapefruit
*Equals 2 vegetables, 1 fruit, 2 starches,
4 ounces protein, 2 fats*

Snack
1 cup lowfat plain yogurt
Equals 1 milk

Dinner
Whole-Grain Bruschetta Pizza, 2 servings
(Chapter 14)
1 cup salad tossed with 2 tablespoons
balsamic vinegar and 1 teaspoon olive oil
*Equals 3 vegetables, 4 starches, 2 ounces
protein, 3 fats*

Gradual-Change Plan, Level 2: Sample Week Meal Plan for Women

Day 1

Breakfast
Banana-Almond Breakfast Toast
(Chapter 12)
1 cup fat-free or lowfat milk
Equals 1 fruit, 1 milk, 1 starch, 1 ounce protein, 1 fat

Snack
Baked Apple (Chapter 15)
1 cup lowfat plain yogurt
Equals 1 fruit, 1 milk

Lunch
2 ounces flounder, grilled or broiled
1 cup frozen spinach, thawed and sautéed
in 2 teaspoons olive oil
1 cup cooked whole-grain pasta
1 cup fruit salad
Equals 2 vegetables, 1 fruit, 2 starches, 2 ounces protein, 2 fats

Snack
1 cup celery sticks topped with
4 teaspoons natural peanut butter
Equals 1 vegetable, 2 fats

Dinner
Low-Calorie Chicken Parmesan
(Chapter 14)
1 cup Brussels sprouts, sautéed in
1 teaspoon olive oil
Equals 2 vegetables, 0.5 starch, 5 ounces protein, 1 fat

Snack
4½ cups air-popped popcorn
Equals 1½ starches

Day 2

Breakfast
Waistline-Slimming Omelet (Chapter 12)
½ cup Mandarin oranges
2 slices 100% whole-grain toast topped
with 1 teaspoon olive oil-based spread
Equals 1 vegetable, 0.5 fruit, 2 starches, 3 ounces protein, 2 fats

Snack
Belly-Blasting Trail Mix (Chapter 15)
Equals 0.5 fruit, 1 starch, 2 fats

Lunch
Shockingly Healthy (and Easy!) Calzone
(Chapter 13)
1 medium apple
Equals 1 vegetable, 1 fruit, 1 starch, 2 ounces protein

Snack
Smoothie made with 1 cup lowfat yogurt,
1 cup mixed berries, and 1 tablespoon
flaxseed
Equals 1 milk, 1 fruit, 1 fat

Dinner
3 ounces pork tenderloin, grilled or broiled
½ cup carrots, steamed and topped with
1 teaspoon olive oil-based spread
½ cup zucchini, steamed
1 cup fat-free or lowfat milk
½ cup cooked quinoa
Equals 2 vegetables, 1 milk, 1 starch, 3 ounces protein, 1 fat

Day 3

Breakfast
Quick and Belly-Friendly Cold Cereal with
Fruit (Chapter 12)
Equals 1 fruit, 1 milk, 2 starches

Snack
1 cup raw carrot sticks topped with
4 tablespoons hummus
Equals 1 vegetable, 2 fats

Lunch
Spicy Shrimp Kabobs (Chapter 14)
2 cups salad tossed with 2 tablespoons
vinaigrette dressing
1 cup fruit salad
Equals 3 vegetables, 1 fruit, 4 ounces protein, 2 fats

Snack
1 cup lowfat plain yogurt topped with
1 cup raspberries
Equals 1 milk, 1 fruit

Dinner
4 ounces flounder, sautéed in 1 teaspoon
olive oil
1 cup frozen kale, thawed and sautéed
in 1 teaspoon olive oil and 1 teaspoon
minced garlic
1½ cups cooked whole-grain pasta
Equals 2 vegetables, 3 starches, 4 ounces protein, 2 fats

Day 4

Breakfast
Bean, Ham, and Cheese Breakfast Burrito (Chapter 12)
Equals 2 starches, 4 ounces protein, 1 fat

Snack
1 cup diced papaya
12 almonds
Equals 1 fruit, 2 fats

Lunch
2 ounces chicken breast, grilled or broiled
1 cup chopped vegetables (onions, peppers, and mushrooms), stir-fried in 2 teaspoons olive oil
1 medium peach
Equals 2 vegetables, 1 fruit, 2 ounces protein, 2 fats

Snack
1 cup lowfat plain yogurt
1 cup grapes
Equals 1 milk, 1 fruit

Dinner
2 ounces London broil, grilled or broiled
1 cup green beans, sautéed in 1 teaspoon olive oil
1 cup fat-free or lowfat milk
1 cup cooked wild rice
Equals 2 vegetables, 1 milk, 3 starches, 2 ounces protein, 1 fat

Day 5

Breakfast
1 cup blackberries
¾ cup lowfat cottage cheese
1 cup cooked steel-cut oatmeal (prepared with water)
Equals 1 fruit, 2 starches, 3 ounces protein

Snack
1 small banana
1 cup lowfat plain yogurt or lowfat milk
6 almonds
Equals 1 fruit, 1 milk, 1 fat

Lunch
Hummus and Avocado Sandwich (Chapter 13)
1 cup lowfat plain yogurt
Equals 1 vegetable, 1 milk, 2 starches, 3 fats

Snack
1 hard-boiled egg
1 slice 100% whole-grain toast topped with 2 teaspoons almond butter
Equals 1 starch, 1 fat, 1 ounce protein

Dinner
Pepper Steak with Fresh Vegetables (Chapter 14)
1 cup strawberries
2 cups shredded cabbage, steamed
Equals 3 vegetables, 1 fruit, 4 ounces protein, 1 fat

Day 6

Breakfast
Veggie-Egg Muffin (Chapter 12)
1 cup lowfat plain yogurt
12 almonds
Equals 0.5 vegetable, 1 milk, 2 ounces protein, 2 fats

Snack
Chocolate-Drizzled Strawberries (Chapter 15)
Equals 1 fruit, 0.5 starch

Lunch
Hot and Spicy Vegetarian Chili (Chapter 13)
1 cup blueberries
Equals 1.5 vegetables, 1 fruit, 1.5 starches, 2 ounces protein, 1 fat

Snack
¼ cup lowfat cottage cheese
½ cup pineapple
6 rye crisps
Equals 1 fruit, 1 starch, 1 ounce protein

Dinner
3 ounces chicken breast, grilled or broiled
1 cup chopped bell peppers, ½ cup chopped mushrooms, ½ cup chopped onions, stir-fried in 1 tablespoon soy sauce and 1 tablespoon olive oil
⅔ cup cooked brown rice
1 cup fat-free or lowfat milk
Equals 2 vegetables, 1 milk, 2 starches, 3 ounces protein, 3 fats

Day 7

Breakfast
½ cup liquid egg substitute (or 4 egg whites), scrambled
Yogurt parfait made with 1 cup lowfat yogurt, 1 cup mixed berries, and 2 tablespoons chopped walnuts
Equals 1 fruit, 1 milk, 2 ounces protein, 2 fats

Snack
1 medium plum
1 stick lowfat string cheese
Equals 1 fruit, 1 ounce protein

Lunch
Herb-Roasted Salmon (Chapter 14)
1 cup frozen spinach, thawed and sautéed in 1 teaspoon olive oil
1 cup cooked kidney beans
Half a grapefruit
Equals 2 vegetables, 1 fruit, 2 starches, 4 ounces protein, 2 fats

Snack
1 cup lowfat plain yogurt topped with ½ cup whole-grain cereal
Equals 1 milk, 1 starch

Dinner
Whole-Grain Bruschetta Pizza, 1 serving (Chapter 14)
2 cups salad tossed with 2 tablespoons balsamic vinegar and 1 teaspoon olive oil
Equals 3 vegetables, 2 starches, 1 ounce protein, 2 fats

Chapter 9

Easing Yourself into Exercise

In This Chapter

▶ Understanding how exercise can help fight belly fat

▶ Getting ready for your workout routine

▶ Making walking your exercise of choice

*E*xercise is an essential piece of the belly-flattening puzzle. To help fight belly fat and keep it away for good, you must make adjustments to both your dietary habits as well as your physical activity patterns. Staying active isn't just important for shrinking your waistline; it's also vital to your health. Exercise can help reduce your risks of many diseases, including heart disease, type 2 diabetes, and even certain cancers.

In this chapter, I show you simple ways to get started with your Belly Fat Diet Workout plan. (I cover the actual exercise routines in Chapter 10.) This chapter shows you what you need to do to prepare to exercise, how to motivate yourself to get started, and how to tailor your workout plan to ensure you're burning belly fat quickly and easily!

Why Exercising Is Vital

Exercise is an all-around great habit to pick up and maintain. It benefits your body is so many ways, including helping you achieve a flat stomach, improving your health, and giving your metabolism a jolt. I explain each of these benefits in the following sections.

The belly-blasting workout routines in Chapter 10 help you ease into exercise. These workout routines provide something for everyone. If you haven't exercised in the past, you can work slowly into the abdominal exercises and walking routines. If you already exercise on a regular basis, adding interval training can help you target abdominal fat, allowing you to shed it once and for all.

Flattens your abs

You can lose weight and even achieve your ideal weight through diet alone, but if you really want to flatten your belly and keep it that way, you have to exercise as well. Part of what makes up your belly is your abdominal muscles. If you start to strengthen these muscles, they work like an internal girdle, pulling your stomach in, flattening it, and showing those abs you've worked so hard to achieve.

However, you can't just perform abdominal exercises day after day and assume you'll get flat, sculpted abs. Even if you make your abdominal muscles as strong as an Olympic athlete's, you won't be able to see definition if you have a layer of fat covering your muscles. That's why cardiovascular exercise is a critical piece.

The combination of cardiovascular and strength exercises can help you increase your caloric burn and can keep your metabolism fired up all day from the additional muscle mass you build. In combination with your Belly Fat Diet plan, which helps boost your metabolism and provide a calorie deficit, you'll be shedding those layers of abdominal fat in no time!

Improves overall health

In addition to slimming your waistline and flattening your abs, exercise also improves your overall health and well-being in a number of ways. Exercise can help you

- ✔ Decrease blood pressure
- ✔ Decrease blood sugar levels (if diabetic) and prevent insulin resistance
- ✔ Improve cardiovascular health
- ✔ Lower cholesterol levels
- ✔ Prevent diseases like heart disease, diabetes, and certain cancers

Boosts your metabolism

Exercising while losing weight is important because it boosts your metabolism. By following a regular exercise routine while you make dietary changes, you maintain more muscle mass, which ensures that your metabolism is as good as or better than when you started. A good metabolism makes weight maintenance easier.

If you perform little to no physical activity while trying to lose weight, you'll start to lose both fat and muscle mass. Although everyone loses a bit of muscle mass when losing weight, you want to maintain as much muscle mass as possible, because it makes up the majority of your metabolism.

Preparing For Your Workout Routine

Before you start or change a workout routine, you need to do a few things to prepare. It's neither healthy nor efficient to simply start exercising without considering the many factors involved. If you start exercising willy-nilly, you're bound to either hurt yourself or set yourself up for failure. I explain everything you need to think about in the following sections.

Checking in with your doctor

The most important exercise preparation is to consult your physician. She can determine whether you're healthy enough to engage in an exercise routine. Also make sure she approves the workout routine you intend to do, and ask her whether you need to avoid or modify any exercises to protect yourself from injury or health risk. No matter what your age or medical history, getting medical clearance before starting or changing an exercise routine is essential. Doing so ensures you aren't participating in an exercise that may increase your risk of illness or injury.

Even though I recommend that everyone receive medical clearance before starting or changing an exercise routine, the following groups of individuals absolutely must check in with their doctors before getting started:

- Those with a history of heart disease
- Those on medication for high blood pressure
- Those with diabetes
- Those with mobility problems
- Those diagnosed with osteopenia or osteoporosis
- Those with a history of bone or joint surgeries (such as spinal surgery, knee surgery, and so on)
- Those older than 50
- Obese individuals of any age
- Pregnant women
- Women who gave birth within the last three months

If you fall into any of these categories, don't feel that you can't exercise. In fact, you'll likely be cleared for almost any physical activity. But having an examination by your physician before starting an exercise routine ensures that if you have any restrictions, such as keeping your heart rate below a certain level or avoiding a specific exercise or form of movement to prevent injury, you can be sure to follow these instructions. As a result, you'll be able to start your exercise routine and stick with it.

Penciling yourself in

Before getting started, you need to schedule your exercise routine. Just saying you'll exercise every day or every other day is great, but it's easy to get sidetracked and forget or to be unable to fit it in. So just like with any appointment you make, take out your calendar and figure out a time in your day that's best to exercise and write it down as an appointment with yourself.

When scheduling your workout, keep the following factors in mind:

✔ **What location will you exercise in?** Will you be exercising at home, at a gym, at a local park, or even at work? Determining where you plan to exercise can help you consider what time of day may be best to do so. It can also help you figure out whether you need to schedule time to drive to and from your place of exercise.

✔ **What equipment, if any, do you need access to before you can work out?** Depending on what you'll be doing for exercise, you may need some equipment. For instance, if you'll be walking, you need proper footwear. If you'll be performing abdominal exercises, you may need an exercise mat.

✔ **If you'll be working out with an exercise partner, what time of day and what place is best for you both?** An exercise partner is a great way to help you stay motivated, but you need to make sure you pick a time and place that works best for both of you.

✔ **Do you have an alternate time and place to exercise if your planned time frame or location can't be used?** For example, if you plan to walk outside, but it's raining, do you have access to an indoor location where you can walk or use a treadmill? Or can you perhaps work out at a different time?

If you've figured out exactly when you'll exercise, where you'll exercise, and what your backup plan is, you'll be much more likely to stick with your workout routine.

Choosing the right gear

Before starting any exercise routine (even walking), ensure that you have the right equipment on hand to make your workouts effective and to prevent injury. The most important (and most basic) gear you need to consider includes shoes, clothes, and a pedometer. I discuss each of these in the following sections.

It's also important to make sure you stay hydrated when exercising, so consider investing in a reusable water bottle to carry with you during your workout. And, if you'll be exercising outdoors, don't forget to use sunscreen!

Footwear

The most important piece of equipment you need when exercising, especially when following a walking routine (which is the focus of the belly-blasting workout routines in Chapter 10), is to have supportive footwear.

The right footwear can help prevent injury and discomfort while exercising. But there's no one-size-fits-all approach when it comes to selecting the right shoe. Because every foot is different, the right shoe for you depends on what fits your particular feet the best. Consult with an expert shoe fitter to determine the best shoe for your needs.

When picking footwear for your workout routine, consider these factors:

- **Flexibility:** The shoe you choose should be flexible. Hold the shoe and see whether you can bend and twist it. If you can't, it may be too stiff and may not allow your foot to bend, flex, and roll from heel to toe with each step.

- **Heel size and height:** Look for a shoe with a slightly undercut heel size. As you walk, your heel is the first area to hit the ground, so it's important not to have a shoe with a flared heel. The wider heel is better for running than walking. And keep in mind that a shoe used for brisk walking needs to have a flat heel rather than a raised one.

- **Purchase location:** To be sized correctly for the shoes that are best for you, try shopping at a store that specializes in walking or running rather than at a department store or generalized sporting goods store. Specialized stores have more experience in analyzing your needs and helping you select the best shoe for your foot.

Clothing

You need the correct attire for working out. Loose-fitting clothes or body-hugging clothes with stretch are the best bet because they're comfortable and allow you to have increased range of movement.

Make sure your clothing is appropriate for the weather as well. For instance, if you'll be exercising outdoors, make sure to have attire made with material that's appropriate for all kinds of weather, including wet, hot, and cold days. For instance, dressing in layers is key in cold weather. Clothes that help wick away moisture are helpful on hot and humid days. And waterproof coverings can help you stay dry during rainy day workouts.

Pedometer

A *pedometer* is a tool that counts every step you take during the day. When you take 2,000 steps, you have walked approximately 1 mile. You can start by wearing the pedometer for a few days to get your average number of daily steps. After you have this average, work to increase the number of steps you take daily. Every 2,000 steps equals an extra mile of walking per day. The goal is to achieve at least 10,000 to 15,000 steps per day.

According to the Harvard Health Letter, a summary of 26 unique studies showed that individuals who used a pedometer walked at least 2,000 additional steps daily when compared to individuals who didn't use the device. That's an extra mile each and every day! And in the course of a year, all that extra walking can really help you shed those pounds.

When choosing a pedometer, keep the following tips in mind:

- ✔ **Focus on the basic models.** Many pedometers offer tons of features, such as telling you how many calories you've burned, distinguishing between elevated walking and walking on flat surfaces, and talking to you! But before you get too wrapped up in all the additional bells and whistles, remember that all you really need is a pedometer that accurately counts your steps.

- ✔ **Select a brand with a cover.** Some pedometers have a reset button on the outside. If your pedometer has one and you accidentally bump into something, it may reset all your steps for the day. If you choose a pedometer with a reset button, make sure it includes a cover (or a locking mechanism) so you can avoid accidentally resetting your steps.

- ✔ **Purchase a brand with a safety strap.** If your pedometer falls off, a safety strap acts as a backup so you don't lose the device. Try to purchase a pedometer with this additional strap to cut down on your risk of losing it.

Motivating yourself to exercise

Getting up off the couch and talking yourself into starting an exercise routine can be challenging and requires a good amount of motivation. If you aren't feeling the motivational vibes, try the following to get yourself moving:

✔ **Remind yourself why you wanted to achieve your goal in the first place.** The stronger your reason for wanting to do something, the more energy you will put into achieving it. And once you're working toward your goal, it's easier to stay motivated.

✔ **Focus on the rewards.** Staying motivated to continue with an exercise routine over a period of weeks or months can be challenging, but it helps to look at how you stay motivated in other parts of your life. For instance, what motivates you to stay late at work? Perhaps you're aiming for a raise and the financial rewards that this raise will bring. You can apply this technique to your fitness routine as well. Just like you may not enjoy every minute of staying late at work, you may also not love staying on the treadmill for an extra 15 minutes. However, when you focus on the rewards this extra time will bring you (a flatter belly, increased energy levels, and so on), you can glean some motivation to continue.

✔ **Write down your life and fitness goals and prioritize them.** As you're compiling your goals, keep in mind that maintaining your health by achieving physical and mental fitness helps you achieve your other life goals. After you have your list of goals, write out a plan of action to achieve them. Seeing your list and plans on paper is one of the best ways to help you achieve success.

✔ **Don't be discouraged by past failures.** Have you tried to improve your fitness levels in the past and subsequently failed? If so, remember that you aren't destined to fail. Instead, focus on why you weren't successful in the past. After you understand what kept you from being successful, you can work on making changes.

✔ **Understand the impact exercise has on your life.** When you're physically fit, how do you feel? Do you have more energy? Can you multitask better? Does your mental clarity improve? Identifying how much better you function in other areas of life when you're physically fit can help you to stay on track with your exercise goals.

✔ **Find an exercise buddy.** When you don't feel like exercising, you may "self-talk" yourself out of it. However, if you know someone else is relying on you to work out, you're more apt to stay on track with your routine and show up for your scheduled exercise session. So find someone whose goals are similar to yours and meet regularly.

Deciding on the type of exercise that's appropriate for you

The best exercise for you is the exercise you enjoy and can stick with. To determine your ideal exercise, take a look at your current activity level, your goals, and your current health. Some options include walking, running, biking, tennis, aerobics, soccer, basketball, and swimming. The list goes on and on. Just find something you enjoy and go with it.

Walking is a fantastic form of exercise, and I recommend it for everyone. It's great because to get started you don't need much equipment (just a place to walk, a comfy outfit, and some shoes). You can walk almost anywhere, and the best part is that it has no learning curve. You've been walking since your first birthday, so you're now a pro at it!

Running is a great form of exercise, too, but you have a much greater chance of injury due to the increased pounding on your joints. Walking provides less impact, so you have less chance of injury. Walking is also a bit easier and great for those at all fitness levels. Sure, you can burn more calories per minute running, but if you're winded and have to stop after running just five or ten minutes, you aren't able to fit in much exercise. Even for most beginners, walking for at least ten minutes without getting too out of breath is easier.

As you become more accustomed to walking and begin to improve your endurance levels, you can increase your speed, change terrain to add incline or stairs, and increase your overall walking time, making it a perfect form of exercise for weight loss.

Walking is also an excellent way to keep the weight and belly fat off after you've reached your goals. Studies have shown that individuals who lose weight and keep it off long term include exercise on a regular basis, so why not pick an exercise that has a low injury rate and can be done anywhere at any age!

Determining your target heart rate

It's important to work within the appropriate intensity level to gain the maximum benefit from your workout. To determine the intensity at which you need to work out, use the following formula, which tells you your target heart rate zone:

1. Subtract your age in years from 220 = _____.

2. Multiply the number from Step 1 by 0.65 = _____.

3. Multiply the number from Step 1 by 0.85 = _____.

The numbers from Steps 2 and 3 represent your target heart rate zone, or the range of how fast your heart should beat per minute when exercising.

For example, here's how this calculation works for a 30-year-old:

1. $220 - 30 = 190$
2. $190 \times 0.65 = 123$
3. $190 \times 0.85 = 161$

The target heart rate zone for this person is between 123–161 beats per minute.

If you're under your respective target heart rate zone, you need to increase the intensity of your workout. If you're above it, you're working at too high an intensity and should decrease it. Continue to monitor your heart rate throughout your exercise program. You'll notice as you become more and more conditioned that raising your heart rate becomes more difficult. Vary your exercise routine every six to ten weeks to continue to elevate your heart rate to within the target zone to get the best benefit from your workout.

This formula for determining a target heart rate while exercising is an estimate. Make sure to consult your physician for the most appropriate heart rate goals for you when exercising. Certain medications, such as blood pressure medication, may lower your heart rate, so your target range may vary.

Knowing your limits

Exercise has many positive health benefits, including weight loss and improved energy levels. But when you increase your amount of exercise, you have the added risk of injury. So slowly easing into your workout routine is essential. If you push too hard too quickly, you can suffer from setbacks due to injury.

You may be tempted to shoot for an intense, long workout right out of the gate, especially if you used to do this in the past. However, it's better to start slowly and increase your speed and time over the course of a few weeks. Pushing too fast not only increases injury risk, but it also can increase muscle soreness and stiffness, which can make staying motivated to stick with your workout routine difficult.

Listen to your body, always warm up and cool down, and make sure to stretch regularly. If you have any joint or bone issues or have a history of injury, you need to consult your physician or physical therapist about the forms and types of exercise that are most appropriate for you.

Walking Away Your Belly Fat

I focus on walking as the main cardiovascular exercise of the belly-blasting workout routines in Chapter 10 because it's not only something that almost everyone can do, but also because it's great for melting away belly fat.

If you're thinking "Walking is fine, but if I could run daily I would lose weight faster and more effectively," don't worry. Running is fantastic exercise, but it's not appropriate for everyone. Walking is safe for almost everyone, and it's something you can do on a regular basis. And as long as you cover the same distance, whether you walk two miles or jog them, you'll burn the same number of calories (according to research done by the Mayo Clinic). It may take a bit longer to cover the same distance walking briskly versus running, but the result is the same!

The following tips can help you maintain correct walking form:

✔ **Watch how you step.** How you step is important to your foot health when walking. Stepping incorrectly can result in overuse injuries and pain. When taking a step, start by pushing off from the heel of your rear foot, and then push off with your toes. As you bring that foot forward, land on the heel of your foot and then roll through the foot as you walk. So you land on your heel, roll through the ball of your foot, and then push off with your toes to begin the next step.

✔ **Keep good posture, especially on uneven terrain.** When walking, stand upright and make sure your feet are pointing forward. Keep your back straight, and pull your shoulder blades back to ensure you aren't slouching. Your abs should be pulled in and held tight while walking as well. As you walk uphill or downhill, resist the tendency to lean forward or backward. Instead of leaning, use your arms to propel you up steep inclines. Leaning can increase the pressure on your back and joints, possibly causing injury.

✔ **Use your arms.** You want to pump your arms and engage your arm muscles while walking. Especially at high speeds or when climbing steep terrain, your arms can help propel you. As you walk, keep your arms near your sides and bend your elbows 90 degrees. As you move, allow your arms to move from your shoulders, not your elbows, and try not to let your arms rise higher than your chest. Resist the urge to clench your fists; relax your hands instead.

✔ **Keep your core tight.** As you walk, think about tightening your abdomen and pulling your stomach muscles in toward your spine. Doing so helps engage your abdominal muscles while walking. As you walk, allow your pelvis to move forward, but don't allow it to turn from side to side as you step. Keeping your toes forward and knees in line with your hip help to prevent this side-to-side swaying.

Chapter 10

Belly-Blasting Workout Routines

· ·

In This Chapter

▶ Identifying the best abdominal exercises

▶ Understanding the two phases of a belly-blasting workout

▶ Planning your pre- and post-workout snacks and meals

· ·

*Y*ou need cardiovascular exercise like walking, running, or swimming to help burn up the fat surrounding your belly. But as this fat burns, you also want to reveal sexy abdominal muscles by including toning exercises. This added muscle tissue also boosts metabolism, helping to keep belly fat away for good!

So in this chapter, I provide workout routines that include both cardiovascular and toning exercises. Your belly-blasting workouts contain two parts: Phase 1 and Phase 2. Phase 1 starts with basic abdominal exercises to help you build strength in your core. This phase also starts out by incorporating regular cardiovascular exercise in the form of walking. Phase 2 picks up the pace by increasing both the speed and duration of cardiovascular exercise to help increase belly fat burn. This phase also introduces you to more challenging abdominal exercises that use a combination of balance and resistance to rapidly tone and tighten abs. Finally, I explain how to fuel your body before and after working out and how to get motivated and stay the course.

Mastering Some Abdominal Exercises

The toning exercises I cover in this section help to strengthen your *core,* or abdominal muscles. These muscles surround your belly and act as an internal girdle. The stronger your abdominal muscles, the easier it is for these muscles to hold your stomach in, giving the appearance of a lean and toned tummy. Building stronger muscles also has a fat-burning benefit. Muscle actually burns more calories than fat. So the more muscle you build, the more calories you burn daily. As a result, you reduce body fat and lose weight.

In this section, I lead you through two separate abdominal workouts. The first workout consists of the exercises you use to get started. You should start with this exercise routine (which includes core strengtheners and cardiovascular exercise) for the first two weeks of the Belly Fat Diet plan. Later in the section, I show you more advanced exercises — the ones I like to call *super belly blasters*.

Don't be discouraged if you can't master the basic exercises after just two weeks. It can take a bit of time to build core strength, so don't start the advanced exercises too early if you aren't yet mastering the basic exercises. The worst thing you can do is try to perform an exercise you aren't ready for. Doing so can make you perform the exercise with poor form, causing an injury.

Your form is *very* important in all exercises, but it's especially vital with core exercises. If you have poor form, you won't be working the right muscles. And if you aren't working the right muscles, you won't be getting the results you want. Make sure to carefully follow the exercise instructions, and watch yourself in a mirror as you perform every exercise. If you notice your form beginning to waiver, take a break. Poor form can be a sign that your muscles are getting tired. Building core strength isn't a race. It's okay if you need to go at a slower pace. Your strength will improve over time. And doing exercises correctly, with good form, is what's going to help you build that strength. Rushing through exercises or letting form suffer just to get in an extra rep won't help you. In fact, it can hurt your progress, so don't do it!

Basic exercises to get you started

Ready to start working your abs? The exercises in the following sections are great, basic moves that can help you begin to melt inches off your waistline and give you that strong, toned core you've been longing for.

Basic Plank

This exercise is the foundation for advanced core exercises and helps to build strength in your core, back, and even chest and shoulders.

1. **Put your body in a plank position with hands and toes on the floor and body outstretched.**

   Your midsection should be straight. No arching or sagging of your back, and don't stick your butt in the air! You should be one straight line from your nose to your toes. You can see what the plank position looks like in Figure 10-1.

2. **Concentrate on keeping your core tight, hold this position for 30 seconds, and then relax.**

   Repeat these steps five times.

Advanced: Challenge yourself to hold this position for a longer period of time. Build to 45 seconds and finally to 60 seconds per hold.

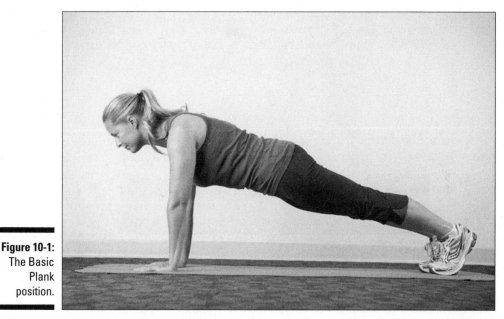

Figure 10-1:
The Basic
Plank
position.

Photo by Matt Bowen

Arm Circles

Core exercises don't always need to be done on the floor. This exercise helps you get up off the floor and works your obliques, upper and lower abs, and your shoulders and arms.

1. **Stand with your legs slightly wider than shoulder width apart. Hold a 5-pound dumbbell (or use a filled water bottle if a dumbbell isn't available) with both hands in front of your body and straight arms.**

   Keep your back straight and your core tight. See Figure 10-2 to get an idea of the position you should be in. If you prefer, you can start with no weight and gradually build up.

2. **While keeping both hands on the weight and your arms straight, slowly make a large circle with your arms to the right, above your head, to the left, and back to the starting position.**

   Keep your core tight the whole time you're making the circle.

3. **Repeat the preceding step 15 times to the right and 15 times to the left for one set. Rest for 30 seconds.**

   Perform three full sets with 30 seconds of rest in between each set.

Advanced: Over time, build up to an 8- or 10-pound dumbbell.

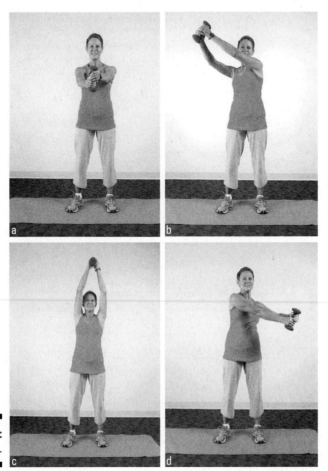

Figure 10-2:
Arm Circles.

Photos by Matt Bowen

Swingin' Abs

By using your own body weight for resistance, this exercise helps you focus on toning the lower abs and obliques.

1. **Stand perpendicular to a chair with your legs slightly spread at shoulder width apart (left side toward the chair), and place your left hand on the chair.**

2. **While keeping your core tight (pull your belly button into your spine), lift your right leg straight in front of you to hip level, as shown in Figure 10-3.**

3. **In a controlled swing, lower your right leg down to the front, and then swing it to the right, bringing it straight out to your right side at hip level. Then swing your leg back in a controlled motion first down to the front and then up to the left at hip level.**

   Remember to always keep your core tight and your back straight as you complete this exercise.

4. **Repeat the steps ten times, and then turn to the right and repeat with the left leg for one set. Rest for 30 seconds, and then repeat.**

   Perform three full sets.

Advanced: Add 1- or 2-pound ankle weights as you complete the exercise.

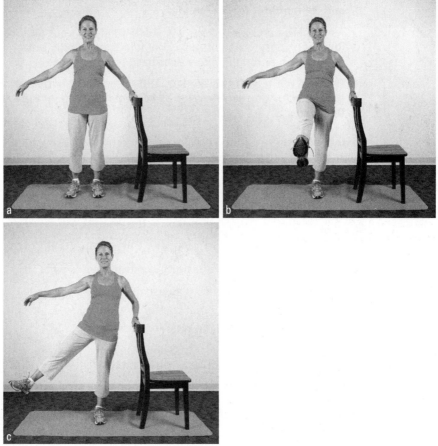

Figure 10-3:
Swingin'
Abs.

Photos by Matt Bowen

Chair Leg Raises

This exercise allows you to focus on your form to target both lower and upper abdominals. Your quadriceps and hip flexors also are challenged. For this exercise, use a sturdy chair with an upright back and no armrests.

1. **Sit in the chair with your back flat against the chair back.**

   Make sure your whole back is pushing against the chair back. No arching! (You can see the correct position in Figure 10-4.)

2. **Place your arms by your sides with your palms facing down, grasping either side of the chair. Stretch out your left leg so it's parallel with the seat of the chair.**

3. **While pushing down on the chair with your hands, raise your left leg up off the chair. Try to raise your thigh at least 2 inches off the chair, and then hold it for 5 seconds.**

   As you raise and lower your leg, you should feel your abdominals engaging. Keep your core tight (envision pulling your belly button toward your spine), and don't allow your back to arch.

4. **Perform ten leg lifts on the left, and then repeat with your right leg ten times for one set. Rest for 30 seconds and repeat for a total of three sets.**

Advanced: If you're up for a challenge, work toward raising both legs together at the same time for an intense belly-burner.

Laying Leg Raises

This exercise helps to tone and tighten your midsection by using your own body for resistance. Form is essential in this exercise, so pay close attention to how you perform it. Slow, controlled movements are what you want here.

1. **Lay on the floor with your body outstretched.**

   Your arms should be at your sides, and your legs and ankles should be together.

2. **Place one hand under the small of your back.**

   Your back should be flat throughout the entire exercise, so this hand placement helps you notice if you begin to arch at any point.

3. **Slowly raise your left leg (keeping your knee straight) until your toes are pointed to the ceiling and your leg is perpendicular with your torso. Then slowly lower your leg back down to the floor, as shown in Figure 10-5.**

The slower you do this exercise, the more difficult it is, so don't rush the move. Count to five on the way up and five on the way down. Perform the exercise ten times with the left leg, and then switch to the right leg and perform ten times for one set.

If you find you can't do this exercise without arching your back, you may need to build a bit more strength first. Try this modified version in the meantime: Bend your knees while laying on the ground. Raise and lower your legs while bent. Check out Figure 10-6 to see the modified version.

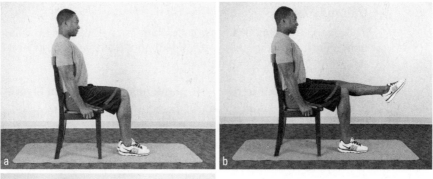

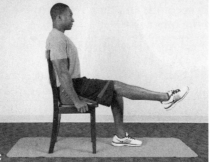

Figure 10-4:
Chair Leg
Raises.

Photos by Matt Bowen

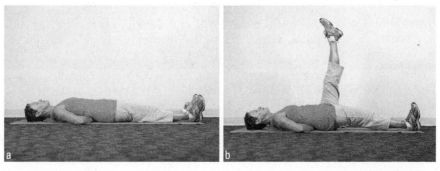

Figure 10-5:
Laying Leg
Raises.

Photos by Matt Bowen

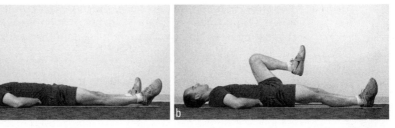

Figure 10-6:
Modified
Laying Leg
Raises.

Photos by Matt Bowen

Oblique Planks

This exercise is similar to the basic plank in that it relies on balance and body control to help tone your midsection. However, in this exercise, you will be focusing on the obliques.

1. **Place yourself in the basic plank position shown in Figure 10-1.**

2. **Raise your right hand up to the ceiling and slightly turn your body so your right hip and side are facing the ceiling, as shown in Figure 10-7.**

   Don't allow your body or left hip to sag. Push your left hip toward the ceiling to keep your body in a straight line.

3. **Hold the position for 20 seconds, and then return to the basic plank position and repeat on the other side.**

   This counts as one set. Perform three full sets.

Advanced: Work to build from holding each side for 20 seconds to 60 seconds as you get stronger.

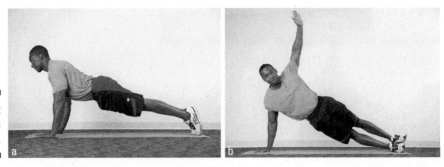

Figure 10-7:
Oblique
Planks.

Photos by Matt Bowen

Crunchy Sits

This fun variation to the traditional floor crunches provides a greater challenge to your core as it incorporates balance and resistance from your body weight.

1. **Sit on the floor with your legs stretched out away from your body with your feet together.**

   Your arms should be straight out at your sides, forming a straight line from your shoulders to your fingers.

2. **Slowly lift your legs off the floor, bending and pulling your knees toward your stomach, as shown in Figure 10-8.**

   As you bring your legs into your body, your arms should bend to wrap around your knees.

3. **Return to the starting position, and repeat 15 times.**

Advanced: As you get stronger, build slowly until you can perform 25 times at once.

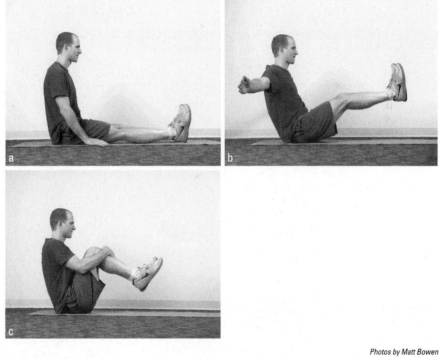

Figure 10-8:
Crunchy
Sits.

Photos by Matt Bowen

Wall Hollow Hold

This exercise uses specific body positioning to activate and challenge your abdominal muscles. Form is vital to performing this exercise correctly, so make sure you closely follow the upcoming steps.

When doing this exercise correctly, your lower back should be pushing flat against the wall with no arch. If you don't feel your abdominal muscles working, you aren't doing it correctly.

1. **Stand with your back flat against a wall. Walk your feet about 1 foot away from the wall, and raise your arms over your head.**

2. **Tilt your pelvis so your hips are tucked under, your abs are engaged, and your back is pushing against the wall, as shown in Figure 10-9.**

   Your glutes should be slightly removed from the wall, and you should feel your abdominals working. And remember: No arching!

3. **Hold this position for 30 seconds, relax, and then repeat twice.**

Advanced: Build from holding this position for 30 seconds to holding it for 60 seconds.

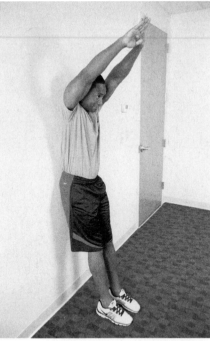

Figure 10-9:
Wall Hollow
Holds.

Photo by Matt Bowen

Grab That Leg

Unlike a traditional floor crunch, where you may not lift your shoulders high enough off the floor to be effective, this exercise challenges you by helping you reach higher and farther, providing a greater abdominal challenge and, therefore, greater results!

1. **Lay on the floor with your body outstretched.**

   Your arms should be at your sides, and your legs and ankles should be together.

2. **Bend your left knee, and then lift your shoulders off the floor while at the same time raising your right leg, as shown in Figure 10-10.**

   Raise your leg and shoulders high enough that you can touch your toes.

3. **Slowly lower your shoulders and legs back to the floor.**

   Repeat the steps with your right leg ten times. Keep your back flat on the floor throughout the exercise, making sure not to arch.

4. **Perform the steps with the other side by bending your right knee and raising your left leg and shoulders.**

   Repeat the steps with the left leg ten times.

If this exercise is difficult initially, reach for your knee at first, and then as you get stronger, reach for your toes.

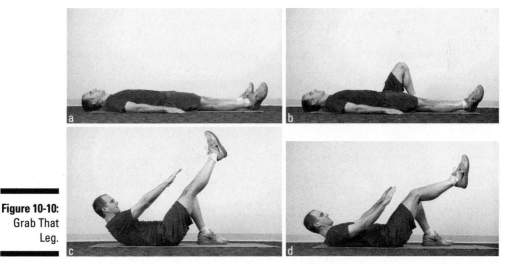

Figure 10-10:
Grab That
Leg.

Photos by Matt Bowen

Super belly blasters

After you have mastered the basic belly-blasting exercises, the super belly blaster exercises in this section provide you with an even greater challenge. You perform toning exercises that incorporate balance, resistance, and dynamic movements to get every muscle in your midsection engaged for even faster results.

These exercises are advanced, so don't move on to this section of exercises unless you have mastered the basic exercises with good form.

Spider Walk

This exercise will have you walking like Spider-Man and gaining abs of steel like Superman! Make sure to keep your core tight throughout the exercise.

1. **Place your body in the plank position with your hands shoulder width apart and feet together.**

   You can see the basic plank position in Figure 10-1, earlier in the chapter.

2. **Lower yourself to a half-finished push-up position. Hold this position, bring your left knee toward your left elbow, and then return your left leg to its starting position (see Figure 10-11).**

3. **Bring your right knee to your right elbow and return it to its starting position.**

4. **Push back up to the plank position, walk each hand a few inches forward, and then repeat.**

   Do ten repetitions so you travel across the floor.

Advanced: To really challenge yourself, do ten repetitions in reverse.

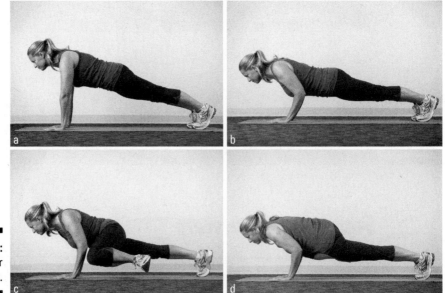

Figure 10-11:
Spider
Walk.

Photos by Matt Bowen

Slidin' Abs

For this exercise, you need to be on a solid surface (wood or linoleum, for example) using a towel. If you only have access to a carpeted area, use carpet sliders or a cardboard square instead of a towel to help you achieve the sliding motion.

1. **Kneel down on the floor, and place a towel (or carpet sliders) a few feet in front of you.**

   The towel should be shoulder length in size. If using sliders, make sure your arms are shoulder width apart.

2. **Lean forward and rest your hands on the towel/carpet sliders so you're in a crawling position.**

3. **Keeping your knees in place, push on the towel/carpet sliders, sliding yours arms and upper body away from your knees, as shown in Figure 10-12.**

   As you perform this step, keep your core muscles tight.

4. **Slide the towel/carpet sliders away from your body as far as you can, and then engage your abdominals and pull back to the starting position.**

   This equals one repetition. Start by performing 15 repetitions. Over time, as you build strength, aim to perform 25 repetitions.

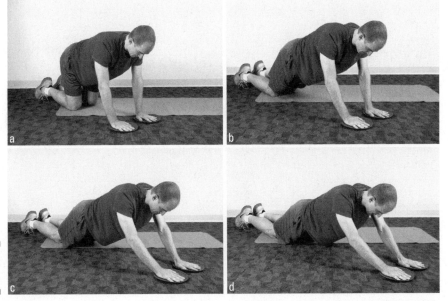

Figure 10-12:
Slidin' Abs.

Photos by Matt Bowen

Biking Away Your Belly

This variation of a traditional crunch helps involve not only your upper and lower abdominals, but also your obliques. And it's almost as simple as riding a bike!

1. **Lay face up on the floor, and place your hands behind your head.**

2. **Slowly lift your shoulder blades off the floor while pulling your knees in toward your chest.**

3. **Rotate your torso to the right and bring your left elbow toward your right knee. As you do this, straighten your left leg.**

   As you perform this step, your legs will be cycling like riding a bike. See Figure 10-13.

4. **Repeat on the other side by rotating your torso to the left, bringing your right elbow to your left knee, and straightening your right leg.**

   This completes one full repetition.

5. **Keep cycling your legs and alternating sides.**

   Complete eight to ten repetitions, and then rest for 30 seconds. Then repeat for a total of three sets.

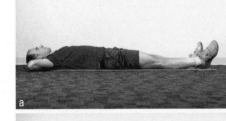
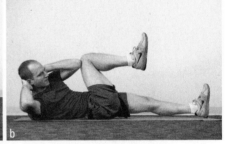
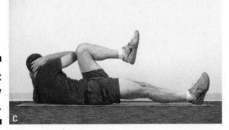

Figure 10-13:
Biking Away
Your Belly.

Photos by Matt Bowen

V-Sit Leg Switches

The V-Sit exercise is challenging on the abdominals. It engages your abs by using your body weight for resistance as well as your core to improve your balance throughout the exercise. But for an added challenge, I add leg switches at the top of the V, which electrifies your abs and tones them in no time!

1. **Sitting on the floor, stretch your arms straight over your head so your elbows are by your ears.**

2. **Create a V with your body by raising your legs.**

   Your ankles should be together and your knees should be straight.

3. **While keeping your core tight and balancing, lower your left leg until your left ankle hovers 1 inch above the floor, and then return it to the V position, as shown in Figure 10-14.**

4. **Repeat with the right leg, lowering it to 1 inch above the floor and then returning to the V position.**

   Lowering and raising each leg once counts as one repetition. Repeat ten repetitions for one set. Perform three sets.

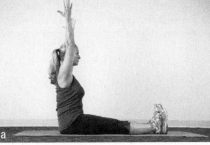
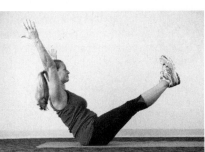
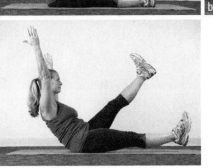

Figure 10-14:
V-Sit Leg
Switches.

Photos by Matt Bowen

Double Leg Raises

This exercise looks easy, but it's a tough one. Form is of the upmost importance in this exercise. Poor form can lead to injury as well as decreased effectiveness of the exercise. Make sure to perform this exercise slowly (the slower the better) and be very careful not to allow your back to arch.

1. **Lay on the floor with your body outstretched.**

   Your arms should be at your sides, and your legs and ankles should be together.

2. **Place one hand under the small of your back.**

   Your back should be flat throughout the entire exercise, so this hand placement helps you notice if you begin to arch at any point.

3. **Keeping your ankles together and your knees straight, slowly raise your legs until your toes are pointed to the ceiling and your legs are perpendicular with your torso (as shown in Figure 10-15). Slowly lower your legs back down to the floor.**

   The slower you do this exercise, the more difficult it is, so don't rush the move. Count to five on the way up and five on the way down. Perform ten repetitions for one set. Complete three sets.

If you find you can't do this exercise without arching your back, you may need to build a bit more strength first. Try this modified version in the meantime: Bend your knees while laying on the ground. Raise and lower your legs while bent.

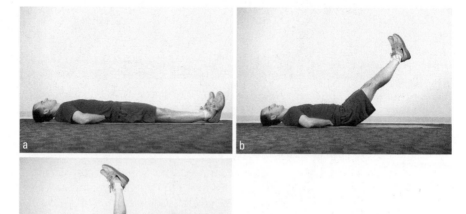

Figure 10-15:
Double Leg
Raises.

Photos by Matt Bowen

Elbow Planks

This exercise is similar to the basic plank. However, performing it from your elbows instead of your hands brings on an extra challenge. And not only does this exercise help to tone your core, but it's a great way to tone your shoulders, back, and chest as well.

1. **Lay face down on the floor, resting on your elbows (see Figure 10-16).**

   Your toes should be on the floor, and your knees should be straight. Just like in the basic plank (refer to Figure 10-1), you want to keep your back flat and your body straight in this exercise. In other words, don't allow your hips and buttocks to raise into the air. To prevent this, tilt your pelvis and contract your abs (just like in the Wall Hollow Hold exercise earlier in the chapter).

2. **Hold this position for 30 seconds and then relax.**

   Repeat the steps two times. Build up to holding each rep for 60 seconds.

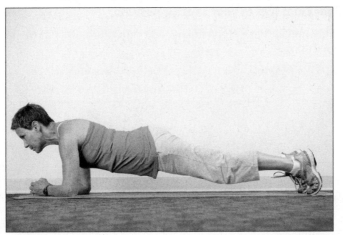

Figure 10-16: Elbow Planks.

Photo by Matt Bowen

Roll-Tuck-V-Surprise

This exercise has it all! It takes movements from multiple exercises to become one of the most challenging (and most effective) exercises in this book. Get ready to feel your belly fat burning away.

1. **Lay on the floor face up.**

   Your arms should be at your sides, your ankles should be together, and your legs should be straight.

2. **Slowly roll your shoulder blades off the floor until your chest is perpendicular to the floor and you're seated upright. Tuck in your legs so your knees are pulled into your chest.**

   Your knees should be bent, and your ankles and toes should be perpendicular to the floor.

3. **Raise your arms so your elbows are next to your knees and your arms are straight. Straighten your knees so you're in a V shape.**

4. **Hold the V shape and join your hands together. Slowly lower your arms to your left hip while lowering your legs toward the right, as shown in Figure 10-17.**

   Don't allow your legs or feet to touch the ground. You should feel your abs engaging.

5. **Return to the V shape and repeat on the other side by lowering your arms to the right hip while lowering your legs to the left. Return to the V shape.**

6. **Slowly roll your spine down against the floor, lowering your shoulder blades and legs to your starting position.**

   Following all these steps equals one repetition. Repeat the steps for ten repetitions.

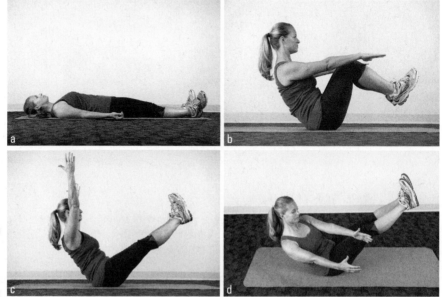

Figure 10-17:
Roll-Tuck-V-
Surprise.

Photos by Matt Bowen

Laying Leg Flutters

This exercise is great for targeting the upper and lower abs. Pay close attention to form here, because proper form makes this exercise effective. Poor form limits the challenge to your abs, and, therefore, limits your results.

1. **Lay on the floor face up.**

   Your arms should be at your sides, and your ankles should be together.

2. **Slowly lift your shoulder blades and ankles off the floor about 1 to 2 inches. Tilt your pelvis so your back is pushing against the floor.**

   You shouldn't be arching, and your abs should be engaged.

3. **Quickly flutter your ankles back and forth for 30 seconds (as shown in Figure 10-18), and then relax.**

   Remember to breathe throughout the exercise. Repeat three times.

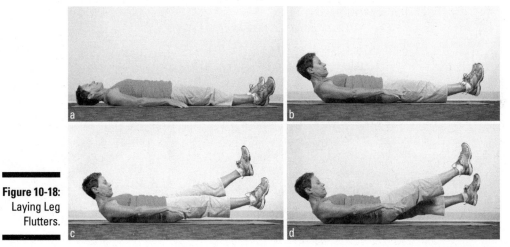

Figure 10-18: Laying Leg Flutters.

Photos by Matt Bowen

Spinning Planks

This exercise is a full body workout. It challenges your body by engaging your core, shoulders, triceps, chest, and glutes. Carefully watch your form throughout the exercise; don't allow your back to arch or your belly to sag.

1. **Place yourself in the basic plank position.**

   You can see what this position looks like in Figure 10-1, earlier in the chapter.

2. **Raise your right hand up to the ceiling and slightly turn your body so your right hip and side are facing the ceiling. Hold for 5 seconds.**

3. **Continue to rotate by dropping your right arm back to the floor so your stomach/front side is facing the ceiling and you're supporting yourself in a reverse plank (see Figure 10-19). Hold for 5 seconds.**

   Keep your core very tight. Push your hips toward the ceiling, and don't allow them to drop.

4. **While supporting yourself on your right arm and leg, lift your left leg to the ceiling and rotate so your left side is now facing the ceiling. Continue to rotate toward your left so you're back to the basic plank position.**

   One full rotation back to starting position is one repetition. Repeat for ten repetitions.

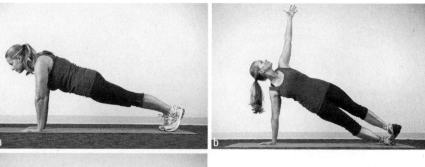

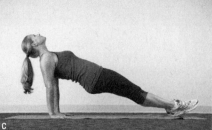

Figure 10-19:
Spinning
Planks.

Photos by Matt Bowen

Belly-Blasting Workouts Phase 1: The First Two Weeks

The Phase 1 workout starts you on your way to a flat stomach and a strong, toned core. This phase helps you slowly increase your cardiovascular and abdominal strength exercises over time.

Keep the following guidelines in mind:

- ✔ **With toning exercises, form is key.** If you can't perform the exercise with good form, you may not be ready for it. Instead, perform the modified versions or focus on the exercises you can perform with correct form. As you build strength, you'll build the ability to complete the more advanced exercises.

- ✔ **With cardiovascular exercise, your starting level of endurance may vary.** If you haven't exercised in a while or have never exercised before, you may need to reduce the walking times a bit until you can comfortably increase them. However, by the end of Week 2, you should be ready to include some sprint walking intervals in your daily walk. A *sprint walk* means simply walking as quickly as you can.

The point is that if at any time the listed exercise is too challenging or the cardio duration is too long, scale back until you're ready.

It's extremely important to consult your physician before starting or changing any exercise routine. If you have any preexisting medical conditions, such as high blood pressure or heart disease, or any joint problems, make sure your physician approves your exercise routine. And follow your doctor's orders on exercise modifications.

Tables 10-1 and 10-2 show the cardio and abdominal workouts you should aim for during the first two weeks of your new exercise regimen. You can get details about the belly-blasting exercises in the earlier section "Mastering Some Abdominal Exercises." If you prefer a cardiovascular exercise other than walking (such as jogging, swimming, or biking), you may substitute this exercise for the walking listed in the schedules.

Table 10-1	Week 1 Workout Schedule	
Day	*Walking Schedule*	*Belly-Blasting Exercises*
Day 1	Walk duration: 10 minutes Pace: Brisk	Basic Plank: Hold plank for 30 seconds. Repeat 2 times. Swingin' Abs: Perform 2 sets. Arm Circles: Perform 2 sets.
Day 2	Walk duration: 15 minutes Pace: Brisk	None
Day 3	Walk duration: 10 minutes Pace: Brisk	Wall Hollow Holds: Hold for 30 seconds. Repeat 2 times. Laying Leg Raises: Perform 3 sets. Oblique Planks: Hold for 20 seconds on each side. Repeat 1 time. Grab That Leg: Perform 10 leg reaches on each side. Repeat 1 time.
Day 4	Walk duration: 18 minutes Pace: Brisk	None
Day 5	Walk duration: 15 minutes Pace: Brisk	Chair Leg Raises: Perform 2 sets. Crunchy Sits: Perform 10 crunches, rest for 30 seconds, and then perform 10 more. Arm Circles: Perform 3 sets. Basic Plank: Hold plank for 30 seconds. Repeat 3 times.
Day 6	Walk duration: 20 minutes Pace: Brisk	None
Day 7	None	Rest or light stretching

Table 10-2	Week 2 Workout Schedule	
Day	*Walking Schedule*	*Belly-Blasting Exercises*
Day 1	Walk duration: 20 minutes Pace: Brisk	Swingin' Abs: Perform 3 sets. Wall Hollow Holds: Hold for 30 seconds. Repeat 3 times. Oblique Planks: Hold for 30 seconds on each side. Repeat 1 time. Laying Leg Raises: Perform 10 leg lifts on the left leg and 10 on the right. Repeat 2 times.
Day 2	Walk duration: 25 minutes Pace: Brisk	None
Day 3	Walk duration: 22 minutes Pace: Brisk	Chair Leg Raises: Perform 2 sets. Basic Plank: Hold plank for 45 seconds. Repeat 2 times. Arm Circles: Perform 3 sets. Grab That Leg: Perform 10 leg reaches on each side. Repeat 2 times.
Day 4	Walk duration: 30 minutes Pace: Brisk	None
Day 5	Walk duration: 25 minutes Pace: Brisk	Oblique Planks: Hold for 45 seconds on each side. Repeat 1 time. Crunchy Sits: Perform 15 crunches, rest for 30 seconds, and then perform 15 more. Laying Leg Raises: Perform 10 leg lifts on the left leg and 10 on the right. Repeat 3 times. Swingin' Abs: Perform 3 sets.
Day 6	Walk duration: 30 minutes Pace: Brisk Every 10 minutes, add a 15-second sprint walk, and then return to a normal brisk pace.	None
Day 7	None	Rest or light stretching

Belly-Blasting Workouts Phase 2: Increasing Intensity to Increase Results

Phase 2 of your belly-blasting routine picks up the pace of your cardiovascular exercise by increasing the length and speed of your walking. For the first two weeks of Phase 2, the incline remains at zero. However, as you get stronger, you can slowly increase your incline as you walk. The abdominal exercises in Phase 2 are more advanced as well, helping to further challenge your core.

Just like in Phase 1 (see the earlier section "Belly-Blasting Workouts Phase 1: The First Two Weeks"), you should only perform these exercises if you can do so with good form. When your form starts to decline, you need to stop. If you need to, go back to the Phase 1 exercises until you build enough core strength to complete the Phase 2 exercises with perfect form. Good form is how you get results!

As you continue with your Belly Fat Diet plan and workout routine, you can continue to challenge yourself in different ways to see increased strength and results. In other words, you can go beyond Phase 2 of the workouts. Here are some suggestions for adding to your workouts:

✔ Increase the speed and duration of your walks to burn extra fat and calories.

✔ Add inclines like hills or stairs to your walks for added intensity.

✔ Continue to tone your core and increase strength by increasing the number of repetitions and sets of the abdominal exercises you do. For some exercises, such as Swingin' Abs and Leg Flutters, you may add very light ankle weights (1 to 2 pounds per ankle) to further build strength and resistance. However, if you do add additional weight, make sure not to sacrifice form!

✔ If you'd like, you can substitute walking with another form of cardiovascular exercise, such as jogging, biking, swimming, or even cardio-based dancing or kickboxing.

Tables 10-3 and 10-4 show the cardio and abdominal workouts you can do after you finish Phase 1. You can get details about the belly-blasting exercises in the earlier section "Mastering Some Abdominal Exercises."

Table 10-3	Week 3 Workout Schedule	
Day	*Walking Schedule*	*Belly-Blasting Exercises*
Day 1	Walk duration: 30 minutes Pace: Brisk	Elbow Planks: Hold for 30 seconds. Repeat 1 time.
	Every 10 minutes, add a 15-second sprint walk, and then return to a normal brisk pace.	Laying Leg Flutters: Flutter for 30 seconds. Rest for 30 seconds. Repeat 1 time.
		Oblique Planks: Hold for 45 seconds on each side. Repeat 2 times.
		Grab That Leg: Perform 15 leg reaches on each side. Repeat 2 times.
Day 2	Walk duration: 30 minutes Pace: Brisk	None
	Every 10 minutes, add a 30-second sprint walk, and then return to a normal brisk pace.	
Day 3	Walk duration: 30 minutes Pace: Brisk	Spider Walks: Perform 10 walks forward.
	Every 10 minutes, add a 15-second sprint walk, and then return to a normal brisk pace.	Swingin' Abs: Perform 3 sets.
		Sliding Abs: Perform 15 repetitions.
		Wall Hollow Hold: Hold for 45 seconds. Repeat 3 times.
Day 4	Walk duration: 35 minutes Pace: Brisk	None
	Every 7 minutes, add a 30-second sprint walk, and then return to a normal brisk pace.	
Day 5	Walk duration: 30 minutes Pace: Brisk	Biking Away Your Belly: Perform 2 sets.
	Every 10 minutes, add a 30-second sprint walk, and then return to a normal brisk pace.	Arm Circles: Perform 4 sets.
		V-Sit Leg Switches: Perform 1 set.
		Chair Leg Raises: Perform 3 sets.

(continued)

Table 10-3 *(continued)*

Day	Walking Schedule	Belly-Blasting Exercises
Day 6	Walk duration: 30 minutes Pace: Brisk Every 5 minutes, add a 30-second sprint walk, and then return to a normal brisk pace.	None
Day 7	None	Rest or light stretching

Table 10-4 **Week 4 Workout Schedule**

Day	Walking Schedule	Belly-Blasting Exercises
Day 1	Walk duration: 30 minutes Pace: Brisk Every 5 minutes, add a 30-second sprint walk, and then return to a normal brisk pace.	Spider Walks: Perform 10 walks forward and 10 walks back. Biking Away Your Belly: Perform 3 sets. Double Leg Raises: Perform 2 sets. Elbow Plank: Hold for 30 seconds. Repeat 2 times.
Day 2	Walk duration: 35 minutes Pace: Brisk Every 5 minutes, add a 60-second sprint walk, and then return to a normal brisk pace.	None
Day 3	Walk duration: 30 minutes Pace: Brisk Every 5 minutes, add a 45-second sprint walk, and then return to a normal brisk pace.	Slidin' Abs: Perform 20 repetitions. Repeat 1 time. V-Sit Leg Switches: Perform 2 sets. Spinning Planks: Perform 5 repetitions. Laying Leg Flutters: Flutter for 45 seconds. Rest for 30 seconds. Repeat 2 times.

Day	Walking Schedule	Belly-Blasting Exercises
Day 4	Walk duration: 35 minutes Pace: Brisk Every 5 minutes, add a 60-second sprint walk, and then return to a normal brisk pace.	None
Day 5	Walk duration: 30 minutes Pace: Brisk Every 5 minutes, add a 45-second sprint walk, and then return to a normal brisk pace.	Roll-Tuck-V-Surprise: Perform 2 sets. Spider Walks: Perform 10 walks forward and then 10 walks back. Repeat 1 time. Double Leg Raises: Perform 3 sets. Elbow Planks: Hold for 45 seconds. Repeat 2 times.
Day 6	Walk duration: 40 minutes Pace: Brisk Every 5 minutes, add a 60-second sprint walk, and then return to a normal brisk pace.	None
Day 7	None	Rest or light stretching

Fueling Your Body for Workouts

Think of your body as a car. If you don't put gas in a car, it can't go anywhere. Your body is the same way. If you don't fuel it, you'll have trouble finding the energy to get moving. As I discuss earlier in the chapter, exercise is important for shrinking fat around your midsection as well as toning and tightening your muscles to give you the flat, sexy abs you desire. In order to have the energy and strength to perform the exercise routines I lay out for you earlier in the chapter, you have to understand how to properly fuel your body before workouts and how to eat and rehydrate after for muscle recovery.

In the following sections, I show you which nutrients impact your workout, what to eat and when to eat it for the best results from your exercise routine, and how to recover properly so your body has the energy reserves it needs to get up and get moving the next day.

Pre-workout snacking basics

In the workout routines I outline for you earlier, you perform both cardiovascular and abdominal exercises. Cardio exercise, which includes your walking routine, relies mainly on carbohydrate energy. For this reason, you need to take in an adequate amount of healthy carbohydrates throughout the day, but particularly before your workout. If you take in too few, you'll have less energy readily available for your body for exercise, which can make you feel sluggish during and after your workout. You may also notice that your endurance begins to decline.

On days when you'll be doing cardio exercise, make sure you consume healthy sources of carbohydrates (which include vegetables, fruit, milk, yogurt, and whole-grain starches) throughout the day and also at specific times to help your body perform at its peak. For instance, you want to consume an adequate number of carbohydrates before your workout so you have energy while you exercise, and then you also want to consume some within a short period of time after your workout to replenish the energy stores you used up.

Eating carbs at these specific times is important because if you fail to replenish your energy stores, your energy level will slowly decrease throughout the week, making it more challenging to stick with your exercise routine.

An abdominal or strength-training workout also requires a large amount of energy, so consuming a good source of carbohydrates beforehand is important as well. Because the duration of your abdominal workout may be less than your cardiovascular workout, you may not need as many grams of carbohydrates, but you should consume at least one serving.

To help you plan your pre-workout snack, follow these rules:

- ✔ **For cardio or abdominal workouts lasting at least 15 minutes but less than 40 minutes,** consume one carbohydrate serving 60 minutes before your workout.

- ✔ **For aerobic or strength-training workouts lasting 40 to 60 minutes,** consume two carbohydrate servings 60 minutes before your workout.

- ✔ **For high-intensity workouts or workouts lasting longer than 60 minutes,** consume up to three carbohydrate servings 60 minutes before your exercise routine.

Some one- and two-serving carbohydrate snack suggestions include 1 cup of low-fat yogurt, 1 cup of berries, a slice of 100 percent whole-grain toast with half a banana, or a smoothie made with 1 cup fat-free or lowfat milk and 1 cup berries. Refer to Chapter 6 for a detailed listing of carbohydrate sources and their serving sizes.

Each of the preceding snack options contains a healthy source of carbohydrates. Just as it's important to choose whole-grain carbohydrates to help reduce belly fat, it's equally important to choose these before and after exercise. Whole grains give consistent, steady energy during exercise, whereas refined carbohydrate sources give a spike in energy followed by an energy crash, which can significantly decrease your endurance.

Prior to a workout, I don't recommend a large amount of protein or fat. These foods provide your body with energy, but they take much longer to digest. Eating a large amount of protein or fat before a workout can cause you to feel weighed down during your exercise routine. It also can lead to those pesky side cramps, which can make it difficult to continue with your exercise session. These nutrients are better reserved for after a workout session.

Post-workout snacking basics

After completing a workout, your body needs two things:

- ✔ **Protein:** After a workout, especially an abdominal or strength-training workout, your body needs adequate protein to build and repair muscle. Eating protein within 30 to 60 minutes after a workout has been shown to promote muscle growth and strength because that's the time when the body is most able to use protein. I recommend consuming 1 to 2 ounces of protein within 30 to 60 minutes after cardio or light abdominal workouts and 3 ounces after more intensive workouts.

- ✔ **Carbohydrates:** Your body's energy stores, which are made up of glucose, are depleted during exercise. The longer and more intense your workout, the more your glucose stores are depleted. You need to replenish these stores after a workout so you have the energy and endurance you need to exercise again tomorrow. Carbohydrates, when digested, are converted into glucose and stored in your body for energy. So after completing a workout, you need to consume an adequate source of healthy carbohydrates to replenish your glucose stores and refuel for your next workout.

The more intense your workout, the more carbohydrates you need to replace. Here are the general carbohydrate guidelines:

- ✔ **For a light cardiovascular workout that's 30 minutes in duration or less, or a light abdominal or strength-training workout that's 60 minutes or less,** aim to consume one serving of carbohydrates within 30 to 60 minutes after completing your workout.

- ✔ **For high-intensity cardio or abdominal workouts, or cardio workouts lasting 30 to 60 minutes,** consume two carbohydrate servings.

- ✔ **For intense cardio exercise lasting longer than 60 minutes,** consume three carbohydrate servings.

Planning meals and snacks around your workouts

Protein and fat can take up to three hours to be digested, whereas carbohydrates can be digested within one hour. To prevent cramping and decreased performance, only carbohydrate sources should be consumed within an hour prior to cardiovascular exercise or intensive abdominal or strength training. Protein and fat can be consumed three to four hours prior to a workout and anytime following an event. To help improve your endurance, as well as get an added metabolism boost, consume five to six small, frequent meals throughout the day to help maintain energy levels as well as aid in digestion.

A carbohydrate serving includes fruit, starches, milk, yogurt, and starchy vegetables. The following are some healthy post-workout snack ideas:

- 1 ounce low-fat string cheese and a medium apple
- Half a turkey breast sandwich on 100 percent whole-grain bread
- 1 cup low-fat plain Greek yogurt
- Smoothie (refer to Chapter 12 for the Belly-Blasting Berry Smoothie recipe)
- ½ cup lowfat cottage cheese and ½ cup pineapple

Refer to Chapter 6 for a detailed listing on other carbohydrate sources and their serving sizes.

Hydration basics

Hydration is a key ingredient to a successful workout. Dehydration can lead to many nasty side effects, including decreased energy levels, electrolyte imbalances, and, in extreme circumstances, heat exhaustion and heat stroke. Adequate hydration is also essential to your Belly Fat Diet plan, because the more fluid you drink, the less you retain, helping to promote a slim, toned belly.

The amount of fluid you need per day depends on many factors:

- Length of your workout
- Intensity of your workout
- Temperature in which you're working out
- Hydration status before starting your workout

The more intense your workout, the longer your workout, and the hotter it is outside when you're exercising, the more fluid you need. In general, without exercise, you need approximately 8 cups (64 ounces) of fluid per day. This fluid should come from caffeine-free, calorie-free beverages. (Caffeine is a diuretic, so if all your fluid comes from caffeinated sources, it may not be as hydrating as you think!) When you add in exercise, your fluid needs go up. Use the following guidelines to make sure you drink enough when you work out:

- ✔ During cardiovascular exercise, drink an additional 1 cup (8 ounces) of fluid for every 20 minutes of exercise. Increase this amount by ½ cup (4 ounces) if you're working out on a very warm day.

- ✔ During abdominal or strength-training exercise, drink an additional 1 cup of fluid for every 30 minutes of exercise. Increase this amount by ½ cup if you're working out on a very warm day.

- ✔ Within 30 minutes of completing your workouts, make sure to drink an additional 1 cup of fluid.

Water is the best choice for hydration. Sports drinks aren't needed unless you're performing a long endurance exercise (think a half or full marathon) or working out in extreme heat. Juice and sugary drinks, such as soda, shouldn't be consumed during exercise because the excess sugar in these beverages can lead to cramping. (And they should be avoided on a regular basis anyway because they promote increased belly fat storage!)

Want an easy way to judge whether you're hydrated? Look at your urine! Urine should be clear to pale yellow. If it's darker, you need to drink more!

Making Exercise a Priority

Fitting yet another activity into what I'm sure is a jampacked schedule is really difficult. But the truth is, if you make exercise a priority, you can always find the time. And you don't need to find hours in your day to schedule it in. Even 10 to 15 minutes to start can make a huge difference in not only your belly-fighting efforts, but also your health.

I would love to snap my fingers and give you results in a flash, but that isn't realistic. However, throughout the Belly Fat Diet plan, I show you many ways to save time and make the plan as easy as possible. And it's the same with exercise. I make it as easy as possible with just a few simple exercises that target your abs in just minutes per day (see the earlier sections for details). But you need to do these exercises and stick with your routine to achieve your desired results.

Fitting exercise into your day requires strategy. To help with this process, ask yourself the following questions:

- ✔ **What time of day would I like to work out?** Am I a morning person who enjoys working out as soon as I wake up, or would I enjoy exercising later in the day?

- ✔ **When do I have a little down time during the day?** Do I have a few minutes at lunch time or maybe when I first get home from work?

- ✔ **Where will I be exercising?** Will I be walking outside? If so, what is my bad weather backup plan? Will I be working out at a gym? If so, what are the gym's hours of operation? Will I be working out at home? If so, do I have to share my exercise space with anyone else?

- ✔ **What do I need to have with me to be ready to work out?** For instance, if you're walking during lunch at work, you'll want to make sure to pack your walking shoes and bring them to work each day.

When you've answered all these questions, sit down and write out a workout schedule for yourself. Write down the days you'll exercise, the time of day you'll exercise, where you'll exercise, and what, if anything, you need to have with you to exercise. This is your action plan. Put this summary somewhere you can see it and refer to it every day. This action plan can help keep you on track so that you can make sure to fit in your belly-blasting workout routine on a regular basis, thus, getting you the results you want quickly and keeping them permanently!

Part III
Cooking Up Some Healthy and Tasty Recipes

The 5th Wave

By Rich Tennant

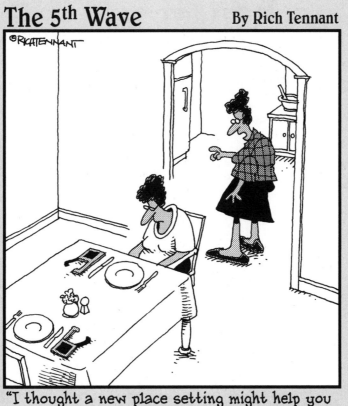

"I thought a new place setting might help you lose some belly fat. It's a knife, a fork, and a BMI caliper."

In this part . . .

Think losing weight and belly fat means giving up the foods you love or eating foods that are bland and boring? Think again! In this part, I provide you with delicious and easy-to-make recipes — fantastic, belly-friendly alternatives to old favorites. I also show you just how to stock and prepare your pantry and kitchen so you'll have belly-burning foods and seasonings on hand at all times.

Chapter 11

Planning and Stocking a Flat-Belly-Friendly Kitchen

*H*ave you ever been at the grocery store and started picking up products to look at the labels and been left wondering what it all means? Have you spent hours wandering aimlessly through the store aisles wondering which foods are actually healthy and promote weight loss only to get so frustrated you give up and go home empty-handed? Well if so, you're not alone. Reading a food label can be like learning a new language. But don't despair! With these tips and hints, you'll be an expert at reading food labels in no time! And then you'll be able to fill your home with those foods that help you achieve a flatter belly.

In this chapter, I review the Nutrition Facts panel on food packaging and identify what components make a food a fat fighter. I also break through the mystery of the ingredient list and reveal which ingredients help to burn belly fat and which ingredients promote fat storage so you can work to avoid them. I also take a look inside your home pantry and refrigerator and identify foods that may be sabotaging your flat belly efforts. I show you simple solutions to get rid of these items and replace them with healthy, delicious alternatives your whole family will enjoy.

If you need help generating healthy grocery shopping lists, check out dummies.com/go/bellyfat. There you'll find articles with great ideas for stocking both your fridge and pantry.

Decoding the Food Label and Ingredient List

The mysterious food labels on packages of processed foods make many dieters feel anxious, confused, and defeated before they ever leave the grocery store. But not you. No, those feelings are all going to change today! Here I show you the ins and outs of the Nutrition Facts panel, including what to look at, what to ignore, and, most importantly, what to buy to help you achieve your flat belly goals. I start from the top and break the food label down section by section.

Reading the Nutrition Facts panel

The food label is the window that looks into the food you're about to consume. It discloses everything from the suggested serving size to the good and bad ingredients contained in the food. After you understand exactly how to read a food label and what to look for, you'll be on your way to easily identifying whether a food is a belly buster or a belly flattener!

You can see an example of a typical Nutrition Facts panel in Figure 11-1.

Figure 11-1:
Nutrition
Facts panel
for a com-
mon snack
food.

Nutrition Facts
Serving Size 2 crackers (14g)
Servings Per Container About 21

Amount Per Serving	
Calories 60	Calories from Fat 15

	% Daily value*
Total Fat 1.5g	2%
Saturated Fat 0g	0%
Trans Fat 0g	
Cholesterol 0mg	0%
Sodium 70mg	3%
Total Carbohydrate 10g	3%
Dietary Fiber Less than 1g	3%
Sugars 0g	
Protein 2g	

Vitamin A 0%	•	Vitamin C 0%
Calcium 0%	•	Iron 2%

*Percent Daily Values are based on a 2,000 calorie diet. Your daily values may be higher or lower depending on your calorie needs:

	Calories:	2,000	2,500
Total Fat	Less than	65g	90g
Sat Fat	Less than	20g	25g
Cholesterol	Less than	300mg	300mg
Sodium	Less than	2400mg	2400mg
Total Carbohydrate		300g	375g
Dietary Fiber		25g	30g

TECHNICAL STUFF

Nutrition claims on packaging

Nutrition claims like "lowfat" and "high fiber" can be seen on all sorts of food product packaging throughout the grocery store. Today, government standards require a food to meet certain requirements before the distributors can boast claims on their packaging labels. Here are common claims seen on product packaging and what they really mean:

✔ **Calorie-free:** Fewer than 5 calories (per serving size)

✔ **Low calorie:** 40 calories or fewer (per serving size)

✔ **Lite or light (in calories):** ⅓ fewer calories than the original product

✔ **High fiber:** 5 grams of fiber or more per serving

✔ **Fat-free:** Less than ½ gram of fat per serving

✔ **Lowfat:** 3 grams of fat or less per serving

✔ **Lite or light (in fat):** 50 percent less fat than the original

✔ **Sodium-free:** Less than 5 milligrams of sodium per serving

✔ **Very low sodium:** 35 milligrams or less of sodium per serving

✔ **Lite or light (in sodium):** 50 percent less sodium than the original product

✔ **Low sodium:** 140 milligrams or less of sodium per serving

✔ **Low cholesterol:** 20 milligrams or less of cholesterol and 2 grams or less of saturated fat

Here's a breakdown of the most important parts of a Nutrition Facts panel:

✔ **Serving size:** Before you can determine whether a food will positively or negatively affect belly fat, you first need to find out how much of the particular food you can eat. This amount is referred to as the *serving size.* Looking at the serving size is important because the nutritional information (calories, fat, and sodium, for example) is based on that serving size. So if the serving size on the label is listed as ½ cup and you consume 1 cup of the food, you must double the calories and nutrients to determine how much you're truly taking in.

✔ **Calories:** In order to lose weight, including belly fat, you have to take in fewer calories than you burn each day. The weight loss meal plans in this book are based on a calorie range of 1,200–1,500 calories per day for women and 1,600–1,800 calories per day for men. When choosing a food, follow these guidelines to prevent yourself from taking in too many calories per day: Keep snacks around 50–200 calories each and meals to 200–400 calories each.

✔ **Saturated and trans fats:** Both good fats and bad fats exist in diets today. Bad fats, which include saturated fats and trans fats, can increase inflammation in your body, promoting unwanted fat storage in the abdomen. The good fats include monounsaturated fats, some polyunsaturated fats, and omega-3 fatty acids. Monounsaturated fats and omega-3 fatty acids have been shown to help blast belly fat. The Nutrition Facts panel only has to include saturated and trans fat, but occasionally it may also list monounsaturated fats and polyunsaturated fats.

REMEMBER

Regardless of the total fat grams listed, focus on the saturated and trans fats. You want to select a food with absolutely no trans fats and as few grams of saturated fat as possible. You want to keep your total intake of saturated fat per day to 15 grams or less.

✔ **Sodium:** Because sodium can trigger fluid retention, causing the stomach to look distended and bloated, you want to limit sodium intake for a flatter, firmer belly. The goal here is to keep your daily sodium intake to 2,000 milligrams or less per day. An easy trick for determining whether a food is high in sodium is to look at the "% Daily Value" column on the right-hand side of the food label. Aim to keep snack foods to 0–15 percent of your daily recommended sodium amount and meals to 25 percent or less to prevent exceeding your daily sodium allotment.

✔ **Fiber:** Fiber is a powerful nutrient and is a key component to reducing belly fat for two main reasons: It helps to decrease appetite and slows the insulin response. Try to consume at least 30 to 35 grams of total fiber per day with at least 8 grams coming from soluble fiber. When looking at the Nutrition Facts panel, aim to choose foods with at least 3 grams of fiber or more per serving (for foods where fiber should naturally occur, such as in breads, pastas, and cereals).

TIP

When reviewing food labels for fiber, keep in mind that fiber occurs naturally in vegetables, fruit, and grains like cereals, breads, and pastas. Fiber occurs naturally in limited amounts or not at all in proteins, fats, and dairy products.

✔ **Sugar:** Foods high in sugar and low in fiber may cause a spike in insulin levels, resulting in increased fat storage in the abdomen as well as increased hunger and cravings. Aim to select foods with as little added sugar as possible. Use the rule of thumb of eating foods with only 10 grams of sugar or less per serving. To put this in perspective, just one chocolate chip cookie contains 10 grams of sugar!

Avoiding unhealthy foods in the ingredient list

Did you know that the Nutrition Facts panel doesn't tell the whole story about whether a food is a healthy choice? You may have never realized this, but the Nutrition Facts panel can at times be misleading or even deceptive! It takes a bit more detective work to identify whether a food is truly a belly fat blaster or a belly buster in disguise. The good news is you can use the ingredient list on the food label to identify the truly healthy foods from the foods that are just marketed that way.

Here are the most common belly-busting ingredients that may be lurking in your food, along with some ways to identify and avoid them:

✔ **Trans fats:** If a food has less than half a gram of trans fat, it can be listed as having zero grams on the Nutrition Facts panel. If you eat multiple servings of a food with less than half a gram of trans fat, you may actually be eating multiple grams without ever realizing it. Research has shown that having as little as 2 grams of trans fats per day can increase your risk of heart disease as well as increase the amount of belly fat you have. So you can see how dangerous this ingredient can be!

If you see the words "partially hydrogenated oil" in the ingredient list for a food, you know it contains a source of trans fats. Because even small amounts of trans fats can be damaging to both your health and your waistline, try to avoid all foods with partially hydrogenated oils.

✔ **Refined carbohydrates:** Foods with refined carbs can trigger a large insulin response (and therefore increased belly fat storage) even when they aren't high in sugar. Refined carbohydrates, which are in grain products like breads, cereals, and pastas, have a majority of the outer grain removed (the part of the grain highest in fiber and nutrients). Because the outer grain is removed, these carbs are digested rapidly by the body and quickly increase blood sugar levels.

When choosing a grain product, not only do you want to look at the grams of fiber and sugar on the Nutrition Facts panel, but you also want to look at the ingredient list. A whole grain (for example, whole-wheat flour, brown rice flour, oat flour, or rye flour) should be listed as the first ingredient. If the first ingredient is enriched flour or white flour, the majority of the food is a refined grain, which can damage your belly-blasting efforts.

✔ **Added sugars:** The Nutrition Facts panel doesn't differentiate between naturally occurring sugars, such as those in fruit, and added sugars, such as high-fructose corn syrup. Some foods with large amounts of added sugars can trigger a larger insulin response than foods that contain only naturally occurring sugars.

Be on the lookout for ingredients that indicate that sugar has been added to your food. These ingredients include high-fructose corn syrup, honey, dehydrated cane juice, malt syrup, maltodextrin, molasses, and any ingredient that contains "-ose" on the end.

Evaluating Your Kitchen and Chucking the Junk

After you're familiar with the basics of evaluating a food using the label and ingredient list (refer to the earlier section "Decoding the Food Label and Ingredient List"), you're ready to get down to business. Start by going through your kitchen. Check out the refrigerator, the pantry, and anywhere else you store food. Determine which foods are the best bet for your belly and which foods are belly busters. After you identify all the belly-busting choices currently in your house, get rid of them!

Some foods can be donated or given away to family and friends because they may be healthy and appropriate for other people even though they aren't ideal for someone on a Belly Fat Diet plan. However, other foods aren't good for anybody and should be pitched. In the following sections, I help you dive in and determine which foods should stay in your kitchen and which should go to a new home or in the trash.

Determining which foods to donate or give away

As I'm sure you know from past experience, having a less-than-healthy food in the house is a sure bet in sabotaging your weight-loss efforts. You can say to yourself, "I'll put it in the back of the cabinet and forget about it," but you still know it's there. And in times of stress, extreme hunger, or even boredom, you may find yourself reaching for these belly busters that can blow all your efforts. So once and for all, you need to get rid of those foods!

When ridding your kitchen and pantry of these unhealthy foods, you can pitch the things that are half eaten, but if you come across fresh things that haven't been opened, consider donating or giving away these items to family and friends. These foods that aren't helping your weight loss and belly-flattening efforts may still be healthy for someone else. It would be wasteful to just toss these foods, especially when someone around you may benefit from them. These foods may be perfect for a growing child, for instance, and would make a wonderful donation to families in need.

Here are some of the less-than-friendly-to-your-belly foods to consider donating to a food pantry, shelter, or soup kitchen (or to family and friends who may be able to use them):

✔ **Canned vegetables:** These vegetables are still rich in many essential vitamins and minerals, but the high sodium content may be a belly-buster. If you must purchase canned vegetables for their convenience, pick up the ones that have no salt added (but don't be heavy handed with the salt shaker at the table!).

✔ **White rice/flavored rice/white pasta:** These products are a rich source of carbohydrates (energy) and are usually fortified with nutrients; however, because they're made with refined grains, they trigger an increased insulin response and should be avoided when you're on a Belly Fat Diet plan. Pre-flavored rice products are also high in sodium, which adds to the bloat.

✔ **Instant oatmeal:** Slow-cooked oatmeal, such as steel-cut oats or old-fashioned rolled oats, is higher in fiber, especially the cholesterol-lowering soluble fiber, than the fast cooking, instant varieties. So send the instant stuff packing.

Don't worry if you don't have time to prepare slow-cooked oatmeal in the morning. Here's an easy trick: Soak the steel-cut or rolled oats in water the night before and then pop them in the microwave in the morning. They'll cook just as quickly as the instant and keep you full much longer.

✔ **Fruit juice:** A cup of 100 percent fruit juice contains just as many vitamins and minerals as whole fruit, but it lacks fiber. The simple sugars in juice may also trigger an increased insulin response. And if you have juice cocktails that aren't 100 percent fruit juice, you definitely need to remove them from your fridge. Because these contain added sugars, instead of just naturally occurring sugar, they're lower in nutrients and can cause a greater insulin response.

✔ **Carbonated beverages:** Carbonated drinks, including seltzer, club soda, and diet soda, contain no calories, but the increased gas production can be bloating, causing your belly to look and feel larger.

✔ **Low-fiber cereals:** In order to achieve the flat belly of your dreams, you want to avoid grains that are highly processed or low in fiber. Cereals with less than 5 grams of fiber per serving aren't appropriate for your belly-flattening plan. However, these may be just fine for a growing child who could benefit from a food fortified with nutrients. So definitely put those products in the donate box!

✔ **Canned meats:** Canned lean meats, such as tuna and shrimp, are great sources of omega-3 fatty acids, but they're high in sodium. And, of course, canned mystery meat is a big no-no because of its high fat and sodium content. Your best bet on the Belly Fat Diet plan is to choose fresh tuna or shrimp to reduce your sodium intake. If you do prefer canned options, just make sure to choose no-sodium-added varieties.

- ✔ **Canned soups:** Many canned soups are a great source of carbohydrates and protein, but the increased sodium content and refined grains can wreak havoc on your belly-flattening efforts. If you do opt for canned soup, choose a low-sodium or no-salt-added option made with whole grains like barley or brown rice.

- ✔ **Butter:** Butter is very high in saturated fat, which may increase visceral fat in the abdomen. However, young children need saturated fat for brain development. So donate it to a shelter or pantry that caters to families with young children.

- ✔ **Vegetable oil:** On your Belly Fat Diet plan, you want to focus on consuming healthy, belly-flattening fat sources like olive oil. Replacing vegetable oil with an oil rich in monounsaturated fats is a better choice.

- ✔ **High-fat dairy products (whole milk, full-fat cheese, and full-fat yogurts):** Because these items are high in saturated fat, they aren't appropriate for belly flattening. However, they are healthy options for young children who still need a good source of saturated fat in their diet on a daily basis. So be sure to pass them on.

Deciding what foods to toss

Some foods just aren't healthy for anyone to consume. Donating these foods to a shelter or pantry wouldn't be as appropriate, because consuming these foods on a regular basis can have detrimental side effects for anyone, regardless of age or size. It's best to take the following foods and throw them away once and for all:

- ✔ **Snack foods containing partially hydrogenated oils:** If a food contains partially hydrogenated oils in its ingredient list, it contains a source of trans fats. Because even 2 grams of trans fat can have a negative impact on health, toss foods containing these. You see these oils in everything from crackers and sweets to margarines and convenience foods, so make sure to carefully read the ingredient list.

- ✔ **Processed, high-fat meats:** Meats that are highly processed and high in fat, such as sausages or hot dogs, contain not only saturated fat but also a significant amount of nitrates, which are a known carcinogen. Unless you have processed meats that are labeled nitrate-free, I would recommend tossing these products.

- ✔ **Pre-fried frozen foods:** Pre-fried frozen foods like french fries and mozzarella sticks are typically high in saturated fat, refined starches, and sodium. Many times, these foods also contain a large amount of preservatives and trans fats. Check the ingredient list carefully, and if you see partially hydrogenated oils, toss 'em.

  ✔ **Candy:** Candy is typically pure sugar or sugar and fat combined. Because it has little or no nutritional value, toss it.

  ✔ **Soda:** Soda is just liquid sugar. It causes a very high insulin response and provides absolutely no nutritional value. Pitch it!

Shopping for Belly-Friendly Foods

After you've cleaned house and removed all the foods that could potentially hurt your belly-busting efforts, you can stock your house with all the belly-friendly foods that keep you on track and help you successfully reach your flat belly goals.

Before you run out to the grocery store, consider a few things first. Ask yourself these questions:

  ✔ **What are the foods I absolutely can't live without?** If you crave certain foods all the time, ask yourself whether these foods are those that promote belly fat or help to shrink it. If they shrink belly fat, plan to stock up on them. However, if the foods promote the storage of belly fat, don't panic! Later I help you come up with healthy alternatives to these foods so you can enjoy them more often.

  ✔ **Are there certain foods that my family loves to have on hand?** Chances are your family has its favorites, whether it's chips, ice cream, or pickles. If these tempting foods sabotage your belly-flattening efforts, don't despair. Later I help you come up with healthy alternatives to these as well.

  ✔ **Which of the belly-flattening foods that I discuss in Chapter 6 and later in this chapter are your favorites?** Keep these foods in mind as you start to build your belly-flattening shopping list.

Making your list by food group

A shopping list is a must. If you want to lose weight and flatten your belly, you can't go shopping unprepared (or hungry). Shopping without a list is like trying to write a check when your account balance is zero — it's not a good idea, and it can get you into a lot of trouble! Creating a shopping list helps you to stay organized in the store, buy just what you need, avoid tempting foods you don't need, and prevent the frustrating feeling of realizing you forgot an important food item when you're already home.

When making your list, first plan out the meals and snacks you and your family will eat during the week. This way, you know exactly what ingredients and what foods you need to put on your list. (For instance, you can follow the advice and meal plans in Chapters 7 and 8.)

I find the easiest way to create a shopping list is to go by food groups. Doing so helps prevent you from forgetting any essential foods, and it also helps ensure you're buying a good balance of foods. The following sections break up the foods into groups for you.

Vegetables

You want to stock up on both fresh and frozen varieties. Select a good variety by aiming to pick vegetables from every color of the rainbow to maximize your nutrient intake.

If choosing frozen vegetables, select plain frozen vegetables, not the ones with seasonings and sauces (unless the total fat is less than 2 grams per serving and the sodium is less than 140 milligrams per serving).

Organic is the best choice when buying produce, but if you have to pick and choose to fit your budget, try to always purchase organic varieties for at least the following vegetables, because they tend to be the "dirtiest":

- ✔ Bell peppers
- ✔ Celery
- ✔ Lettuce
- ✔ Spinach

Fruit

Selecting fresh and frozen varieties of fruit is a great idea. I especially love frozen berries because they last longer, have just as much nutrition, and are great for adding to recipes and smoothies. Canned fruit can also be a great choice — if you're careful. Avoid fruit canned in syrup. Instead, choose fruit canned in 100% fruit juice.

Watch out for dried fruit. If selecting dried fruit, monitor the ingredients carefully and select the ones whose ingredients are mainly fruit and not added sugars and colorings.

Just like with vegetables, organic is best, but if you have to pick and choose what organic produce you buy, choose the following, which are the "dirty" fruits:

- ✔ Apples
- ✔ Cherries

✔ Grapes (imported)

✔ Nectarines

✔ Peaches

✔ Pears

✔ Strawberries

Milk and yogurt

Dairy products are good for you because they provide calcium and protein. However, you do have to be choosy. Here are the general guidelines to follow:

✔ **Milk:** Select any variety of fat-free (skim) or lowfat (1%) milk, such as cow's milk, soy milk, or almond milk. If you choose soy or almond milk, avoid the flavored milks that have sugar or corn syrup as one of the first five ingredients. When choosing cow's milk, opt for organic milk that's free of hormones and antibiotics.

✔ **Yogurt:** When selecting yogurt, avoid options with added sugar. Because yogurt has naturally occurring sugar as well, it's more important to focus on the ingredient list rather than the grams of sugar on the label. Avoid options where sugar and corn syrup are in the first five ingredients. Choose yogurts that are fat-free or lowfat (3 grams of total fat or less per 6-ounce serving).

Starches

When choosing any type of starch, which includes foods like bread, cereal, and pasta, select only whole-grain varieties. Before purchasing, always look at the first ingredient and make sure it lists a whole grain, such as whole wheat, rye, or bran. Avoid starches with more than 10 grams of sugar or less than 3 grams of fiber per serving. Be adventurous and try some new grains you may not have had before, such as quinoa. It's high in protein and fiber, so it keeps you quite satisfied for a long time.

Proteins

The leaner the protein, the leaner your belly. Make sure to select lean protein options, such as fish, white-meat poultry, pork tenderloin, and vegetarian-based proteins like edamame and tofu. Don't forget to pick up some whole eggs and liquid egg whites; both are great in recipes, and hard-boiled eggs make a fine snack. If you purchase cheese, make sure to select lowfat varieties with 3 grams of fat or less per ounce. Aim to have fish at least twice a week, because the omega-3 fatty acids can be powerful belly fighters.

Fats

Fats aren't all bad. Some are good for you! You want to stock up on those good belly-blasting monounsaturated fats, including healthy oils (like olive oil) and nuts (especially almonds, walnuts, and pistachios). Pick up some natural almond or peanut butter for a delicious belly-friendly treat. Seeds, such as sunflower seeds, make a great snack option and are full of healthy fats. You can also venture a bit outside the box and try some fat sources that are great for your belly and that you may not have had before, such as chia seeds. They're rich in belly-flattening omega-3 fatty acids.

Snacks

You didn't think I would tell you to leave the store without snacks, did you? Of course not! Snacking is essential to your belly-flattening plan. Many of the foods already on your list, such as raw vegetables, fresh fruit, nuts, and hard-boiled eggs make great snack options, but you may want to have more options on hand.

Foods from any food group can be snacks, so use the preceding guidelines for each food group when choosing snack options. For instance, if you choose a starchy snack, make sure it's made with whole grains and contains at least 3 grams of fiber per serving.

Popcorn is my favorite belly-flattening snack, especially because you can have so much of it! Buy the loose kernels instead of the packaged microwave varieties to help reduce your sodium intake. Use an air-popper or my easy popcorn recipe in Chapter 15 for a salt-free and fat-free snack. If you do choose microwave popcorn, opt for only lowfat and low-sodium options.

If you're looking for something sweet, pick up some dark chocolate. That's right! I am telling you to buy chocolate! Why? Because cocoa has been found to increase blood flow in the arteries, which may in turn help decrease blood pressure and lower the risk of blood clots. But make sure it contains at least 70 percent cocoa, and limit it to no more than one ounce per day.

Beverages

Water is the best beverage choice on your Belly Fat Diet plan. However, if you're looking for something with more flavor, you have options. For instance, skip the soda aisle all together, and pick up some green tea. Its belly-fighting ingredients, such as the compound epigallocatechin gallate (EGCG), make green tea a delicious and slimming drink. And you can drink it hot or cold.

If you really miss soda, you can pick up some naturally flavored seltzer, but try to limit it to 12 ounces per day or less, because carbonation can be bloating to your belly. And, although water and naturally flavored beverages, such as tea, are the best choice, artificially sweetened, calorie-free beverages are also acceptable for your Belly Fat Diet plan.

The best belly-fighting foods for your pantry

The pantry is a great place to stock up on nonperishables with belly-flattening benefits. Start stocking up on the following foods so you can stay on track with your weight-loss plan at all times:

- ✔ **Steel-cut oats:** Loaded with heart-healthy soluble fiber, this great breakfast option helps keep you feeling full and satisfied without bloating your belly. Old-fashioned rolled oats are also a good option here as well.

- ✔ **Whole grains (whole-wheat pasta, brown rice, and quinoa, for example):** These high-fiber options provide a great taste without the belly-bloating side effects of refined grains. A study by the American Journal of Clinical Nutrition found that dieters who ate five servings of whole grains every day for 12 weeks lost two times as much belly fat as people who ate refined carbohydrates instead. How's that for motivation?

- ✔ **Green tea:** Catechins in green tea help your body burn fat more effectively, thus flattening your belly one cup at a time.

  Select green tea that you brew yourself. Premade green tea, such as bottled iced green tea, is often high in sugar and contains less of the belly-fighting compound EGCG.

- ✔ **Almonds or almond butter:** A terrific source of heart-healthy monounsaturated fats, almonds were found in a study to help reduce insulin resistance and lower unhealthy LDL cholesterol levels. Raw almonds make a great snack, and almond butter can be smeared on whole-grain toast or celery sticks for a mini meal.

- ✔ **Beans and lentils:** Beans are great for you because they're rich in filling fiber and protein.

  Look into stocking up on cannellini beans. These beans contain one of the highest levels of *resistance starch,* which is a fiber that resists digestion. This high level of resistance starch means your body has to work harder to digest it, and, in turn, burn more calories, which helps promote weight loss.

- ✔ **Olive oil:** You want to transition from cooking with fats high in unhealthy, saturated fat, such as butter, and instead use oils with a high level of heart-healthy and belly-flattening monounsaturated fats, such as olive oil. Peanut oil, grapeseed oil, and canola oil are also rich sources of monounsaturated fats.

- ✔ **Apple cider vinegar:** Try adding a small amount of apple cider vinegar to some recipes or even to a drink. Why? A study out of Japan found overweight individuals who consumed a drink with 1–2 tablespoons of apple cider vinegar daily for 12 weeks lost more body weight and visceral fat, helping to decrease waist circumference and body mass index (BMI).

Navigating the store

You have your list and are ready to start shopping. But first, make sure you know the simple tricks that can help you make the healthiest choices while you're at the grocery store. Consider the following:

- **Don't go grocery shopping hungry.** When you're hungry, *everything* looks good, especially the foods that can expand your belly. So you'll more than likely come home with way more food than you planned to buy and very likely with many more unhealthy choices. Your best bet is to ward off hunger, cravings, and temptation by having a snack before heading to the store.

- **Shop the perimeter.** The perimeter of the store is where you find fresh vegetables and fruit, lean proteins like fish and chicken breast, and yogurt, milk, and eggs. Belly expanders, such as cookies, cakes, and chips, reside in the center aisles, so skip these if you can.

- **Don't forget to read the labels while you're in the store.** You may have written whole-wheat bread on your shopping list, but make sure when you go to purchase it, it's truly whole grain and not just enriched wheat flour or loaded with added sugars like high-fructose corn syrup. Flip the bread over, look at the label, and make sure the first ingredient is whole-wheat flour. Also, watch out for overly processed foods that seem healthy. Aim to select foods with five ingredients or less. At the very least, select foods that only contain ingredients you can pronounce and recognize.

Chapter 12

Waking Up to Healthy Breakfast Options

In This Chapter

▶ Understanding breakfast's role in weight loss and metabolism

▶ Identifying delicious and easy breakfast options to fight belly fat

*1*f you want to make a huge impact on fighting belly fat, you have to start first thing in the morning. Breakfast is truly the most essential meal of the day. After all, it boosts your metabolism and helps you make better food choices throughout the day. However, to many people, breakfast is no more than an afterthought as they're running out the door. If you're serious about banishing belly fat for good, you have to get started as soon as you wake up.

Luckily, breakfast doesn't have to be difficult or time consuming. In this chapter, I show you the importance of breakfast and provide you with easy-to-make recipes that you can enjoy. I even show you what recipes you can make in advance, freeze, and pop in the microwave for a super-fast breakfast solution.

Revving Your Engine with a Tasty and Nutritious Breakfast

Your body is similar to a car: If you don't put gas into it, you can't expect it to go anywhere. As you sleep overnight, your body hasn't received any "fuel" (food) for a long period of time. Depending on how long you sleep and when your last meal was, this period of time can be anywhere from 8 to 12 hours or more.

During this extended period of time, your body relies on stored energy in your cells for fuel. To protect you from running out of stored energy, your body also slows down your energy needs by slightly slowing your metabolic rate. This process puts your body in a fasting state. So if you wake up, start your day, and don't fuel your body with food, your body continues to stay in that fasting state. Because your metabolic rate is slightly slowed during a state of fasting, you won't burn as many calories throughout the morning. And burning fewer calories means you have to eat even less or exercise even more during the rest of the day to help promote weight loss. I doubt you want to do that! Instead, you want to rev up your metabolism so you burn more calories every minute of every day, helping to quickly (and permanently) burn away unwanted fat and pounds.

So to avoid slowing down your metabolism and making weight loss more difficult, you only have to do one simple thing: Eat! And who doesn't want to eat? I know I do! You should eat breakfast within an hour of waking up. Keep in mind, however, that you don't have to eat an elaborate breakfast. You just need a small amount of belly-friendly food in your system to break the fasting state.

"But I'm not hungry in the morning . . ."

I know what all of you non-breakfast-eaters are saying right now: "I'm just not hungry in the morning. But when I do eat breakfast, my appetite increases, and I feel hungry all morning." If this happens to you, I understand why you would be hesitant to start eating breakfast, especially if you feel you're going to start feeling hungrier and eating more all day long.

But get this: What's really happening here is that when your body is in that prolonged fasting state, all of your body systems slow down. Your body — which can't tell whether you're purposefully fasting or whether the grocery store ran out of food due to a mass famine — decreases hunger signals in the body to protect you. When you do start eating, the fasting stage is over, metabolism is increased, and your body goes back to normal functioning, including normal hunger and satiety signals.

Because you aren't used to eating breakfast, feeling these hunger signals in the morning may seem new to you, and it will seem as though having eaten breakfast is what made you feel hungry. In reality, however, you became hungry because your metabolism revved up, which is a good thing. If you begin eating breakfast on a regular basis, for at least a week or two, this hunger after eating will start to subside.

Why breakfast affects your choices throughout the day

Breakfast helps you make better meal choices throughout the day and allows you to better control your portions, promoting weight loss. If you skip breakfast entirely, you don't feel hungry because your body is in the fasting state I discuss earlier in the chapter. However, your body can go only so long suppressing hunger cues. So at some point you start feeling hungry. But maybe you're at work or rushing around taking care of the kids and you ignore this hunger signal. The signal gets stronger and stronger, and eventually you can't ignore it anymore. Now you're ravenous and ready to devour anything and everything you can find.

As you probably know, when you get really hungry, you aren't exactly looking for the healthiest food choices. You grab whatever is the easiest and quickest — maybe a bag of chips or a burger from a fast-food joint — and you end up eating too much of it and way too fast. This cycle of eating can promote weight gain rather than weight loss. And what's worse is that not only did you just eat too many calories, but your body was also already burning fewer calories because you skipped breakfast. You just set yourself up for a double whammy that fuels weight gain and belly fat storage.

To prevent this cycle from happening, you need to eat a healthy, filling breakfast. But you also need a breakfast that is realistic and works for your lifestyle. If you have time in the morning to make an elaborate breakfast, that's terrific! But if you're like many people who just need to grab something as you run out the door, there's still hope. This chapter provides some excellent options. You can even prepare some of them on a day when you have more time and then refrigerate or freeze them so you can simply reheat for a superfast breakfast on those busy days.

Breadless Breakfast Quiche

Prep time: 10 min • **Cook time:** 30 min • **Yield:** 4 servings

Ingredients	Directions
Nonstick cooking spray	*1* Preheat the oven to 375 degrees and spray a 10-x-10-inch glass baking pan with nonstick cooking spray.
2 cups fresh spinach	
1 cup chopped mushrooms	*2* In a large sauté pan, sauté the spinach and mushrooms in the olive oil until tender.
1 tablespoon olive oil	
4 eggs	*3* Beat the whole eggs along with the liquid egg whites. Pour half the egg mixture into the prepared baking pan.
1 cup liquid egg whites (or 8 egg whites)	
½ cup fresh or no-salt-added canned diced tomatoes	*4* Evenly spread the spinach and mushroom mixture on top of the egg mixture and then top with the diced tomatoes. Sprinkle the feta cheese on top of the tomatoes.
½ cup part-skim feta cheese	
	5 Pour the remaining egg mixture on top, covering the cheese and vegetables.
	6 Place the baking pan in the oven and cook for 30 minutes, or until a toothpick comes out clean.

Meal plan servings: *1 vegetable, 2 ounces protein, 1 fat.*

Per serving: *Calories 172 (From Fat 90); Fat 10g (Saturated 3g); Cholesterol 188mg; Sodium 369mg; Carbohydrate 5g (Dietary Fiber 1g); Protein 16g.*

Tip: I recommend you make this recipe on the weekend (or your day off work), refrigerate it, and then just slice a serving and microwave it for a quick breakfast any day. This recipe can stay in the fridge for up to 3–4 days.

Tropical Yogurt Parfait

Prep time: 5 min • **Yield:** 1 serving

Ingredients	*Directions*
1 cup fat-free plain or vanilla Greek yogurt	*1* Place ¼ cup of the yogurt in a clear glass. Top with 1 tablespoon of chopped walnuts and ¼ cup papaya.
¼ cup chopped walnuts	
1 cup chopped papaya	*2* Repeat in layers to make an attractive and tasty parfait.

Meal plan servings: *1 milk, 1 fruit, 4 fats.*

Per serving: *Calories 371 (From Fat 178); Fat 20g (Saturated 2g); Cholesterol 0mg; Sodium 90mg; Carbohydrate 27g (Dietary Fiber 5g); Protein 25g.*

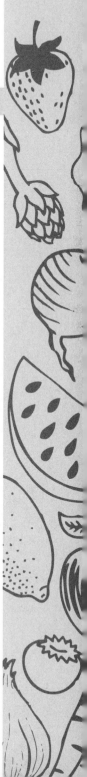

Waistline-Slimming Omelet

Prep time: 5 min • **Cook time:** 10 min • **Yield:** 1 serving

Ingredients	*Directions*
Nonstick cooking spray	*1* Spray a large sauté pan with nonstick cooking spray and sauté the onions and chili peppers until tender. Remove from the pan and keep warm. (If you prefer crunchy vegetables, leave the onions and peppers uncooked.)
¼ cup chopped onion	
¼ cup chopped chili peppers (canned or fresh)	
1 egg	*2* Spray the pan with nonstick cooking spray again and place over medium heat.
¼ cup liquid egg whites (or 2 egg whites)	
¼ cup grated Parmigiano-Reggiano cheese	*3* Whisk together the whole egg and the liquid egg whites (or egg whites). Add the egg mixture to the prepared sauté pan.
	4 Allow the eggs to slightly firm, and then top with the onions, peppers, and grated cheese.
	5 Gently fold over the egg to create an omelet. Flip once to allow for even cooking.

Meal plan servings: 1 vegetable, 3 ounces protein, 1 fat.

Per serving: Calories 226 (From Fat 100); Fat 11g (Saturated 5g); Cholesterol 198mg; Sodium 548mg; Carbohydrate 8g (Dietary Fiber 1g); Protein 23g.

Banana-Almond Breakfast Toast

Prep time: 10 min • **Cook time:** 10 min • **Yield:** 2 servings

Ingredients	Directions
½ cup liquid egg substitute (or 4 egg whites) 1 tablespoon vanilla extract 3 tablespoons ground cinnamon ¼ cup crushed almonds Nonstick cooking spray 2 slices 100% whole-wheat bread 1 large banana, sliced	**1** Place the liquid egg substitute (or egg whites) in a large bowl. Add the vanilla extract and 2 tablespoons of the cinnamon and whisk together. On a plate, spread out the crushed almonds. **2** Spray a small sauté pan with nonstick cooking spray and place over medium heat. **3** Dip one slice of bread into the egg mixture until fully coated. Remove the bread from the egg mixture and dip it into the crushed almonds, flipping to evenly coat both sides. **4** Place the bread in the prepared sauté pan and allow to cook for 1 to 2 minutes on each side, or until the egg mixture firms and no liquid is present. **5** Remove the toast from the pan and place it on a clean plate. Repeat Steps 1–4 with the second slice of bread. **6** Top each piece of toast with sliced banana and then sprinkle with the remaining cinnamon.

Meal plan servings: 1 starch, 1 ounce protein, 1 fruit, 1 fat.

Per serving: Calories 289 (From Fat 71); Fat 8g (Saturated 1g); Cholesterol 0mg; Sodium 261mg; Carbohydrate 41g (Dietary Fiber 11g); Protein 13g.

On-the-Go Breakfast Sandwich

Prep time: 5 min • **Cook time:** 5 min • **Yield:** 1 serving

Ingredients	Directions
Nonstick cooking spray 1 egg (or ¼ cup liquid egg whites) 2 slices 100% whole-grain bread 1 ounce Canadian bacon 1 ounce part-skim provolone cheese	*1* Spray a small sauté pan with nonstick cooking spray and place over medium heat. Add the egg (or liquid egg whites) to the pan. *2* Allow the egg to firm in one solid piece as you would when making an omelet, making sure the egg maintains the size of a bread slice. Flip the egg once to ensure adequate cooking. *3* Once firm, remove the egg from the heat. Place the cooked egg on top of one slice of bread. Top with Canadian bacon and cheese, and then cover with the other slice of bread to create a sandwich.

Meal plan servings: 2 starches, 3 ounces protein.

Per serving: Calories 322 (From Fat 128); Fat 14g (Saturated 6g); Cholesterol 211mg; Sodium 885mg; Carbohydrate 25g (Dietary Fiber 3g); Protein 25g.

Tip: This sandwich can be frozen and reheated for 30 to 45 seconds in your microwave for a quick and easy breakfast option.

Vary It! Try adding belly-flattening veggies, such as cooked spinach, tomato, or peppers, to your egg sandwich for an added benefit.

Belly-Blasting Berry Smoothie

Prep time: 5 min • **Yield:** 1 serving

Ingredients	Directions
1 cup fat-free plain Greek yogurt	*1* In a blender, combine the yogurt, berries, vanilla, ground chia seeds, and ice.
1 cup frozen organic berries (blueberries, strawberries, or açai berries make great choices)	*2* Blend on high for 1 minute, or until desired consistency is reached.
1 tablespoon vanilla extract	
1 tablespoon ground chia seeds	
½ cup ice	

Meal plan servings: 1 milk, 1 fruit, 1 fat.

Per serving: Calories 294 (From Fat 42); Fat 5g (Saturated 2g); Cholesterol 0mg; Sodium 92mg; Carbohydrate 35g (Dietary Fiber 8g); Protein 23g.

Tip: Ground chia seeds can be found in many grocery stores in the organic/health food sections as well as in most natural food stores. If you can't find chia seeds, you can substitute with the same amount of ground flaxseed.

Cinnamon Oatmeal with Almonds

Prep time: 2 min • **Cook time:** 35 min • **Yield:** 4 servings

Ingredients	*Directions*
3 cups water 1 cup steel-cut oats	*1* Place the water in a saucepan and bring to a boil over high heat.
2 tablespoons cinnamon ¼ cup chopped almonds	*2* Stir in the oats and allow the mixture to come back to a boil.
1 teaspoon stevia extract or zero-calorie artificial sweetener (optional)	*3* When the oatmeal reaches a boil, cover and reduce the heat to medium-low. Let it simmer for 20 to 30 minutes, or until the oats reach desired consistency, stirring occasionally.
	4 Sprinkle cinnamon and almonds on top, and add stevia or zero-calorie artificial sweetener, if desired.

Meal plan servings: 1 starch, 1 fat.

Per serving: Calories 140 (From Fat 45); Fat 5g (Saturated 1g); Cholesterol 0mg; Sodium 3mg; Carbohydrate 21g (Dietary Fiber 4g); Protein 5g.

Tip: When cooking oatmeal, shorter cooking time leads to chewier oats and longer time leads to softer oats.

90-Second Omelet

Prep time: 1 min • **Cook time:** 1½ min • **Yield:** 1 serving

Ingredients	*Directions*
Nonstick cooking spray	*1* Spray a 12-ounce coffee mug with nonstick cooking spray.
2 eggs (or ½ cup liquid egg substitute), whisked	
½ cup cooked broccoli	*2* Pour half of the whisked egg into the prepared mug, and then add the broccoli and cheese. Pour the remaining egg on top.
¼ cup shredded part-skim cheddar cheese	
	3 Microwave for 90 seconds, or until firm, and remove.

Meal plan servings: 3 ounces protein, 1 vegetable, 2 fats.

Per serving: Calories 239 (From Fat 145); Fat 16g (Saturated 7g); Cholesterol 385mg; Sodium 137mg; Carbohydrate 4g (Dietary Fiber 1g); Protein 21g.

Vary It! You can add any cooked vegetables you like to this one-cup omelet. Try onion, red pepper, mushrooms, or tomatoes (or a mix!). Steaming is the best option for cooking the veggies, but if you're short on time, using flash-frozen and microwaving is fine as well.

Bean, Ham, and Cheese Breakfast Burrito

Prep time: 5 min • **Cook time:** 5 min • **Yield:** 4 servings

Ingredients	*Directions*
Nonstick cooking spray	*1* Spray a sauté pan with nonstick cooking spray and place over medium heat.
4 eggs (or 1 cup liquid egg whites)	
4 ounces chopped lean ham	*2* In a small bowl, whisk the eggs (or egg whites). Add to the prepared pan along with the ham and beans.
2 cups cooked cannellini beans (or one 16-ounce can, rinsed and drained)	*3* Stir the mixture occasionally until the eggs are fully cooked and scrambled.
Four 6-inch 100% whole-grain tortillas	*4* Place ¼ of the mixture onto each tortilla and top with 1 ounce of the shredded cheese.
4 ounces shredded part-skim cheddar cheese	*5* Wrap the tortilla into a burrito shape and allow the cheese to melt.

Meal plan servings: 2 starches, 4 ounces protein, 1 fat.

Per serving: Calories 389 (From Fat 118); Fat 13g (Saturated 6g); Cholesterol 217mg; Sodium 445mg; Carbohydrate 45g (Dietary Fiber 8g); Protein 30g.

Tip: If selecting canned beans, aim to choose no-sodium-added or low-sodium options whenever possible.

Vary It! You can personalize this burrito by adding some cooked vegetables, such as green pepper and onion, and by using different kinds of cheese and beans. Experiment with black beans, pinto beans, lowfat hot pepper cheese, or lowfat Monterey Jack, for example.

Veggie-Egg Muffins

Prep time: 10 min • **Cook time:** 15–20 min • **Yield:** 8 servings

Ingredients	Directions
Nonstick cooking spray 1 tablespoon olive oil 4 eggs 1 cup liquid egg whites (or 8 egg whites) ¾ cup broccoli, chopped 1 cup grated fresh mozzarella cheese ¾ cup mushroom, diced 1 cup onion, chopped ½ cup tomato, diced ¾ cup crumbled part-skim feta cheese ½ cup spinach, chopped ¾ cup bell pepper, chopped	*1* Preheat the oven to 375 degrees, and then spray an 8-count muffin tin with nonstick cooking spray. Set aside. *2* In a sauté pan, heat the olive oil over medium heat. Cook each of the vegetables separately in the oil until they're tender. *3* Meanwhile, in a bowl, whisk together the whole eggs and the liquid egg whites. Pour ¼ cup of the egg mixture into each muffin cup. *4* Add in one of the following varieties of vegetables and cheese to each muffin cup to make a variety of muffins: ½ cup broccoli and ¼ cup mozzarella cheese ¼ cup mushroom, ¼ cup onion, and ¼ cup mozzarella cheese ¼ cup tomato, ¼ cup onion, and ¼ cup feta cheese ¼ cup spinach, ¼ cup mushroom, and ¼ cup feta cheese ¼ cup bell pepper, ¼ cup mushroom, and ¼ cup onion ¼ cup tomato, ¼ cup spinach, and ¼ cup mozzarella cheese ¼ cup broccoli, ¼ cup onion, and ¼ cup feta cheese ½ cup bell pepper and ¼ cup mozzarella cheese *5* Place the muffin tin in the oven and bake for 15 to 20 minutes.

Meal plan servings: 2 ounces protein, 0.5 vegetable.

Per serving: Calories 125 (From Fat 68); Fat 8g (Saturated 4g); Cholesterol 106mg; Sodium 281mg; Carbohydrate 2g (Dietary Fiber 0g); Protein 13g.

Vary It: The vegetables listed here are just a starting point. You can get creative by substituting with different vegetables, different varieties of lowfat cheese, and even lean proteins such as low-sodium ham or turkey bacon.

Quick and Belly-Friendly Cold Cereal with Fruit

Prep time: 1 min • **Yield:** 1 serving

Ingredients	Directions
1 cup whole-grain cereal	*1* Pour the cereal in a small bowl and top with milk.
1 cup fat-free or 1% milk (or substitute with almond or soy milk)	*2* Serve along with ½ cup of grapefruit on the side.
½ cup grapefruit	

Note: You probably don't need a recipe for cereal, but I wanted to make the point that it is a viable and quick option for breakfast. You're better off throwing together some whole-grain cereal and milk than skipping the meal altogether. If you think cold cereal is boring, make it more exciting with your favorite fruit.

Meal plan servings: 2 starches, 1 milk, 1 fruit.

Per serving: Calories 238 (From Fat 20); Fat 2g (Saturated 1g); Cholesterol 5mg; Sodium 385mg; Carbohydrate 69g (Dietary Fiber 10g); Protein 14g.

Making cereal a healthy breakfast option

Cereal can make a quick and filling breakfast option when even the quickest of the recipes I provide you earlier in this chapter isn't quick enough. I realize that most of you aren't going to make your own cereal; you're going to go to the grocery store and buy a box. You have to be careful about what cereal you select, however. You want to use these guidelines:

✔ The first ingredient of the cereal needs to be a whole grain (for example, whole wheat, oat bran, or brown rice).

✔ The cereal should contain at least 5 grams of fiber per ½ cup serving.

✔ The cereal should contain 110 calories or less per ½ cup serving.

Make sure to use a fat-free or lowfat dairy-based milk for your cereal. If you select a non-dairy option, such as soy or almond milk, make sure it contains 10 grams of sugar or less per 1 cup serving.

Chapter 13

Whipping Up Lunches That Fight Belly Fat

. . . .

In This Chapter

▶ Understanding the importance of eating lunch

▶ Preparing tasty lunch options that help you slim your tummy

. . . .

*T*he key to losing weight and keeping it off is to eat regularly throughout the day. Doing so not only helps boost your metabolism, but it also helps control your appetite. When you get too hungry, it can be difficult to ward off the temptation to overeat or fight cravings for foods that are less than friendly to your belly. That's why lunch is so critical to your success with the Belly Fat Diet plan. If you skip lunch, you set yourself up for mid-afternoon fatigue, cravings, and overeating at dinner and later on in the evening.

I know lunch can be hard to fit in at times. Maybe you were rushing out to work in the morning and didn't have time to pack anything. Or maybe you were so busy caring for the kids that you didn't have a chance to make lunch for yourself. So that you don't stop at the nearest fast-food joint to pick up a sandwich that will pack fat on your belly, I show you some quick (and really tasty!) lunches you can make in a hurry. I also point out my favorite belly-blasting lunches that are nice to make in advance. You can make these lunches in bulk on a day when you have some free time, and then you can freeze them and reheat them for a super-fast lunch anytime.

This chapter shows you that you have no excuse to not have a healthy lunch every day. And after you taste the recipes, you'll look forward to lunch so much that you won't be able to skip it!

Preparing Belly-Shrinking Lunches

Not just any old meal will do for lunch. You want to make sure you take time at lunch to make it a belly-burning opportunity. So throughout the recipes in this chapter, you see some key ingredients that help you burn belly fat. These include ingredients like avocado, apple cider vinegar, and cannellini beans. Research has shown that these ingredients help you more effectively burn fat (see Chapter 11 for a detailed explanation on why). And the best part? They also taste great, which is a real win-win for your belly and your taste buds!

Do you have a typical lunch staple? What's your go-to meal on a busy day? Is it a healthy choice? Is it rich in belly-blasting ingredients, such as monoun- saturated fats, omega-3 fatty acids, and antioxidants? Or is it a belly-bloater rich in refined grains, saturated fat, and sodium? If your typical lunch is more of a belly-bloater than a belly-burner, the good news is that it just takes a few simple changes to revamp it to a belly-friendly meal. Consider the following examples:

- If your typical lunch contains white bread, Italian bread, or a white-flour wrap, simply switch to a 100 percent whole-grain alternative, such as a 100 percent whole-wheat wrap or 100 percent rye bread.

- If your normal lunch contains a high amount of saturated fats from lunch meats like liverwurst and salami or full-fat cheese, try switching to low- fat, reduced-sodium ham or turkey breast and opt for reduced-fat cheese made with 1 percent milk instead.

- Is your lunch lacking in antioxidant rich foods? No problem! Add slices of fresh tomato, onion, or roasted red peppers on top of your sandwich. Have a side of fresh berries or a side salad with your meal. Or switch from mayonnaise to hummus as a spread on your wrap.

- If you eat out for lunch, your meal may be packed full of sodium, refined carbohydrates, and unhealthy fats without you even realizing it. Make sure to visit Chapter 17 for healthy lunch alternatives when eating out at any restaurant or fast-food establishment.

As you can see, just a few simple adjustments can take almost any meal from a belly-bloater to a belly-blaster! Throughout this chapter, I show you how to transform some typical lunches into powerful belly fat fighters. I also introduce you to some quick and easy lunch options you may have never even considered (but will love!).

Grilled Chicken Salad

Prep time: 35–40 min • **Cook time:** 15–20 min • **Yield:** 4 servings

Ingredients	*Directions*
½ cup apple cider vinegar, divided	*1* Preheat the oven to 400 degrees.
½ cup balsamic vinegar, divided	*2* In a small bowl, mix together ¼ cup of the apple cider vinegar, ¼ cup of the balsamic vinegar, and 1 tablespoon of the garlic. Place the chicken tenderloins in the mixture and let them marinate in the refrigerator for 30 minutes.
2 tablespoons minced garlic, divided	
1 pound chicken tenderloins, trimmed of fat	*3* Place the marinated chicken in a shallow baking dish (along with the marinade) and cook 15 to 20 minutes, or until the internal temperature reaches 165 degrees.
1 tablespoon olive oil	
1 head of lettuce, cut or torn into pieces	
1 large tomato, sliced	*4* While the chicken is cooking, mix together the remaining ¼ cup of the apple cider vinegar, ¼ cup of the balsamic vinegar, and 1 tablespoon of garlic along with the olive oil to create your salad dressing.
1 large cucumber, sliced	
1 avocado, sliced	
1 cup black olives	*5* When the chicken is done cooking, cut it into small slices.
	6 In a large bowl, toss together the lettuce, tomato, cucumber, avocado, olives, and chicken along with the salad dressing.

Meal plan servings: 1.5 vegetables, 4 ounces protein, 2.5 fats.

Per serving: Calories 224 (From Fat 128); Fat 14g (Saturated 3g); Cholesterol 18mg; Sodium 330mg; Carbohydrate 17g; Dietary Fiber 7g; Protein 11g.

Hot and Spicy Vegetarian Chili

Prep time: 5 min • **Cook time:** 60 min • **Yield:** 6 servings

Ingredients	*Directions*
2 tablespoons olive oil	*1* In a large stockpot, add olive oil over medium heat. Add the garlic, bell peppers, onion, and celery, and cook until the vegetables are softened, about 8 to 10 minutes.
3 garlic cloves, finely chopped	
1 green bell pepper, chopped	
1 red bell pepper, chopped	*2* Add the tomatoes, Chili Seasoning (see the following recipe), and 4 cups of water and stir. Allow to simmer over medium heat for 20 minutes.
1 medium green onion, finely chopped	
3 large celery ribs, chopped	*3* Stir in the kidney beans, cannellini beans, black beans, and the jalapeño (seed the jalapeño if you want less heat to the chili), and allow to simmer for an additional 30 minutes.
One 28-ounce can no-salt-added diced tomatoes	
1 recipe Chili Seasoning (see the following recipe)	
4 cups water	
2 cups red kidney beans, cooked and drained (or one 16-ounce can, rinsed and drained)	
2 cups cannellini beans, cooked and drained (or one 16-ounce can, rinsed and drained)	
1 cup black beans, cooked and drained (or one 8-ounce can, rinsed and drained)	
1 jalapeño, chopped	

Chili Seasoning

1 tablespoon chili powder

1 teaspoon turmeric

2 teaspoons black pepper

1 tablespoon crushed red pepper flakes

1 teaspoon garlic powder

1 teaspoon onion powder

2 teaspoons ground cumin

1 teaspoon salt

1 teaspoon paprika

1 teaspoon dried oregano

1 In a small bowl, combine the chili powder, turmeric, black pepper, red pepper flakes, garlic powder, onion powder, cumin, salt, paprika, and oregano.

Meal plan servings: 1.5 starches, 1.5 ounces protein, 1.5 vegetables, 1 fat.

Per serving: Calories 302 (From Fat 55); Fat 6g (Saturated 1g); Cholesterol 0mg; Sodium 488mg; Carbohydrate 50g; Dietary Fiber 15g; Protein 16g.

Black Bean Quesadilla

Prep time: 5 min • **Cook time:** 10–15 min • **Yield:** 4 servings

Ingredients	*Directions*
1 teaspoon olive oil	*1* In a sauté pan, heat the olive oil over medium heat. Add the black beans, tomato, bell pepper, and onion, and cook for 5 to 7 minutes, or until the onions are tender.
1 cup canned black beans, rinsed and drained	
1 medium tomato, chopped	
1 large green bell pepper, chopped	*2* Add the cilantro, jalapeños, and cayenne pepper. (Seed the jalapeño if you want the quesadillas to be less spicy.) Stir and cook for 1 minute, and then remove the vegetables and beans from the pan and set aside.
1 red onion, chopped	
3 tablespoons fresh chopped cilantro	
¼ cup chopped jalapeño pepper	*3* In a small bowl, mix together the Monterey Jack and cheddar cheeses to create a Mexican blend.
1 teaspoon ground cayenne pepper	*4* Spray the sauté pan with nonstick spray and place back on medium heat. Put a tortilla in the bottom of the pan and top with ¼ of the bean vegetable mixture and ¼ cup of the cheese mixture on one side.
½ cup part-skim shredded Monterey Jack cheese	
½ cup part-skim shredded cheddar cheese	
Nonstick cooking spray	*5* Fold tortilla to create a quesadilla. Cook the quesadilla for 1 to 2 minutes on each side, or until the tortilla becomes crispy and the cheese melts.
Four 100% whole-wheat tortillas (12-inch diameter)	*6* Follow Steps 4 and 5 for the remaining quesadillas. Serve warm with a side of fresh salsa.
1 cup fresh salsa	

Meal plan servings: *2.5 starches, 2 ounces protein, 1 vegetable, 1 fat.*

Per serving: *Calories 416 (From Fat 106); Fat 12g (Saturated 4g); Cholesterol 18mg; Sodium 583mg; Carbohydrate 67g; Dietary Fiber 10g; Protein 18g.*

Quick and Easy Turkey Wrap

Prep time: 3 min • **Yield:** 1 serving

Ingredients	*Directions*
2 tablespoons hummus	*1* Spread the hummus evenly over the tortilla.
One 12-inch 100% whole-grain tortilla	*2* Layer lettuce, tomato, and turkey on the tortilla.
½ cup shredded lettuce	
½ cup sliced tomato	*3* Roll the tortilla to create a wrap sandwich.
3 ounces low-sodium, nitrate-free turkey breast cold cut	

Meal plan servings: 2 starches, 1 vegetable, 3 ounces protein, 1 fat.

Per serving: Calories 356 (From Fat 59); Fat 7g (Saturated 2g); Cholesterol 71mg; Sodium 251mg; Carbohydrate 42g; Dietary Fiber 5g; Protein 37g.

Tuna and Salsa Stuffed Pepper

Prep time: 10 min • **Cook time:** 5 min • **Yield:** 4 servings

Ingredients	*Directions*
4 large green bell peppers	*1* Bring a large stockpot of water to a boil.
8 ounces low-sodium canned tuna, packed in water	*2* Slice off the tops of each pepper and remove the seeds.
1 cup fresh salsa	*3* Place the peppers in boiling water and cook for 5 minutes. Drain and set aside.
	4 In a small bowl, mix together the tuna and salsa. Stuff each pepper with equal parts of the mixture. Serve the peppers chilled.

Meal plan servings: *1 vegetable, 2 ounces protein.*

Per serving: *Calories 144 (From Fat 12); Fat 1g (Saturated 0g); Cholesterol 51mg; Sodium 259mg; Carbohydrate 10g; Dietary Fiber 3g; Protein 24g.*

Tip: If you prefer a creamier taste, add mashed avocado or lowfat plain Greek yogurt to the tuna mixture.

Tortilla Pizza

Prep time: 5 min • **Cook time:** 10 min • **Yield:** 4 servings

Ingredients	Directions
¾ **cup tomato paste**	**1** Preheat the oven to 350 degrees.
2 **tablespoons minced garlic**	
1 **tablespoon olive oil**	**2** Make the tomato sauce by bringing the tomato paste to a simmer in a small saucepan. Add the minced garlic and olive oil, and allow it to simmer for 2 minutes. Remove from the heat and set aside.
2 **teaspoons dried basil**	
Four 8-inch 100% whole-wheat tortillas	
1 **cup sliced fresh mozzarella cheese**	**3** Lay the tortillas on a baking sheet. Cover each one with ¼ cup of the tomato sauce. Top each one with ¼ cup of the cheese along with some of the mushrooms and onions. Sprinkle dried basil over the tops of the pizzas.
½ **cup sliced mushrooms**	
½ **cup sliced sweet yellow onion**	
	4 Place the baking sheet in the oven and bake for 6 to 8 minutes, or until the cheese is melted. Cook slightly longer for a crispier crust.

Meal plan servings: 1 starch, 1 ounce protein, 1 vegetable, 1 fat.

Per serving: Calories 275 (From Fat 113); Fat 13g (Saturated 5g); Cholesterol 20mg; Sodium 181mg; Carbohydrate 34g; Dietary Fiber 4g; Protein 12g.

Shockingly Healthy (and Easy!) Calzone

Prep time: 3 min • **Cook time:** 1½ min • **Yield:** 1 serving

Ingredients	Directions
8-inch 100% whole-wheat tortilla	**1** Place the mozzarella cheese on one side of the tortilla. Top with the spinach, tomato, and ricotta cheese.
¼ cup shredded fat-free mozzarella cheese	
¼ cup cooked spinach	**2** Fold over the tortilla to create a calzone shape. Pinch the edges together to seal the calzone. You can use a toothpick to hold the tortilla closed.
2 tablespoons diced tomato	
2 tablespoons fat-free ricotta cheese	**3** Microwave on high for 1½ minutes, or until the cheese melts. Serve warm with a side of tomato sauce for dipping, if desired.
¼ cup canned tomato sauce (optional)	

Meal plan servings: 1 starch, 1.5 ounces protein, 1 vegetable.

Per serving: Calories 226 (From Fat 20); Fat 2g (Saturated 0g); Cholesterol 15mg; Sodium 577mg; Carbohydrate 34g; Dietary Fiber 5g; Protein 19g.

Vary It! Mix it up by adding different veggies and even different lean protein options. For instance, you can make one calzone with spinach and tomato and another with peppers and onions. The choices are limitless! Chapter 6 provides some lean protein options to consider.

Turkey Burger and Sweet Potato Fries

Prep time: 15 min • **Cook time:** 45–60 min • **Yield:** 4 servings

Ingredients	Directions
1 pound ground 98% fat-free turkey breast 1 tablespoon minced garlic 1 tablespoon olive oil 2 tablespoons diced shallots ¼ cup whole-wheat breadcrumbs 2 tablespoons apple cider vinegar 2 teaspoons black pepper 1 tablespoon dried rosemary Four 100% whole-wheat hamburger buns	**1** In a large bowl, mix together the ground turkey, garlic, olive oil, shallots, breadcrumbs, vinegar, black pepper, and rosemary. Use your hands to evenly mix the seasonings throughout the meat. **2** Heat a sauté pan over medium heat. In the meantime, create four even-sized patties with the meat mixture. **3** Add the patties to the pan and cook for 8–10 minutes, or until they reach an internal temperature of 180 degrees. Flip the patties halfway through cooking. **4** Place the cooked patties on hamburger buns and serve warm with the Sweet Potato Fries (see the following recipe).

Sweet Potato Fries

Ingredients	Directions
Two 6-ounce sweet potatoes 1 tablespoon olive oil 2 tablespoons cinnamon	**1** Preheat the oven to 400 degrees. **2** Slice each potato into 15 skinny fries and place on a large baking sheet. Drizzle the olive oil over the fries and top with cinnamon. **3** Bake for 30 minutes, and then flip the fries over. Bake for an additional 15 to 30 minutes, or until the fries are the desired texture (longer cooking time for crispier fries).

Meal plan servings: *3 starches, 4 ounces protein, 1 fat.*

Per serving: *Calories 375 (From Fat 88); Fat 10g (Saturated 2g); Cholesterol 74mg; Sodium 269mg; Carbohydrate 41g; Dietary Fiber 8g; Protein 32g.*

Tip: Top your burger with belly fighters like avocado, or add a metabolism kick by tossing spices like cayenne pepper into your burgers before cooking.

Belly-Beating Bean Burrito

Prep time: 5 min • **Cook time:** 15 min • **Yield:** 4 servings

Ingredients	Directions
4 teaspoons olive oil	**1** Heat the olive oil in a large sauté pan over medium heat.
1 medium red onion, diced	
3 cloves of garlic, minced	**2** Sauté the onion, garlic, and mushrooms until tender, about 7 to 8 minutes.
1 cup sliced fresh mushrooms	
1 cup cannellini beans, cooked and drained (or one 8-ounce can, rinsed and drained)	**3** Add the kidney beans, cannellini beans, balsamic vinegar, red wine vinegar, apple cider vinegar, basil, thyme, oregano, cilantro, and pepper. Sauté for 5 to 7 minutes, or until heated through, and then remove from the heat.
1 cup kidney beans, cooked and drained (or one 8-ounce can, rinsed and drained)	
2 tablespoons balsamic vinegar	**4** Top each tortilla with ¼ cup shredded lettuce, ⅛ cup shredded carrots, and ¾ cup cooked bean mixture.
1 tablespoon red wine vinegar	
1 tablespoon apple cider vinegar	**5** Wrap each tortilla and serve warm.
1 teaspoon dried basil	
1 teaspoon dried thyme	
1 teaspoon dried oregano	
1 tablespoon fresh chopped cilantro	
1 teaspoon black pepper	
1 cup shredded romaine lettuce	
½ cup shredded carrots	
Four 8-inch whole-wheat tortillas	

Meal plan servings: *2 starches, 1 ounce protein, 2 vegetables, 1 fat.*

Per serving: *Calories 302 (From Fat 64); Fat 7g (Saturated 1g); Cholesterol 0mg; Sodium 150mg; Carbohydrate 52g; Dietary Fiber 10g; Protein 13g.*

Tip: If you enjoy sour cream on your burrito, top each tortilla with lowfat, plain Greek yogurt instead.

Hummus and Avocado Sandwich

Prep time: 7 min • **Yield:** 2 servings

Ingredients	*Directions*
4 slices 100% whole-grain bread	*1* Toast the bread. While the bread is toasting, mash the avocado with a fork in a small bowl. Mix in the black pepper and cilantro.
1 avocado, pitted and sliced	
1 teaspoon black pepper	
1 tablespoon fresh chopped cilantro	*2* Spread 2 tablespoons of the hummus over two of the slices of bread. Then top each slice with half of the mashed avocado.
4 tablespoons hummus (homemade or store-bought)	*3* Sprinkle the chopped cucumber over the avocado and top with a few slices of tomato. Drizzle balsamic vinegar over the tomato. Top each with a toasted slice of bread.
½ cup chopped cucumber	
1 medium tomato, sliced	
1 tablespoon balsamic vinegar	

Meal plan servings: 2 starches, 1 vegetable, 3 fats.

Per serving: Calories 345 (From Fat 158); Fat 18g (Saturated 3g); Cholesterol 0mg; Sodium 365mg; Carbohydrate 42g; Dietary Fiber 14g; Protein 11g.

Tip: For extra flavor and belly-fighting goodness, try a sprouted bread instead of whole-wheat.

Chapter 14

Deliciously Slimming Dinners

In This Chapter

▶ Understanding dinner's role in weight loss and metabolism

▶ Identifying delicious and healthy dinner options to fight belly fat

Recipes in This Chapter

↺ Whole-Grain Bruschetta Pizza

▶ Low-Calorie Chicken Parmesan

▶ Walnut-Encrusted Flounder

↺ Portobello Mushroom Salad

▶ Chicken Cordon Bleu

▶ Belly-Friendly Chicken Marsala

▶ Roasted Pork Tenderloin with Vegetables

▶ Spicy Shrimp Kabobs

▶ Herb-Roasted Salmon

↺ Sweet and Sour Tofu Stir-Fry

▶ Pepper Steak with Fresh Vegetables

▶ Reformed Spaghetti, Meatballs, and Garlic Bread

↺ Quinoa-Stuffed Eggplant

▶ Shrimp Stir-Fry

🔪 🍴 ↺ 🥄 🌶 🌿

*Y*ou've made it to the the end of the day, and so far you've done a great job sticking with your Belly Fat Diet meal plan and workout routine. Now you want to make sure you stay on track the rest of the night so you don't sabotage all your efforts. Luckily, you've come to the right place!

This chapter is filled with delicious, easy-to-make dinner options that provide you with tons of flavor without wrecking your diet plan. The recipes have no belly-bloating ingredients or additives that can make it harder to reach your weight-loss goals.

Controlling Yourself at Dinnertime

Dinner can be a great time to fill up on belly-fighting nutrients. However, you can easily undo all your hard work from earlier in the day if you aren't careful. The biggest belly-busters that commonly occur in the evening include the following:

✔ Waiting too long to eat dinner, which leads to excessive hunger and overeating

✔ Eating too fast, which results in eating too much

✔ Filling up on belly bloaters, such as saturated fats, sodium, and refined carbohydrates

✔ Eating too large of portions

By keeping these traps in mind and applying the following simple strategies, you can easily stay on track with your Belly Fat Diet at dinner:

✔ **Pile on the veggies.** Fill half your plate with belly-friendly vegetables, such as peppers, tomatoes, kale, spinach, and mushrooms. Doing so keeps you satisfied with filling fiber and gives you a great source of belly-fighting antioxidants. Check out Chapter 6 for a detailed list of vegetables from every color of the rainbow and how they help shrink your belly.

✔ **Watch added fats.** Limit the amount of cooking you do in large amounts of oils and saturated fats like butter and cream. Instead, try cooking in low-sodium broth, wine, nonfat cooking spray, and vinegars.

The recipes in this chapter often call for olive oil. This great source of monounsaturated fat is a potent belly-fat fighter. However, too much of a good thing can still be bad. Too large a portion of oils and other healthy fats can increase your caloric intake and slow weight loss efforts. So make sure to keep your portions in check.

✔ **Change up the china.** Even too large a portion of healthy foods can result in you taking in too many calories and preventing weight loss. To prevent eating too large of portions of anything, use a salad plate instead of a large dinner plate at meals.

✔ **Slow down when eating.** It takes 20 minutes for your stomach to send a signal to your brain letting you know you're satisfied. So if you eat too quickly, you may eat beyond the point of being satisfied and feel stuffed. Check out Chapter 16 for more on defending yourself against mindless eating.

✔ **Pack on the seasonings.** Dinner can be a great time to fill up on belly-fighting seasonings, such as hot peppers, turmeric, garlic, and cinnamon. This chapter provides you with lots of recipes that contain these added belly fighters. But also look at the typical recipes you make at home and think about ways you can squeeze in the additional belly-fat fighters.

✔ **Watch out for hidden belly bloaters.** Sodium, for instance, is a huge belly bloater. And dinner can be an easy meal to pack in the sodium. Sodium holds onto water and can make you look and feel bloated and puffy. So take the salt shaker off the table, and instead season foods with herbs and spices that contain little to no sodium (but lots of flavor).

Added sugars and white flour can also increase insulin response (Chapter 2 explains how this works in more detail), triggering belly-fat storage. So avoid recipes with large amounts of added sugar or refined flour, or adjust these recipes to use belly-friendly options like whole-grain flour.

✔ **Eat regularly.** If you wait too long between your last meal or snack and dinner, you're going to be too hungry. This excessive hunger causes everything from food cravings to eating too fast and eating more with your eyes than your stomach. In other words, you want to fill your plate and pack in more than your stomach needs because you're so hungry and everything looks so great! Don't let this happen to you. Make sure to stick with your regular meals and snacks throughout the day, and eat every three to four hours to prevent excessive hunger at night.

✔ **Make dinner an event.** Sit down, put your food on a plate, and really enjoy it. Take note of the tastes and textures and focus on each bite. Doing so helps you to eat slower, feel satisfied sooner, and prevent cravings right after eating. If you eat dinner in a rush, on the run, or even standing up, you won't feel satisfied, and chances are you'll be rummaging through the pantry for snacks all night. Head to Chapter 16 to read more about mindful eating.

Whole-Grain Bruschetta Pizza

Prep time: 12 min • **Cook time:** 15 min • **Yield:** 8 servings

Ingredients	Directions
¾ cup tomato paste	**1** Preheat the oven to 450 degrees.
2 tablespoons minced garlic	**2** Make the tomato sauce by bringing the tomato paste to a simmer in a small saucepan. Add the minced garlic and olive oil, and allow it to simmer for 2 minutes. Remove from the heat and set aside.
1 tablespoon olive oil	
16 ounces 100% whole-wheat pizza dough	
8 ounces sliced fresh mozzarella cheese	**3** Using a rolling pin, create a 16-inch-diameter pizza from the whole-wheat dough.
1¼ cups fresh bruschetta	
1 cup sliced mushrooms	**4** Spread the tomato sauce evenly over the dough, and then place the fresh mozzarella slices evenly over the sauce. Top the mozzarella with the bruschetta and mushrooms.
	5 Place the pizza on a pizza stone or round pan. Place in the oven, and cook for 15 minutes, or until the edges brown slightly. Slice with a pizza cutter into eight even slices.

Meal plan servings: 2 starches, 1 ounce protein, 1 vegetable, 1 fat.

Per serving: Calories 323 (From Fat 119); Fat 13g (Saturated 5g); Cholesterol 20mg; Sodium 157mg; Carbohydrate 39g; Dietary Fiber 5g; Protein 13g.

Note: You can purchase the bruschetta and whole-wheat pizza dough at most grocery stores. But, if you prefer, you can make them yourself.

Vary It! This recipe only calls for mushrooms, but you can add any toppings you want, such as green pepper, onions, and black olives.

Low-Calorie Chicken Parmesan

Prep time: 15 min • **Cook time:** 35 min • **Yield:** 4 servings

Ingredients	*Directions*
1 cup tomato paste	*1* Preheat the oven to 400 degrees.
2½ tablespoons minced garlic	
1 tablespoon olive oil	*2* Make the tomato sauce by bringing the tomato paste to a simmer in a small saucepan. Add the minced garlic and olive oil, and allow it to simmer for 2 minutes. Remove from the heat and set aside.
1 cup whole-wheat breadcrumbs	
2 tablespoons Parmesan cheese	*3* In a large bowl, mix together the whole-wheat breadcrumbs, Parmesan cheese, garlic, and basil.
1 tablespoon minced garlic	
1 tablespoon dried basil	
Four 5-ounce skinless, boneless chicken breasts	*4* Spray each chicken breast with nonstick cooking spray. Dip each breast into the breadcrumb mixture to cover, and then place into a glass casserole dish that has been sprayed with nonstick cooking spray.
Nonstick cooking spray	
1 cup shredded lowfat mozzarella cheese	*5* Pour the tomato sauce over the chicken breasts to coat evenly. Place the dish in the oven, and bake for 25 minutes.
	6 Remove the chicken from the oven and sprinkle mozzarella cheese evenly over the top of the chicken. Place it back into the oven and cook for another 10 minutes, or until it reaches an internal temperature of 165 degrees.

Meal plan servings: 5 ounces protein, 0.5 starch.

Per serving: Calories 323 (From Fat 104); Fat 12g (Saturated 4g); Cholesterol 92mg; Sodium 338mg; Carbohydrate 15g; Dietary Fiber 2g; Protein 40g.

Tip: To round out this nutritious meal, serve alongside vegetables and whole-grain pasta.

Walnut-Encrusted Flounder

Prep time: 10 min • **Cook time:** 35 min • **Yield:** 4 servings

Ingredients	*Directions*
¼ cup whole-wheat breadcrumbs	**1** Preheat the oven to 325 degrees.
½ cup walnuts, finely chopped	**2** In a large bowl, mix together the breadcrumbs, walnuts, garlic, pepper, basil, rosemary, and salt.
1 tablespoon minced garlic	
½ teaspoon black pepper	**3** Dip each fish fillet in the beaten egg whites, and then dip them into the walnut-breadcrumb mixture to evenly coat. Place the fillets onto a baking sheet greased with nonstick cooking spray or 1 tablespoon olive oil.
½ teaspoon dried basil	
½ teaspoon dried rosemary	
¼ teaspoon salt	
Four 5-ounce flounder fillets	**4** Bake the fish for 35 minutes, or until it's cooked through and flakes easily.
2 egg whites, beaten	
Nonstick spray or olive oil	

Meal plan servings: 4 ounces protein, 1 fat.

Per serving: Calories 265 (From Fat 117); Fat 13g (Saturated 2g); Cholesterol 65mg; Sodium 259mg; Carbohydrate 4g; Dietary Fiber 1g; Protein 35g.

Vary It! Feel free to experiment with other varieties of fish, such as salmon, tilapia, and cod.

Portobello Mushroom Salad

Prep time: 45 min • **Cook time:** 7 min • **Yield:** 4 servings

Ingredients	*Directions*
1 cup balsamic vinegar, divided	*1* In a large bowl, mix together ¾ cup balsamic vinegar and ¼ cup apple cider vinegar. Add the sliced mushrooms, and allow them to marinate for 30 minutes.
½ cup apple cider vinegar, divided	
4 large portobello mushroom caps, sliced	*2* While the mushrooms are marinating, prepare the cabbage, romaine, arugula, spinach, cucumber, and tomato, and then toss together in a large bowl. Set aside.
1 cup purple cabbage, shredded	
2 cups romaine lettuce	*3* Mix together the remaining ¼ cup balsamic vinegar, 1 tablespoon of the olive oil, and the remaining ¼ cup apple cider vinegar to create a salad dressing. Set aside.
2 cups arugula	
1 cup spinach	
1 medium cucumber, sliced	*4* After the mushrooms are finished marinating, place a sauté pan over medium heat and add the remaining 1 tablespoon olive oil and the minced garlic. Add the marinated mushrooms to the pan and sauté for 7 minutes, or until tender.
1 large tomato, sliced	
2 tablespoons olive oil, divided	
1 tablespoon minced garlic	
	5 Top the vegetable mix from Step 2 with the sautéed mushrooms. Top with the salad dressing and toss to evenly coat.

Meal plan servings: 2.5 vegetables, 1.5 fats.

Per serving: Calories136 (From Fat 65); Fat 7g (Saturated 1g); Cholesterol 0mg; Sodium 31mg; Carbohydrate 15g; Dietary Fiber 4g; Protein 5g.

Tip: This hearty salad is perfect for vegans, vegetarians, and veggie lovers!

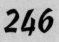

Chicken Cordon Bleu

Prep time: 10 min • **Cook time:** 30 min • **Yield:** 4 servings

Ingredients	*Directions*
Nonstick cooking spray	*1* Preheat the oven to 400 degrees. Spray a baking sheet with nonstick cooking spray.
½ cup whole-wheat breadcrumbs	
2 egg whites, beaten	*2* Place the whole-wheat breadcrumbs in a large bowl or shallow dish and the beaten eggs in a separate bowl or shallow dish.
Four 4-ounce skinless, boneless chicken breasts, pounded to ¼-inch thick	*3* Dip each chicken breast in the beaten egg, and then dip them in the breadcrumbs to evenly coat. Place the chicken on the prepared baking sheet.
4 ounces lowfat, low-sodium, thinly sliced ham	
2 ounces part-skim, low-sodium Swiss cheese	*4* Place 1 ounce of ham and ½ ounce of Swiss cheese on one end of each chicken breast.
	5 Carefully roll the chicken breasts until the ham and cheese are in the middle with the chicken wrapped completely around the outside. Secure with a toothpick if needed.
	6 Bake for 30 minutes, or until the chicken reaches an internal temperature of 165 degrees.

Meal plan servings: 4 ounces protein.

Per serving: Calories 228 (From Fat 66); Fat 7g (Saturated 3g); Cholesterol 88mg; Sodium 404mg; Carbohydrate 3g; Dietary Fiber 0g; Protein 36g.

Belly-Friendly Chicken Marsala

Prep time: 10 min • **Cook time:** 20 min • **Yield:** 6 servings

Ingredients	*Directions*
Nonstick cooking spray	*1* Spray a sauté pan with nonstick cooking spray and place over medium heat.
½ **cup whole-wheat flour**	
½ **teaspoon black pepper**	*2* Mix together the flour and black pepper in a large bowl.
Six 5-ounce skinless, boneless chicken breasts	
1 tablespoon minced garlic	*3* Dip each chicken breast into the flour mixture to evenly coat.
1 tablespoon olive oil	
¼ **cup chopped scallions**	*4* Add 1 tablespoon olive oil to the heated pan. Add the chicken and cook for 3 minutes on each side to slightly brown, and then remove from the pan.
2 cups sliced mushrooms	
½ **cup Marsala wine**	*5* In the same pan, add the garlic, scallions, and mushroom, and sauté for 2 to 3 minutes. Add the wine to the pan and cook until the wine reduces to form a glaze, about 3 to 5 minutes.
½ **cup low-sodium chicken broth**	
¼ **cup fresh parsley, or 4 teaspoons dried**	*6* Add the broth and parsley, and then allow the mixture to cook for 3 minutes.
	7 Place the chicken back into the pan, allowing it to cook for 7 to 10 minutes, or until cooked through (internal temperature should reach 165 degrees).

Meal plan servings: *4 ounces protein, 1 vegetable.*

Per serving: *Calories 203 (From Fat 34); Fat 4g (Saturated 1g); Cholesterol 79mg; Sodium 83mg; Carbohydrate 10g; Dietary Fiber 2g; Protein 31g.*

Note: Marsala wine comes in both sweet and dry varieties. Both are fine on your Belly Fat Diet plan, so choose whichever one suits your taste.

Tip: Serve with a side of fresh vegetables and whole-grain pasta to complete the meal.

Roasted Pork Tenderloin with Vegetables

Prep time: 10 min • **Cook time:** 45 min • **Yield:** 4 servings

Ingredients	*Directions*
Nonstick cooking spray	*1* Preheat the oven to 425 degrees. Spray a 9-x-13-inch pan with nonstick cooking spray.
1 tablespoon minced garlic	
1 teaspoon dried basil	*2* In a small bowl, mix together the garlic, basil, oregano, thyme, salt, and pepper. Set aside.
1 teaspoon dried oregano	
1 teaspoon dried thyme	*3* Arrange the kale (or spinach) on the bottom of the prepared pan. Place the pork tenderloin on top and arrange the sweet potatoes, carrots, and onions around the pork. Drizzle the olive oil over the pork, and then sprinkle with the seasoning mixture. Bake for 30 minutes.
1 teaspoon salt	
1 teaspoon black pepper	
2 cups fresh kale or spinach	
One 1-pound pork tenderloin	
2 medium-sized sweet potatoes, quartered	*4* Turn the pork and cover with foil. Place the pan back in the oven, and cook for an additional 15 minutes, or until the pork is cooked through (internal temperature should be 155 degrees).
2 large carrots, sliced	
2 large sweet onions, sliced	
1 tablespoon olive oil	

Meal plan servings: *4 ounces protein, 1 vegetable, 1 starch.*

Per serving: *Calories 291 (From Fat 80); Fat 9g (Saturated 2g); Cholesterol 65mg; Sodium 662mg; Carbohydrate 28g; Dietary Fiber 5g; Protein 26g.*

Tip: Pork tenderloin is a great lean-protein alternative to the standard chicken dinner, and it contains much less saturated fat than many cuts of beef.

Spicy Shrimp Kabobs

Prep time: 10 min • **Cook time:** 6 min • **Yield:** 4 servings

Ingredients	*Directions*
Nonstick cooking spray	*1* Spray the grill with nonstick cooking spray, and then bring to medium heat. If using wooden skewers, soak them in water to avoid scorching on the grill.
Wooden or metal skewers	
½ teaspoon chili powder	
⅛ teaspoon turmeric	*2* Mix the spices and olive oil in a large bowl. Add the shrimp and toss to evenly coat.
¼ teaspoon black pepper	
¼ teaspoon crushed red pepper flakes	*3* Thread the onions, bell pepper, tomato, and shrimp onto the skewers, and then place on the heated grill. Grill the kabobs for 3 minutes, and then rotate and cook for another 2 to 3 minutes, or until the shrimp are cooked through and the vegetables are tender.
⅛ teaspoon garlic powder	
⅛ teaspoon onion powder	
¼ teaspoon ground cumin	
¼ teaspoon salt	
⅛ teaspoon paprika	
⅛ teaspoon dried oregano	
1 tablespoon olive oil	
16 ounces raw shrimp, peeled, deveined, rinsed, and patted dry	
1 large sweet onion, cut into eighths	
2 large bell peppers, cut into 1-inch pieces	
2 large tomatoes, cut into 1-inch pieces	

Meal plan servings: 1 vegetable, 4 ounces protein.

Per serving: Calories 165 (From Fat 44); Fat 5g (Saturated 1g); Cholesterol 168mg; Sodium 352mg; Carbohydrate 11g; Dietary Fiber 3g; Protein 20g.

Vary It! If you don't want to grill out, you can cook the skewers in a pan over medium heat for 10 minutes (rotating halfway through). Be sure to spray the pan with nonstick cooking spray before cooking.

Herb-Roasted Salmon

Prep time: 15 min • **Cook time:** 25 min • **Yield:** 4 servings

Ingredients	Directions
2 tablespoons lemon juice, divided	**1** Preheat the oven to 400 degrees.
2 tablespoons apple cider vinegar	**2** In a small bowl, mix together 1 tablespoon lemon juice, the vinegar, and the olive oil. Using a basting brush, coat each salmon fillet with a small amount of the olive oil mixture.
1½ tablespoons olive oil	
Four 4-ounce salmon fillets	
1 tablespoon dried basil	**3** Cut four pieces of foil into 8-x-8-inch squares. Place the oiled side of the salmon down on the foil.
1 tablespoon onion flakes	
1 tablespoon dried oregano	**4** In another small bowl, mix together all the seasonings. Sprinkle the seasoning mixture evenly on top of each fillet. Drizzle the remaining 1 tablespoon lemon juice over each fillet.
1 teaspoon black pepper	
1 teaspoon turmeric	
½ teaspoon garlic powder	
½ teaspoon finely grated lemon zest	**5** Fold the sides of the foil over so each fillet is completely sealed in its own foil packet. Place the packets on a baking sheet, and bake for about 25 minutes, or until the salmon is cooked through and flakes easily.

Meal plan servings: *4 ounces protein, 1 fat.*

Per serving: *Calories 244 (From Fat 116); Fat 13g (Saturated 2g); Cholesterol 72mg; Sodium 58mg; Carbohydrate 4g; Dietary Fiber 1g; Protein 26g.*

Tip: Add a side of belly-fighting steamed veggies and some whole-grain rice for a complete meal.

Sweet and Sour Tofu Stir-Fry

Prep time: 10 min • **Cook time:** 12 min • **Yield:** 4 servings

Ingredients	Directions
1 tablespoon olive oil	**1** Heat the olive oil in a large sauté pan or wok over medium heat.
½ cup pineapple juice	
2 tablespoons apple cider vinegar	**2** In a small bowl, whisk together the pineapple juice, vinegars, mustard, tomato paste, brown sugar, and cornstarch to create the sweet and sour sauce. Set aside.
1 tablespoon red wine vinegar	
2 tablespoons mustard	
4 tablespoons low-sodium tomato paste	**3** Add the broccoli, onion, bell peppers, mushrooms, and garlic to the heated pan and stir-fry for 3 minutes.
1 tablespoon brown sugar	
1 teaspoon cornstarch	
2 cups bite-sized broccoli florets	**4** Add the tofu to the pan along with the vegetables and stir-fry for 4 minutes, or until the tofu is golden brown.
1 medium onion, chopped	
1 red bell pepper, sliced	**5** Pour in the sweet and sour sauce and cook, stirring constantly, for another 3 to 5 minutes, or until the sauce slightly thickens.
1 green bell pepper, sliced	
1 cup sliced mushrooms	
1½ teaspoons minced garlic	**6** Place ¾ cup of brown rice onto four individual plates. Top with ¼ of the stir fry.
One 16-ounce package firm tofu, drained and cut into cubes	
3 cups cooked brown rice	

Meal plan servings: 1.5 vegetables, 2 ounces protein, 3 starches.

Per serving: Calories 353 (From Fat 86); Fat 10g (Saturated 1g); Cholesterol 0mg; Sodium 228mg; Carbohydrate 57g; Dietary Fiber 6g; Protein 15g.

Pepper Steak with Fresh Vegetables

Prep time: 10 min • **Cook time:** 17 min • **Yield:** 2 servings

Ingredients	*Directions*
1 tablespoon olive oil 1 cup sliced mushrooms	*1* Set your oven to broil, and heat the olive oil in a large sauté pan over medium heat.
1 medium sweet onion, sliced One 8-ounce flank steak	*2* Add the mushrooms and onions to the pan, and sauté for 5 to 7 minutes, or until tender. Remove from the pan and keep warm.
Steak Seasoning (see the following recipe) 4 cups chopped kale 1 teaspoon minced garlic	*3* Place the steak on a broiler pan, and season the top of it with half the Steak Seasoning. Place the steak in the oven near the broiler for 5 minutes.
¼ cup low-sodium vegetable broth	*4* Remove the steak from the oven, flip it, add the remaining seasoning on top, and place back in the oven for 3 to 5 minutes, or until it reaches desired doneness.
	5 While the steak is broiling, add the kale, garlic, and vegetable broth to the sauté pan used to cook the mushrooms and onions. Cover, and allow to simmer for 5 minutes.
	6 Remove the lid on the kale and cook over medium heat until most of the liquid has evaporated.
	7 After the steak is done, arrange the cooked kale evenly on two separate plates. Top with half of the cooked steak. Top the steak with the cooked mushrooms and onions.

Steak Seasoning

1 tablespoon black pepper

1 teaspoon sea salt

1 tablespoon crushed red pepper

1 tablespoon onion flakes

1 teaspoon garlic powder

½ teaspoon ground cumin

½ teaspoon cayenne pepper

2 teaspoons paprika

1 In a small bowl, mix together the black pepper, salt, red pepper, onion flakes, garlic powder, cumin, cayenne pepper, and paprika.

Meal plan servings: 2 vegetables, 4 ounces protein, 1 fat.

Per serving: Calories 366 (From Fat 160); Fat 18g (Saturated 5g); Cholesterol 54mg; Sodium 1,409mg; Carbohydrate 28g; Dietary Fiber 7g; Protein 30g.

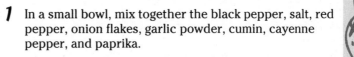

Reformed Spaghetti, Meatballs, and Garlic Bread

Prep time: 10 min • **Cook time:** 20 min • **Yield:** 4 servings

Ingredients	Directions
2 cups tomato paste	*1* Make the tomato sauce by bringing the tomato paste to a simmer in a small saucepan. Add 4 tablespoons minced garlic and 1 tablespoon olive oil, and allow the sauce to simmer for 2 minutes. Remove from the heat.
7 tablespoons minced garlic, divided	
3 tablespoons olive oil, divided	*2* In a large bowl, blend together the ground turkey, breadcrumbs, 2 tablespoons garlic, 2 tablespoons Parmesan cheese, onion, salt, and pepper. Create eight evenly sized meatballs from the mixture.
1 pound ground turkey breast meat	
½ cup whole-wheat breadcrumbs	
6 tablespoons Parmesan cheese, divided	*3* Heat 1 tablespoon of the olive oil in a large sauté pan over medium heat. Add the meatballs, and cook for about 15 minutes, or until the outside of the meatballs is brown and slightly crusted, turning every few minutes.
⅓ cup minced onion	
¾ teaspoon salt	
¼ teaspoon black pepper	*4* While the meatballs are cooking, place the bread slices on a baking sheet and heat the broiler.
4 slices 100% whole-grain bread	
3 cups cooked 100% whole-grain pasta	*5* Sprinkle 1 tablespoon of the Parmesan cheese and 1 tablespoon of the garlic over the slices of bread. Drizzle with 1 tablespoon of the olive oil. Toast in the oven near the broiler for 3 minutes, or until crispy.
	6 Place 1½ cups of the cooked pasta on each plate. Top each plate with ½ cup of sauce, two meatballs, a sprinkling of the remaining Parmesan cheese, and a slice of garlic bread.

Meal plan servings: *3 starches, 4 ounces protein, 1 fat.*

Per serving: *Calories 639 (From Fat 166); Fat 18g (Saturated 4g); Cholesterol 100mg; Sodium 850mg; Carbohydrate 68g; Dietary Fiber 10g; Protein 53g.*

Quinoa-Stuffed Eggplant

Prep time: 25 min • **Cook time:** 50 min • **Yield:** 2 servings

Ingredients	Directions
1 large eggplant ½ cup quinoa 1 cup water 2½ tablespoons olive oil, divided 1 medium sweet onion, chopped 1 red bell pepper, chopped 2 cups fresh spinach 2 tablespoons minced garlic, divided ½ cup grated Parmesan cheese, divided ½ cup part-skim ricotta cheese 1 teaspoon black pepper 3 tablespoons chopped basil 2 tablespoons chopped parsley 1 teaspoon dried oregano 1 medium tomato, chopped ¼ cup tomato paste Nonstick cooking spray	*1* Preheat the oven to 350 degrees. Cut the eggplant in half lengthwise, and scoop out the center. Leave about ¼ inch of eggplant inside the skin. *2* In a small saucepan, mix together the quinoa and water and bring to a boil. Reduce the heat to low, cover, and simmer for 15 minutes. Remove the quinoa from the heat. Let it sit for 5 minutes, and fluff with a fork. *3* While the quinoa is cooking, heat 1 tablespoon of the olive oil in a medium sauté pan. Add the scooped-out eggplant, onion, bell pepper, spinach, and 1 tablespoon garlic, and sauté for 5 minutes, or until tender. *4* In a large bowl, mix together the sautéed vegetables, ¼ cup of the Parmesan cheese, ricotta cheese, prepared quinoa, black pepper, basil, parsley, and oregano. *5* Stuff the hollowed eggplant halves with the vegetable mixture, and top with the chopped tomato. Set aside. *6* Make the tomato sauce by bringing the tomato paste to a simmer in a small saucepan. Add 1 tablespoon minced garlic and ½ tablespoon olive oil, and allow the sauce to simmer for 2 minutes. Remove from the heat. *7* Pour the tomato sauce evenly over the eggplant halves. Sprinkle with the remaining ¼ cup Parmesan cheese, and drizzle the remaining 1 tablespoon of the olive oil on top. *8* Place the eggplant halves in a baking dish that has been sprayed with nonstick cooking spray, and bake for 50 minutes.

Meal plan servings: *3 vegetables, 3 ounces protein, 2 starches, 4 fats.*

Per serving: *Calories 632 (From Fat 271); Fat 30g (Saturated 9g); Cholesterol 35mg; Sodium 532mg; Carbohydrate 69g; Dietary Fiber 13g; Protein 28g.*

Shrimp Stir-Fry

Prep time: 30 min • **Cook time:** 15 min • **Yield:** 4 servings

Ingredients	*Directions*
16 ounces shrimp, peeled, deveined, rinsed, and patted dry	*1* Place the shrimp, black pepper, salt, cayenne pepper, ginger, and 2 tablespoons of the teriyaki sauce into a small bowl. Toss together and cover. Marinate in the fridge for 20 minutes.
¼ teaspoon black pepper	
¼ teaspoon sea salt	
¼ teaspoon cayenne pepper	*2* While the shrimp is marinating, heat the sesame oil in a large sauté pan or wok over high heat.
¼ teaspoon ground ginger	
3 tablespoons low-sodium teriyaki sauce, divided	*3* Add the mushrooms, garlic, broccoli, scallions, and bell peppers to the pan and sauté for 5 minutes, or until the vegetables are tender.
2 tablespoons sesame oil	
1 cup sliced mushrooms	
1 tablespoon minced garlic	*4* Add the remaining 1 tablespoon of teriyaki sauce, edamame, sesame and chia seeds, and the shrimp with marinade to the pan. Cook, stirring occasionally, for 5 minutes, or until the shrimp are opaque in color.
1 cup chopped broccoli	
1 cup chopped scallions	
1 yellow bell pepper, chopped	
1 red bell pepper, chopped	*5* Continue stirring, and add in the broth and cornstarch. Allow the mixture to come to a boil, and then remove from heat.
1 cup shelled edamame	
1 tablespoon sesame seeds	
1 tablespoon chia seeds	*6* Portion the cooked rice onto four plates. Top each with ¼ of the shrimp stir-fry.
¾ cup low-sodium chicken or vegetable broth	
2 teaspoons cornstarch	
3 cups cooked brown rice	

Per serving: 1 vegetable, 5 ounces protein, 2.5 starches, 2 fats.

Per serving: Calories 452 (From Fat 118); Fat 13g (Saturated 2g); Cholesterol 169mg; Sodium 588mg; Carbohydrate 54g; Dietary Fiber 9g; Protein 30g.

Tip: Chia seeds can be found in the organic/health food section of many grocery stores or in most natural food stores. If you can't find chia seeds or don't want to include them, you can substitute flaxseed.

Vary It! This recipe is so versatile! Instead of shrimp, you can make it with tofu, chicken, or even beans.

Chapter 15

Desserts and Snacks

- -

In This Chapter

▶ Understanding the importance of regularly snacking throughout the day

▶ Identifying delicious and easy dessert and snack options to fight belly fat

- -

Recipes in This Chapter

↺ Baked Apples

↺ Mock Ice Cream Sandwiches

↺ Crunchy Peanut Butter Banana Bites

↺ Chocolate-Drizzled Strawberries

↺ Homemade Spicy Microwave Popcorn

↺ Belly-Blasting Trail Mix

↺ Easy Pizza Bites

*W*ho doesn't love dessert or a decadent snack? Luckily, just because you're trying to lose weight, doesn't mean you have to give up these treats. In fact, I want you to have them often! You won't be able to stay on track with your Belly Fat Diet plan if you get too hungry or aren't enjoying the food you're eating. So throughout this chapter, I explain how to enjoy sweet and delicious desserts and show you the best snacks for keeping hunger away while still shrinking your belly!

Desserts and Snacks: They Aren't Evil!

Desserts are an important part of your Belly Fat Diet plan. However, you probably think that they're something you need to avoid. After all, maybe desserts caused your belly fat accumulation in the first place. But, lucky for you, the recipes in this chapter aren't just any desserts. These desserts can satisfy your sweet tooth while actually helping eliminate belly fat (instead of typical desserts, which can store more!). These desserts are just as delicious as the average unhealthy versions and are actually good for your belly.

Snacking on a regular basis is also a vital part of your success with the Belly Fat Diet. Eating small, frequent meals and snacks helps prevent dips in blood sugar, which can not only decrease your energy level but also cause pesky cravings.

The key to losing weight and keeping it off successfully is to prevent hunger. Think about the last time you let yourself get too hungry. You probably started craving high-sugar or high-fat foods. Without being psychic, it's a pretty safe bet to say you weren't craving lettuce and carrots. (If you were, that's great!). Getting too hungry tends to bring on cravings for less-than-healthy foods that can sabotage your belly-flattening efforts. To prevent side-lining your efforts, you have to act before the cravings start. That's where snacking comes in! The goal of a snack is to help carry you from one meal to the next without becoming overly hungry.

I recommend not waiting longer than three to four hours in between a meal or snack. Depending on your schedule, the number of snacks you need may vary. Your snacks should be filling and should contain a large percentage of fiber, lean protein, or healthy fat. These nutrients help slow digestion, allowing you to feel satisfied longer and keep nagging hunger and cravings in check.

Don't panic if you think you don't have time to snack or don't know what to snack on. This chapter shows you quick and easy snack options you can enjoy daily. Whether you prefer a sweet snack, a crunchy snack, or something cheesy, you'll find a snack that suits your fancy.

Your Belly Fat Diet plan really isn't a diet at all. It's a lifestyle change (check out Chapter 4 for more information on how to view your plan as a lifestyle rather than a diet). When you're making any lifestyle changes, you have to be able to implement them for life. So you have to be flexible and realistic. And it isn't realistic to never have desserts and snacks. In fact, the more you avoid desserts and snacks, the more likely you'll crave them. And cravings are exactly what you're trying to avoid.

Baked Apples

Prep time: 3 min • **Cook time:** 10–15 min • **Yield:** 4 servings

Ingredients	*Directions*
4 large apples, cored, peeled, and sliced (any variety) **3 tablespoons cinnamon** **1 tablespoon pure maple syrup**	*1* Preheat the oven to 350 degrees. Place the sliced apples in an oven-safe glass pan or dish and top with cinnamon and maple syrup.
	2 Bake for 10 to 15 minutes (or microwave for 5 minutes on high power).
	3 The apples should be tender. If they're still firm, bake for 3 to 5 additional minutes in the oven (or 1 to 2 minutes in the microwave).

Meal plan servings: 1 fruit.

Per serving: Calories 124 (From Fat 6); Fat 1g (Saturated 0g); Cholesterol 0mg; Sodium 2mg; Carbohydrate 33g; Dietary Fiber 6g; Protein 1g.

Vary It! Top apples with lowfat whipped cream and, for an added belly-flattening bonus, chopped walnuts.

Note: Don't worry about the maple syrup botching your diet. You're only using a small amount, which adds flavor and texture with a minimal blood sugar and insulin response. Aim for pure maple syrup versus brands with high-fructose corn syrup, which may trigger a larger insulin response.

Mock Ice Cream Sandwiches

Prep time: 15 min • **Chill time:** 15–20 min • **Yield:** 6 sandwiches

Ingredients	Directions
12 graham cracker squares	*1* On a cookie sheet or shallow pan, lay out six of the graham cracker squares. Spread each with 1½ tablespoons of the pudding.
Homemade Sugar-Free, Lowfat Chocolate Pudding (see the following recipe)	*2* Layer each with 2 tablespoons of the whipped cream.
¾ cup lowfat whipped cream	*3* Add another layer of 1½ teaspoons of the pudding to each cracker.
	4 Place another graham cracker square on top of each to create sandwiches.
	5 Place the pan in the freezer for about 15 to 20 minutes, allowing the pudding and whipped cream to harden.

Homemade Sugar-Free, Lowfat Chocolate Pudding

1 tablespoon cornstarch	*1* Heat a saucepan over medium heat. Mix together the cornstarch, sugar substitute, cocoa powder, and salt, and add to the saucepan.
¼ cup sugar substitute	
¼ cup cocoa powder	*2* While stirring, slowly add the milk. Cook and stir continuously for 2 to 3 minutes, or until the mixture thickens.
A pinch of salt	
1 cup fat-free milk	*3* Add the beaten egg yolk to the saucepan and stir. Bring the mixture to a boil for 1 minute.
1 egg yolk, beaten	
1 teaspoon vanilla extract	*4* Remove the pan from the heat and stir in the vanilla. Allow the pudding to chill for at least 10 minutes.

Meal plan servings: 1 starch.

Per serving: Calories 89 (From Fat 28); Fat 3g (Saturated 2g); Cholesterol 36mg; Sodium 163mg; Carbohydrate 13g; Dietary Fiber 1g; Protein 3g.

Note: This pudding recipe makes three dessert-sized servings if you want to eat it in a bowl rather than in a sandwich.

Tip: If you're short on time, you may use sugar-free premade pudding from your grocery store. And keep in mind that whole-grain graham crackers are the best option for this recipe.

Crunchy Peanut Butter Banana Bites

Prep time: 10 min • **Chill time:** 60 min • **Yield:** 4 servings

Ingredients	Directions
1 cup 100% whole-grain oats 2 medium bananas 3 tablespoons natural peanut butter	*1* Place the oats in a resealable plastic bag and zip closed. Using a rolling pin, roll over the bag of oats until the oats are small crumbs.
	2 Slice each banana into small, quarter-sized pieces about ½ inch thick. Smear a small coating of peanut butter onto each side of the banana pieces.
	3 Add the peanut butter-coated banana pieces to the plastic bag, and then shake until each piece is coated with the oat crumbs.
	4 Place the coated banana pieces on a plate covered with wax paper. Freeze for 1 hour.

Meal plan servings: 1 fruit, 0.5 starch, 1 fat.

Per serving: Calories 207 (From Fat 65); Fat 7g (Saturated 1g); Cholesterol 0mg; Sodium 46mg; Carbohydrate 31g; Dietary Fiber 5g; Protein 6g.

Vary It! If you'd like, you can skip the freezer and serve immediately at room temperature.

Chocolate-Drizzled Strawberries

Prep time: 10 min • **Cook time:** 5 min, plus 15 min chill time • **Yield:** 7 servings

Ingredients	*Directions*
2 pounds fresh strawberries **¾ cup 70% dark chocolate chips**	**1** Rinse and dry the strawberries, keeping the leaves and stems intact. Cover a plate with wax paper and arrange the strawberries on top.
	2 In a small saucepan, melt the chocolate chips over low heat until they become liquid, about 3 to 5 minutes.
	3 Carefully pour the liquid chocolate into a small, plastic pastry bag or a resealable plastic bag. If using a resealable bag, make a very small cut at the corner of the bag's tip with scissors (or use a skewer to poke a small hole).
	4 Gently squeeze the bag to lightly drizzle the dark chocolate over the strawberries.
	5 Evenly distribute the chocolate over the strawberries, and then allow to cool and harden in the refrigerator for about 15 minutes.

Meal plan servings: *1 fruit, 0.5 starch.*

Per serving: *Calories 115 (From Fat 43); Fat 5g (Saturated 3g); Cholesterol 0mg; Sodium 2mg; Carbohydrate 20g; Dietary Fiber 4g; Protein 1g.*

Note: Be sure to use dark chocolate, which is filled with health-boosting flavonoids that help to decrease inflammation and boost heart health.

Homemade Spicy Microwave Popcorn

Prep time: 5 min • **Cook time:** 3–4 min • **Yield:** 1 serving

Ingredients	*Directions*
4 tablespoons popcorn kernels	*1* Place the popcorn kernels inside a brown paper lunch bag. Fold down the top of the bag about three to four times (use small folds).
½ teaspoon chili powder	
⅛ teaspoon turmeric	
¼ teaspoon black pepper	*2* Lay the bag on its side in the microwave, and cook on high for 3 to 4 minutes, depending on your microwave settings. When the popping sounds begin to slow, stop microwaving.
¼ teaspoon crushed red pepper flakes	
⅛ teaspoon garlic powder	
⅛ teaspoon onion powder	*3* While the popcorn is popping, combine the chili powder, turmeric, black pepper, red pepper flakes, garlic powder, onion powder, cumin, salt, paprika, and oregano in a small bowl to create the seasoning.
¼ teaspoon ground cumin	
¼ teaspoon salt	
⅛ teaspoon paprika	*4* When the popcorn is done, carefully remove the bag from the microwave, pour into a bowl (watch the steam when you open), spray lightly with cooking spray, and top with the seasoning.
⅛ teaspoon dried oregano	
Nonstick cooking spray	

Meal plan servings: 2.5 starches.

Per serving: Calories 120 (From Fat 30); Fat 3g (Saturated 1g); Cholesterol 0mg; Sodium 599mg; Carbohydrate 53g; Dietary Fiber 11g; Protein 8g.

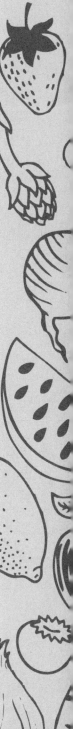

Belly-Blasting Trail Mix

Prep time: 3 min • **Yield:** 8 servings

Ingredients	*Directions*
4 cups high-fiber cereal	**1** In a large bowl, mix together the cereal, peanuts, almonds, dried fruit, and chocolate chips. Store the trail mix in an airtight container.
¼ cup halved unsalted peanuts	
¼ cup sliced unsalted almonds	
½ cup dried cranberries	
½ cup dried blueberries	
4 tablespoons dark chocolate chips (at least 70% cocoa)	

Meal plan servings: 1 starch, 0.5 fruit, 2 fats.

Per serving: Calories 190 (From Fat 58); Fat 7g (Saturated 2g); Cholesterol 0mg; Sodium 131mg; Carbohydrate 44g; Dietary Fiber 17g; Protein 5g.

Tip: This high-fiber, antioxidant-rich mix provides belly-burning monounsaturated fats and is perfect for portioning out into separate containers for an easy, on-the-go snack.

Note: You can use any high-fiber cereal you enjoy. Just make sure it has at least 5 grams of fiber and less than 10 grams of sugar per serving. Fiber One 80 is a favorite of mine as well as Kashi Go Lean Original Cereal and Kellogg's All-Bran.

Easy Pizza Bites

Prep time: 3 min • **Cook time:** 1½ min (microwave), 6–8 min (oven) • **Yield:** 4 servings

Ingredients	*Directions*
2 whole-grain English muffins ½ cup tomato sauce 4 ounces shredded part-skim mozzarella cheese	*1* Open each English muffin, place the four halves on a microwave-safe dish, and evenly cover each of them with the tomato sauce and mozzarella cheese.
	2 Microwave for 90 seconds, or until the cheese melts (or bake in a 400-degree oven for 6 to 8 minutes, or until the muffin edges are slightly browned and crisp).
	3 Cut the English muffin into quarters, and serve as bite-sized pizza snacks.

Meal plan servings: 1 starch, 1 ounce protein.

Per serving: Calories 149 (From Fat 47); Fat 5g (Saturated 3g); Cholesterol 16mg; Sodium 529mg; Carbohydrate 16g; Dietary Fiber 3g; Protein 10g.

Note: You can freeze the halves and reheat as a quick snack option anytime! Frozen bites may need to be microwaved a bit longer (2 minutes), but don't overcook or the cheese may become rubbery.

Tip: To get some extra belly-burning veggies into your snack, top your "pizzas" with toppings like mushrooms, onions, or hot peppers.

Part IV

Overcoming Obstacles and Managing Your Progress

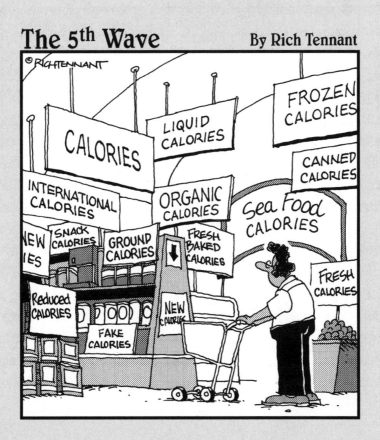

The 5th Wave By Rich Tennant

In this part . . .

I show you the most common pitfalls and challenges you may encounter and exactly how to handle them so you don't get off track with your Belly Fat Diet plan. I even show you how to follow the plan with specific dietary restrictions, such as vegan or vegetarian eating.

And because one of the most difficult parts of losing weight is keeping it off long-term, I devote a large part of this section to explaining weight maintenance. I give you a detailed plan to prevent weight gain and keep your belly flat permanently.

Chapter 16

Common Pitfalls and Challenges

I'm sure you've started out with the best of intentions with your Belly Fat Diet plan, but it isn't unusual to get off track at times. When you're trying to lose weight and make healthy lifestyle changes, many pitfalls and challenges can present themselves along the way. In order to stay on track and not lose sight of your goals, you need to consider upfront the obstacles you may face while on your weight loss journey. By identifying what challenges may come along and developing a strategy to address these obstacles in advance, you can achieve your long-term weight loss goals much easier.

Throughout this chapter, I introduce common issues you may come across that can throw you off track. I help you understand why these challenges occur and the best ways to address them so you can continue with your long-term weight loss and health goals.

Your Belly Fat Diet plan is a lifestyle plan, not a fad diet to go on and off. Fad diets may help you lose weight quickly, but you'll likely gain it all back (plus some) just as quickly. Because the Belly Fat Diet is a lifestyle plan, not just a "diet," you must remember that slip-ups can and will happen — and they're okay. When a slip-up occurs, try to simply accept that it happened and get back on track with your healthy lifestyle at the next meal or the next day. If you let one slip-up get you down and give up, you'll start to gain weight back. But one bad day, or even one bad week, won't undo all your hard work. Just pick right back up where you left off. And don't forget to ask yourself what caused you to get off track and what can you do to prevent it next time.

Managing Your Appetite and Controlling Cravings

One of the main reasons most people get off track with their weight loss efforts is due to cravings. If you constantly desire fatty and sugary foods, it can be hard to always resist them. At a certain point, you may break down and give in. If this breakdown happens occasionally, it's not a problem. However, if it happens every few days, it can certainly impact your weight loss efforts and your health.

But how do you know when you're truly having a craving? Everyone gets passing desires for certain foods now and again. But a craving is typically when you desire the same food or type of food very strongly on a regular basis. For instance, a strong yearning every day at 4 p.m. for something sweet would be considered a food craving.

Cravings and spikes in appetite can occur for a number of reasons. Some of the most common reasons include

- ✔ Emotional cravings
- ✔ Eating foods that trigger cravings
- ✔ Slight dehydration
- ✔ Allowing yourself to become too hungry
- ✔ Dips and spikes in blood sugar levels
- ✔ Seeing, smelling, or hearing about certain foods

Consider whether you experience food cravings. What foods or types of foods do you tend to crave the most? To help you manage your appetite and fight these food cravings, you need to determine the cause. Is it emotional? Do you want food because you're waiting too long to eat? Are you experiencing cravings because you aren't making the right food choices? Your cravings may be caused by one of these reasons or a combination of these reasons. The following sections take an in-depth look at these causes so you can see why you're experiencing them and how to manage them.

Feeding your emotions

Have you ever been so stressed you needed to have something crunchy to calm yourself down? Or maybe you were so upset that the only thing that could cheer you up is the gallon of ice cream in the freezer? If so, you've experienced cravings related to emotions.

Considering certain foods "comfort foods" is quite common. If you get upset, stressed, or anxious, you may often seek out comfort in the form of your favorite foods. When you indulge in comfort foods infrequently, it isn't too big of a deal. However, many people indulge on a regular basis, thus sidelining their weight loss efforts. The following sections help you figure out which emotions are causing you to eat and what you can do besides eating to deal with these emotions.

Recognizing triggers of emotional eating

Emotional eating occurs at different times for everyone. It may occur at night when you're relaxed. It may happen at work due to increased stress. You need to recognize what times of day you eat for reasons other than hunger. After you recognize when your particular emotional eating happens, you can start to realize why it happens.

Some of the most common emotions that drive folks to eat include

- ✔ Boredom
- ✔ Depression
- ✔ Excitement
- ✔ Frustration
- ✔ Loneliness
- ✔ Nervousness
- ✔ Stress

Which of these emotions, or combinations of them, drives you to eat? Think about the emotions you've experienced over the past few days. Were you stressed out? Upset? Very happy? Did you notice a link between what you did or didn't want to eat and the emotions you were feeling? Start monitoring your response, hunger, and food desires based on your emotions, and you may be surprised at the patterns you find.

Keep track of the emotions that trigger food cravings by keeping a journal of what you're eating, the emotions you're feeling, and the cravings you experience. When you keep track of this information, it's easy to pinpoint the emotions that lead to cravings.

To help you identify the emotions that drive you to eat for reasons other than hunger, ask yourself the following questions:

- ✔ Are there certain times of day that I eat when I'm not truly hungry? If so, when are those times?
- ✔ What emotions am I feeling when I eat at these times?

✔ If I eat when I'm not hungry, does this snacking cause me to feel guilty? Does the guilt lead to me eating more?

✔ Do I grab any food that's available or within my sight when I'm emotional?

Think about a time when you went through an entire day without displaying any emotional eating behaviors. What was different about this day than other days? When you felt emotional, what prevented you from reaching for food? What can you do differently on days when you do eat for emotional reasons to help you mirror the day when you didn't?

Creating healthy behaviors to manage emotions

Emotional eating, whether it's due to anxiety, stress, boredom, or excitement, is a learned behavior that becomes a habit. The best way to decrease this behavior is to replace the bad habit with a healthier one. After you recognize the emotions that trigger you to eat, brainstorm ways to deal with these emotions that don't involve food. After you distract yourself from emotional eating with other activities on a regular basis, these activities become a habit and the emotional eating behavior resolves.

Write down the emotional triggers in your daily life that lead you to eat. Then consider some factors or healthy nonfood behaviors that prevent you from emotional eating. For instance, does a brisk walk help clear your mind and get rid of the stress during the day? Does a hot bath allow you to relax at night? Does calling a friend help lift your spirits when you're feeling sad? If so, write these factors down and figure out how you can incorporate them more often to help deter you from eating emotionally. The next time you're experiencing one of these emotions, you can reference this list. The more you can replace emotional eating with a healthy habit that decreases your emotions, the better handle you'll have on emotional eating.

Eating foods that increase cravings

Eating certain foods can bring on strong cravings. For instance, have you ever been in the mood for a sugary food, like candy, had a little bit, and then suddenly wanted a very large amount of the food? If so, you're not alone!

Sugary foods digest rapidly, causing large spikes and drops in both blood sugar and insulin levels. When you eat a food that's high in sugar, your body releases additional insulin to help transport this sugar into your cells. When the extra insulin is then circulating throughout your body, your brain gets the message that you need more sugar and, voilà, you get sugar cravings!

Salty cravings can happen in a similar way. Not only can salt bloat your belly, but it can also make you want to eat more. When you consume a diet high in salt, your taste buds actually become dulled to the taste. As a result, you need to eat that much more sodium for it to taste salty to your tongue, which can cause a pattern of increased salt cravings and increased food and salt intake over time. The good news is that once you decrease your salt intake (and can now taste and enjoy the other flavors food has to offer), your taste buds become sensitive to salt again. In fact, if you go back to eating salty foods you used to enjoy, they may actually taste too salty for your liking.

Here's how to manage cravings caused by choosing the wrong foods:

✔ **Follow the Belly Fat Diet plan.** This plan should help to quash cravings because you'll be avoiding the foods that trigger cravings and consuming foods that help to keep you satisfied. Foods rich in simple sugars, refined carbohydrates, and sodium can increase the cravings you're experiencing. So instead select fresh, whole foods, switch from refined grains to whole grains, and limit foods high in sodium.

✔ **Avoid adding sodium to foods, such as by using the salt shaker at meals.** Instead, select sodium-free seasonings that add tons of flavor but won't increase cravings and belly bloat.

✔ **Get yourself in the mood to eat healthy.** Involve your senses by looking at images of healthy recipes. Or try visiting a farmer's market where you can see, touch, and even smell large amounts of fresh produce. Also, consider watching a healthy cooking show. Before you know it, you'll be craving delicious cooked vegetables.

✔ **Occasionally indulge in your favorites.** If a craving continues to linger on day after day, it's alright to occasionally indulge in the craving to satisfy yourself. However, when indulging, portions do matter. Take just a small piece of the food you desire (the size of a deck of cards or smaller) and eat it very slowly, thoroughly enjoying each bite. Treating yourself every once in a while can be a good way to combat daily cravings.

Becoming too hungry or dehydrated

When you notice you want to eat, is this yearning due to hunger? The most common cause of an increased appetite — your desire for food — is waiting too long in between meals, which can lead to excessive hunger. When you get too hungry, you tend to want many things.

Your body is programmed so that when you're hungry you get a signal that tells you to stop and eat. If you ignore this signal too long, your body increases the signal, which makes you want food, to protect you from starving. What's even worse is that once you finally stop to eat, you're excessively hungry, so you may grab whatever is lying around instead of choosing the healthiest options. You may also find yourself eating too fast, which can lead to overeating.

You can keep your appetite in check by doing the following:

- ✔ **Make sure to eat every three to four hours and avoid skipping meals and snacks.** Eat breakfast within one to two hours of waking up, and have a small snack or light meal at the beginning signs of hunger. Be careful that you aren't eating less than you should be. You need to meet all your meal plan goals each day on your Belly Fat Diet plan. Try incorporating lean protein and vegetables at each meal to help you stay satisfied for a longer period of time.

- ✔ **Watch your fluid intake.** If you haven't waited too long in between meals and are still struggling with cravings, try drinking 8 to 16 ounces of water. If, after waiting about 10 minutes, the cravings are gone or are a lot weaker, you were probably just thirsty. When you're slightly dehydrated, your body can have a difficult time deciphering hunger from thirst. So drink at least 64 ounces of fluid per day and space it out during the day to help combat cravings.

Giving Eating the Attention It Deserves

Have you ever sat down on the couch with a bag of chips while watching TV only to look down later and wonder where all the chips went? If so, you've experienced mindless eating, which is eating without paying attention. In this example, you're distracted by the television and don't even realize that you continue to eat chip after chip until they all disappear. The main problem with mindless eating is that you're ignoring your body's hunger and fullness cues when eating this way. When you ignore these cues, you eat too quickly, eat too much, and regret it later.

Also, when you eat while distracted, you don't really get a chance to enjoy the food. You don't notice the taste or texture; you're just shoveling it in. And when you don't pay attention to what you're eating, you aren't satisfied (even though you're no longer hungry) because you didn't savor your food or enjoy it in any way. When you aren't satisfied, chances are you'll crave and take in more food.

I don't know a single person who hasn't eaten mindlessly at times. With busy schedules, constant distractions, working lunches, and so on, it's bound to happen. But the more it happens, the more unaware you really are about what you're eating, leading you to take in more calories than you need and slowing your weight loss progress. The following sections look at the most common causes of mindless eating so you can recognize and avoid them.

Recognizing mindless eating

Spotting mindless eating after the fact is pretty easy. But to limit it, you need to recognize the situations that increase your risk of mindless eating so you can prevent it all together.

Some of the most common reasons for mindless eating include

- Focusing on distractions, such as the TV or computer, rather than on your food.

- Eating with your eyes rather than your stomach. (People who try to clean their plates rather than just eat until satisfied are guilty of this mindless eating.)

- Picking or grazing on foods throughout the day instead of sitting and focusing on meals and snacks.

- Speed eating, where you eat too fast, not allowing yourself to really taste and enjoy your food.

- Sitting in front of a large bowl of chips or a tray of appetizers at a social event. (This triggers mindless munching, where you eat food just because it's there and in front of you.)

See Chapter 17 for solutions on how to address mindless eating when attending social gatherings and events.

Eating mindfully every day

The focus of mindful eating isn't so much on what you're actually eating; it's more on why and how you're eating. If you're being mindful and really listening to your body, you can recognize whether you're eating due to hunger or for another reason, such as boredom, fatigue, or emotional stress.

When you eat mindfully, you're more in touch with your body so you can determine when you're satisfied and then stop eating as opposed to eating to the point of being stuffed, which can easily happen when you aren't listening to your body's cues. When you eat mindfully, you also recognize the early signs of hunger and act on them instead of waiting until you're excessively hungry (which can lead to eating too fast and eating too much). As you become more mindful, you'll notice that your tendency to crave foods or overeat will slowly fade away.

To become a more mindful eater, try following these guidelines daily:

✔ **Remove distractions so you can focus on your food.** Turn off the TV, get away from the computer, put away any reading material, and sit down at the table with your food on a plate. Before you begin eating, take a few relaxing breaths. As you start to eat, take small bites and ask yourself how aware you are of what you're eating.

To help you slow down and enjoy your food, involve all your senses. Make sure you taste and smell the food. Notice the texture as well. If you're eating too fast, you won't be able to involve all of your senses.

✔ **Make sure you're listening to your body.** Your body wants you to maintain a healthy weight, which is why it's constantly sending out cues to let you know when you need to eat, when you're satisfied, when you've eaten too much, and so on. However, when you're busy, you don't recognize these cues, and you don't give your body what it needs. By taking the time to get to know the signals your body sends to you, you'll start to recognize true hunger versus a food craving or eating due to emotional stress.

Make sure you know what true hunger feels like. Is your stomach rumbling? If so, that's a sign you're truly hungry. At times, the desire for the taste of food is there and makes you want to eat, but if your stomach isn't empty and isn't starting to rumble, chances are you're eating for reasons other than true hunger.

✔ **Don't eat while standing, and don't eat directly from the package.** Sit down at a table to eat; doing so allows you to better focus on your eating. Also, using the meal plan guidelines in Chapter 7, portion out your serving on your plate rather than eating out of the package or dish you cooked in.

✔ **Make sure to chew your food.** Chew each bite at least 10 to 15 times, and make sure you pay attention to the flavor, texture, and aroma of your food.

✔ **Focus on eating with your stomach rather than with your eyes.** It's fine to leave food on your plate. The amount of food on your plate doesn't determine your hunger or fullness — your stomach does. Listen to your body. If you're satisfied, push your plate away. You can always have the leftovers at another meal or as a snack. Or you can freeze them if you don't think you can eat them before they'll spoil.

If you finish your plate and want more, ask yourself whether you're truly hungry. It takes 20 minutes for your brain to get the message that your stomach is satisfied. If you eat your meal in under 20 minutes, you won't really know whether you're still truly hungry. Get up from the table, distract yourself, drink some water, and if you're truly hungry 20 minutes later (your stomach is still rumbling), you can have an additional serving. Vegetables are always unlimited, so if you do have seconds, these would be the best choice.

✔ **Avoid grazing or picking at food throughout the day.** When you graze, you're often eating on the run and not sitting down and focusing on the food, which lead to mindless eating. Grazing and picking at food aren't the same as snacking, however. Snacking is important to prevent excessive hunger. But when you snack, you want to put your snack on a plate, sit down, and eat it slowly and mindfully. Picking or grazing is when you rummage through the refrigerator or pantry and take little bites of this and that. Unfortunately all those little bites can add up in a big way.

Variety, the Spice of Life: Keeping Your Food Interesting

Have you ever eaten the same food so often that finally you couldn't even look at the food without feeling sick? This food boredom can wreak havoc on your waistline. Most people are creatures of habit and often fall into a food rut, eating the same old thing repeatedly. However, if you find yourself eating the same thing too often and for too long, you run the risk of becoming incredibly bored with your food choices. And boredom brings about food cravings, which can make it more challenging to stay on track with your meal plan.

Now before you panic, I'm not saying you can't repeat meals or eat the same lunch daily. If you like the consistency, it's not a problem. But, if you tend to eat the same sort of foods on a regular basis, you need to keep an eye out for signs of boredom with your meal plan. If you start to get bored with what you're eating, change it up before you become burned out and fall off track. I show you how to identify and sidestep food boredom in the following sections.

Recognizing meal plan boredom

How do you know whether you're bored with what you're eating? Ask yourself a few questions:

✔ **Do you look forward to the meals you have prepared?** If you're making meals only to force yourself to eat them, you may need to make a change.

✔ **Do you run out of ideas about what to make and then revert to the same two or three recipes time and time again?** If so, you may need to brainstorm a few new meal options to keep things fresh and interesting. Chapters 12 through 15 provide plenty of belly-friendly recipes to choose from.

✔ **Do you eat a meal and feel satisfied after eating but still have a hankering for something else?** Maybe you need something that would excite your taste buds more? If so, you may be experiencing a sign of meal plan boredom.

Breaking food boredom to stay motivated

If you have recognized that you may be becoming bored with your meal selections, you need to mix things up a bit and add more variety. Doing so can help you enjoy what you're eating, which is important. Remember that the Belly Fat Diet is a lifestyle change, so you want to be eating this way for life. If you want to keep it up, you need to enjoy what you're eating.

Adding variety keeps a meal plan interesting and helps you avoid becoming discouraged with your weight loss plan. If you feel like your meal plan is too limited, you can experience feelings of deprivation, which can cause you to overeat or select foods that are anything but belly friendly.

To add variety to your meal plan, look at what you're currently eating. Are there certain meals or snacks you consume day after day? Are you happy consuming these same foods? Consistency can be helpful with weight loss, so if you're satisfied eating certain foods on a consistent basis, you don't need to change. However, if you're dissatisfied consistently eating the same meals, try finding alternatives to your usual meals. Try some of these simple options to vary your meal plan and make it exciting again:

- ✔ **Add flavor.** Add variety by using various belly-friendly seasonings and sauces to flavor your favorite foods. Examples include garlic, hot pepper, Cajun seasoning, lemon and lime juice, and so on.

  Adding flavor through seasonings can be a great way to mix up your meals, but watch out for seasonings that are high in salt (they can bloat your belly). And if you purchase premade marinades or sauces, make sure to read the labels and watch out for any belly-bloating ingredients. See Chapter 11 for more information on becoming an expert at reading food labels.

- ✔ **Use substitutes.** Use substitutions to help increase variety. For instance, if you consume chicken breast most nights, switch to turkey breast or fish for a change. If your breakfast consists of oatmeal every morning, give dry bran cereals or puffed wheat a try.

- ✔ **Modify your recipes.** Slight modifications to a recipe or meal can add variety. For instance, if you usually have chicken breast with a side of cooked vegetables for dinner, try adding low-fat cheese on top of the chicken with a side of salsa and lowfat sour cream to give your dinner a new southwestern flavor. Or coat the chicken breast in whole-grain breadcrumbs, and top with tomato sauce and lowfat mozzarella. Presto! You now have chicken parmesan!

  Go online and look for recipes and food blogs for inspiration, or pick up a few new cookbooks to help change things up.

✔ **Change up the texture.** Changing texture can also help add variety. If yogurt with fruit is becoming boring, make a smoothie by adding some ice and blending the yogurt and fruit to create a refreshing snack.

✔ **Add another course to your meal.** Treat yourself to a dessert with sugar-free pudding made with skim milk and add some lowfat whipped topping. (See Chapter 15 for a pudding recipe that accompanies the Mock Ice Cream Sandwiches.) Adding a salad or broth-based soup before a meal can also provide you with variety and a feeling of satiety.

Balancing a Vegan or Vegetarian Diet

A well-balanced vegan or vegetarian diet can provide your body with all the essential nutrients needed for health and well-being. But when reducing or eliminating animal products from your diet, a few nutrients may be limited without careful planning. In order to achieve your flat-belly goals and stay as healthy as possible, make sure you achieve balance in your meal plan so you meet all your nutrient needs. The following sections show you how.

Getting your minerals

Nutrients that can be lacking in an unbalanced vegan or vegetarian diet include

✔ **Iron:** This mineral helps transport oxygen in the blood to the cells throughout your body. It's also an essential component to many metabolic reactions. A diet low in iron can lead to iron-deficiency anemia. However, it's possible to get plenty of iron in your diet as a vegan or vegetarian. You just have to carefully plan your meals.

Iron is found in two forms in food: heme and non-heme iron. *Heme iron* is found in animal products, and *non-heme iron* is found in plant-based foods. Non-heme iron is less easily absorbed by the body than heme iron, which means that vegans and vegetarians may absorb slightly less iron from their diets. However, vitamin C increases the absorption of non-heme iron. So combining foods rich in vitamin C (citrus fruits and green peppers) along with plant-based foods rich in iron (whole-grain cereals and flours, leafy green vegetables, beans, and lentils) can help increase the absorption of iron from your diet.

✔ **Zinc:** This mineral plays a major role in wound healing and is also essential for a healthy immune system. Because vegan and vegetarian diets often contain less zinc than diets that include meat, you need to ensure you're taking in enough of this nutrient. Zinc is found in large amounts in animal-based proteins, but many vegetarian sources exist as well, including pumpkin seeds (the most concentrated plant-based source of zinc), dairy products, beans and lentils, yeast, nuts, seeds, and whole-grain cereals.

Taking in vitamin B12

Vitamin B12 is essential for many of your body's functions, including the formation of red blood cells and maintaining a healthy nervous system. Vitamin B12, however, only occurs naturally in animal-based foods like meat and dairy. Because vegans follow a lifestyle that involves no animal products at all, they may find it quite challenging to take in adequate amounts of vitamin B12 daily. Vegetarians who consume few dairy products may have trouble as well.

To prevent a vitamin B12 deficiency while on the Belly Fat Diet plan, you need to regularly consume non-animal-based foods that are fortified with vitamin B12. Consider these fortified foods:

✔ Fortified cereals

✔ Fortified soy or almond milk

✔ Vegan vegetable stock

✔ Veggie burgers and textured vegetable protein

✔ Yeast extracts

If you follow a vegan or vegetarian lifestyle and don't eat many of the preceding foods, consult your personal dietitian or physician to see whether a vitamin B12 supplement may be appropriate for you.

Consuming protein

Many vegans and vegetarians are concerned with meeting their daily protein needs because they avoid animal proteins. But don't worry. You can meet your protein needs each day from plant-based sources and some animal-based sources. If you're comfortable consuming eggs, fish, and dairy as a vegetarian, these can be excellent sources of protein. High-protein plant-based foods that are appropriate for vegans (and, of course, vegetarians) include legumes, soy products, and nuts.

Even though you can take in adequate protein from plant sources daily, you must be careful because some of these protein sources contain a higher volume of carbohydrates or fat than lean animal proteins. Consuming too many of these products can impact your weight loss progress. These products include processed vegetarian options, such as veggie burgers, breaded soy-based "chicken" patties and nuggets as well as beans and lentils.

Because counting protein in ounces (as I do in the Belly Fat Diet meal plans in Chapter 7) may not be appropriate for those following a vegan or vegetarian meal plan, I recommend instead focusing on the grams of total protein you take in throughout the day while keeping the portion sizes of foods from the starch and fat groups within the recommended amounts. Doing so ensures you're taking in adequate protein to maintain lean body mass and keep you full without accidentally taking in too many servings of starch or fat, which can slow your weight loss progress.

For vegans (or vegetarians who choose to count grams of protein), aim to take in the following amounts of protein daily:

- ✔ **Women (Level 1, all plans):** 70 to 95 grams

- ✔ **Men (Level 1, all plans):** 80 to 110 grams

- ✔ **Women (Level 2, all plans):** 60 to 80 grams

- ✔ **Men (Level 2, all plans):** 75 to 95 grams

Table 16-1 shows some vegan foods and their accompanying protein contents. Take note, however, that you need to count many of these foods as servings from other food groups as well, such as fat, milk, starch, and vegetables.

Table 16-1	Protein Content of Vegan Food Sources		
Food	*Portion*	*Protein (grams)*	*Additional Food Group Servings*
Almonds	6 whole nuts	2	+ 1 fat
Black beans	½ cup	8	+ 1 starch
Chia seeds	1 tablespoon	2.5	+ 1 fat
Edamame	¼ cup	5	None
Flaxseed	1 tablespoon	2	+ 1 fat
Lentils	½ cup	9	+ 1 starch
Peanut butter	2 teaspoons	3	+ 1 fat
Quinoa	½ cup	4.5	+ 1 starch
Soy milk, plain	1 cup	11	+ 1 milk
Spinach, cooked	½ cup	2.5	+1 vegetable
Sunflower seeds	1 tablespoon	3	+ 1 fat
Tempeh	¼ cup	8	+ 1 fat
Tofu	¼ cup	10	None
Walnuts	1 tablespoon, chopped	1	+ 1 fat
Whole-grain bread	1 slice	5	+ 1 starch

Chapter 17

Dining Out and Special Occasions

• •

In This Chapter

▶ Understanding how to stay on track when eating out

▶ Determining the best food choices when eating away from home

▶ Identifying strategies when eating socially

• •

*J*ust because you're trying to lose weight, get healthy, and shrink your waistline doesn't mean you can't go out to eat or enjoy a social gathering with friends and family. When people begin their weight loss plans, many tend to shy away from eating anywhere but at home. However, you don't have to become a hermit just because you've changed your diet.

Think about it this way: If you can lose weight and lose your belly while occasionally enjoying a dinner out with friends or while partaking in a holiday meal, maintaining your weight loss will be easy! Let yourself do these things now and gain confidence knowing that you can eat away from home occasionally and still lose weight. If you can do it now, there won't be any stopping you when you reach your goal weight. You'll already be an expert on making healthy meal choices in restaurants and at social events. After all, you aren't going to eat at home for the rest of your life.

Throughout this chapter, I help you understand the simple tips and tricks for making the healthiest selections when eating away from home, whether you're taking a vacation, attending a party, or just having lunch with friends. I also show you the most common mistakes people make when eating out and how you can avoid them.

Basic Strategies for Eating Out

Eating in a restaurant can be a challenge. Temptation crops up everywhere you look, the portions are usually incredibly oversized, and the waiters push sugar-laden desserts that make your mouth water. But don't worry. The following sections give you some tips you can follow the next time you go out to eat. They'll make staying on track with your Belly Fat Diet plan a cinch.

Avoiding going out hungry

The first and most important tip you must always remember is not to go out to eat hungry. This strategy may seem counterintuitive, but it's so important. If you're starved when sitting down to order, do you really think you're going to make a healthy choice? Probably not.

Think about the last time you went out to eat. First you get to the restaurant and wait to be seated. When you're finally seated, you order and then wait for your food. By the time the meal comes out, you're probably so hungry (if you haven't already gobbled up the contents of the bread basket) that you devour your meal in seconds. Eating too quickly leads to you ignoring your body's cues for satiety and causes you to overeat.

Instead of falling prey to the preceding scenario, have a small snack before going out to eat. Doing so helps you avoid excess hunger and overeating. A great option can be a piece of fruit, a lowfat yogurt, a handful of nuts, or even a stick of lowfat string cheese.

Choosing your food wisely

Eating healthfully when eating out is all about making wise choices. If you're not careful, the wrong choice can really sabotage your weight loss efforts. Here are a few rules of thumb you can use when ordering (for cuisine-specific advice, see the later section "Choosing Belly-Flattening Best Bets at a Restaurant"):

- ✔ **Review your choices ahead of time.** One of the best ways to ensure you make a healthy choice when eating out is to prepare. If you're going to a restaurant, try pulling up the menu online before you arrive. Many restaurants offer full menus, or at least partial menus, on their websites.

    Some restaurants, especially chains and fast-food places, provide nutrition data on their meals and sides. Aim to select a meal that's less than 500 calories and less than 20 grams of fat. Remember that these numbers are for the entire meal, including sides, appetizers, and dessert (if you opt for them).

- ✔ **If you plan to get an appetizer, choose a lean protein or vegetable option.** For instance, shrimp cocktail is an excellent appetizer choice; it's typically less than 100 calories for the whole serving. Vegetable soup or roasted red peppers can make a terrific appetizer as well.

- ✔ **A pre-meal salad or cup of soup can be a great way to help you fill up and eat smaller amounts of your entree.** However, if you get a salad before your meal, watch out for toppings that can blow your weight loss efforts. Shredded cheese, croutons, and dressing can add a significant source of fat and calories. Ask for a plain house salad, nix the cheese, and get your dressing on the side. If you opt for a small cup of soup before the meal, make sure it's a broth-based soup, not a cream soup.

✓ **Pay attention to food preparation.** Look for the words "grilled," "broiled," or "steamed" next to entrees instead of words like "sautéed," "fried," or "breaded." The latter provide many more calories and plenty of unhealthy fat.

✓ **Beware of hidden fats in sauces and dressings.** Sauces made with cream and butter, such as Alfredo and vodka sauces, can be loaded with calories and belly-busting saturated fats. Even salad dressing can be a significant source of calories when used in excess. To help control your intake, try choosing dishes prepared in lower-calorie sauces, such as broths, marinara, and wine sauces. When in doubt about the nutritional content, ask for your meal to be prepared without these fats or order sauces on the side so you can control the amount you consume.

✓ **Watch out for sides.** A Cornell University study found that people order 131 percent more calories in side dishes when they feel like they have made a healthy entree selection. Perhaps it's the idea that they have room to splurge on sides, appetizers, or desserts. But be careful. Many times these items can contain just as many or more calories than the entree!

Don't be afraid to ask for substitutions for your sides. Many restaurants offer refined carbohydrates, such as white rice or white pasta, as sides. Because these can bloat your belly, ask whether you can substitute whole-grain options, such as brown rice or whole-grain pasta. Or even better, ask for the starchy side to be replaced with steamed vegetables.

✓ **Occasionally treat yourself.** If you never treat yourself, you're going to start feeling deprived, which can lead to intense food cravings. And intense food cravings can eventually lead to binges. Splurging on the dessert or high-fat meal on occasion is okay. Of course, you don't want to eat these foods on a regular basis, but that doesn't mean you can never enjoy your favorites. Allow yourself to order your favorite meal on special occasions, or limit yourself to doing it once a month. Eating healthy is about being able to enjoy all foods, in limited amounts, on occasion.

Watching portion sizes: Heading out without pigging out

Portion sizes are out of control today. They're not only huge in your home, but they're particularly gargantuan in restaurants. Even healthy foods are served in such large amounts that they can promote weight gain instead of weight loss. In fact, in Chapter 6 you can see the difference in portion sizes of some common meals from 20 years ago to today. The calories have doubled and even tripled in some cases.

If you don't identify when the portions you're eating are larger than you really need, you can trick yourself into thinking you're making a healthy choice, when in reality, you're eating too much.

How can you recognize a true portion when dining out instead of being tricked into overeating? Use the everyday objects in Figure 17-1 as a guide.

 1 cup vegetables = your fist

 1 fat serving = your thumb to the first knuckle
Example: 1 pat of butter (1 teaspoon)

3 oz. of meat, poultry, or fish = a deck of cards

Figure 17-1:
Common
objects
and portion
sizes.

 1 cup of pasta or rice = 1 baseball

 1 ounce of cheese = 1 golf ball

Illustration by Wiley, Composition Services Graphics

Here are a few other ways to make sure you're eating a reasonable amount when eating out:

- ✔ **Wear tight pants or a tight belt when going out to eat.** It may sound silly, but snug-fitting clothes help you recognize when you feel full sooner, preventing you from overeating.

- ✔ **Split it!** Some restaurants give you way more than you need to fuel your body. If you're not careful, you can end up eating with your eyes instead of your stomach. To help with this, order one entree and share it with a friend. Just ask for one entree and two plates and your portion problem is solved! If you're dining alone, cut your entree in half as soon as it arrives and box up that half for lunch or dinner the next day.

- ✔ **Drink water before and after you eat.** Downing a large glass of water before your meal arrives can help to fill you up, allowing you to eat more slowly and better regulate your portions. Sipping on water throughout your meal and at the end of it can also help prevent you from picking at the leftovers on the table that you're planning to take home.

✔ **Watch your eating speed.** Restaurants can be full of distractions that can take away from your ability to eat mindfully. Remember that it takes 20 minutes to recognize your stomach is full. Slow down when eating, sip on a calorie-free beverage, put your fork down between bites, or talk to the folks you're dining with. All these actions allow you to eat your meal more slowly, helping you recognize the body cues of satiety before you overeat.

Eating slowly has another benefit: When you aren't the first one done with your meal, you don't feel pressured to keep eating just because your friends or family still are. The restaurant also won't be in a hurry to free up your table if you're still enjoying your meal, so you get more time to socialize as well.

✔ **If you're eating at a buffet, choose small plates.** One study found that individuals with the highest body mass index (BMI) almost always selected the large plate size at the buffet, eating more because the bigger plate tricks their eye into thinking they aren't eating as much. Choose the smaller salad or dessert plate whenever you have the option.

✔ **If you want a dessert, keep it small.** Instead of the dessert special that's larger than your entree, ask for a small scoop of ice cream. (However, the best choice is a cup of fresh fruit.) And remember that dessert shouldn't be used to fill your stomach or provide you with essential nutrients. Instead you're eating it for enjoyment, so having just a few small bites that you can savor should do the trick.

Drinking alcohol responsibly

One major weight loss sabotage when eating out at restaurants or social events is alcohol. Alcohol is a source of empty calories, meaning it provides your body with a significant source of calories with little to no nutritional value. So too much alcohol can be bloating to your belly and can slow your weight loss progress.

In addition to being a source of calories on its own, alcohol can also stimulate your appetite. So if you go out to eat hungry and then sit down and order a drink, by the time you've consumed your drink you'll be even hungrier. When you finally get a chance to order or eat, you'll be likely to make a healthy choice and more likely to eat too large a portion.

Alcohol, especially wine, can have some health benefits. For instance, resveratrol in red wine has been shown to improve heart health and may have anti-inflammatory properties. So not all alcohol is bad. You just need to be careful with the quantity you take in because too much can negatively impact your waistline.

If you do choose to have alcohol when eating out, follow these guidelines to help you make the best choice:

✔ Choose red or white wine, light beer, or alcohol mixed with sugar-free mixers, such as club soda or seltzer.

✔ Avoid high-sugar mixed drinks with beverages like fruit juice and soda, because they're loaded with belly bloaters.

✔ Aim to drink alcohol toward the middle to end of a meal instead of before the meal, because it can increase your appetite and lead to you eating more.

✔ Limit yourself to one 4-ounce glass of red or white wine per day if you're a woman and no more than two 4-ounce glasses of wine per day if you're a man. For any other form of alcohol (or for more than 4 ounces of wine), count each additional 4-ounce glass as two fat servings. Check out Table 17-1 to see what's considered one serving of alcohol on your Belly Fat Diet plan.

Table 17-1	Portions for Alcohol
Alcohol	*Portion Size (in ounces)*
Beer	12
Light beer	12
Wine, white	4
Wine, red	4
Liquor	1.5

Choosing Belly-Flattening Best Bets at a Restaurant

In this section, I point out the best bets to order when at different types of restaurants. I also tell you which menu options to steer clear of because they can bloat your belly and pack on the pounds.

Your Belly Fat Diet plan is a lifestyle change, so just because an entree is listed as a belly bloater doesn't mean you can't ever order it. Just have it as an occasional treat or for a special occasion, and order the belly-friendly food more often.

Don't be afraid to ask questions. It's normal not to know what goes into every dish on the menu, especially at an ethnic restaurant. Ask questions and ask for questionable ingredients, like unfamiliar sauces, to be prepared on the side.

Family restaurants and diners

Family restaurants and diners tend to have large menus, so they typically have at least a few healthy choices available. These restaurants generally allow for a good deal of substitution as well, such as forgoing cheese, adding vegetables or a side salad in place of a starchy side, and even offering whole grains like whole-wheat pasta and lentils.

When eating at a family restaurant or diner, keep the following tips in mind:

- ✔ **Watch the portion size.** Diners are known for their ultra-large serving sizes. Order lunch-sized portions when possible, or divide your meal in half and box up one half before digging in.

- ✔ **Ask how your food is prepared.** Although meat or seafood may be broiled, the chef may still top it with a pat of butter before serving. So ask that the butter or oil be left off. The same goes for vegetables. Request for them to be steamed instead of sautéed. And ask that they be plain and not topped with butter, sauce, or oil.

- ✔ **If ordering beef, watch the cut.** All cuts of beef aren't created equal. Certain cuts like prime rib are much higher in saturated fat and calories than a lean cut like flank steak. Refer to Chapter 6 for the leanest protein options before you order.

- ✔ **Be wary of appetizers.** Many appetizers at family restaurants and diners are deep fried and not exactly belly-friendly. If you do want an appetizer, order just one for the table and have everyone share to help cut down on the portion size.

Belly-friendly foods

Your best bets at family restaurants and diners are going to be lean proteins that are grilled, broiled, or steamed. And be sure to watch your choice of side dishes. Here's a list of great options:

- ✔ Baked, grilled, or broiled lean protein entrees (seafood, chicken or turkey breast, pork tenderloin, or lean beef) with steamed vegetables

- ✔ Broth-based vegetable soups, such as minestrone, or even French onion soup without the cheese (yes, you can order it that way!)

- ✔ Grilled chicken or turkey sandwiches on whole-grain buns

✔ Lean appetizers, such as shrimp cocktail or broiled clams

✔ Omelets made with eggs or egg whites and stuffed with vegetables (but little or no cheese)

✔ Salads topped with lean grilled proteins, such as chicken breast or shrimp (no cheese or croutons and dressing on the side)

✔ Stir-fry entrees made with lean proteins and brown rice

✔ Vegetable burgers on a bed of lettuce or a whole-grain bun

✔ Whole-grain side dishes, such as baked potatoes or sweet potatoes, brown rice, or whole-grain pasta (If adding butter or sour cream, ask for it on the side.)

Belly-bloating foods

When eating at family restaurants and diners, you most want to avoid fried foods and those doused in fat-laden sauces and cheeses. Here are some definite no-nos:

✔ Appetizers covered in cheese and sour cream, such as potato skins and nachos

✔ Caesar salad (Order salad with vinegar and olive oil instead to make it a lean option.)

✔ Cream-based soups

✔ Coleslaw

✔ Entrees with high-fat sources of meat, including prime rib, short ribs, or ground beef

✔ Fried appetizers, such as deep-fried onions, mozzarella sticks, and buffalo wings

✔ Fried seafood or poultry dishes

✔ Hamburgers or cheeseburgers

✔ High-fat side dishes, including French fries, tater tots, mashed potatoes, and macaroni and cheese

✔ Salads topped with fried proteins, large amounts of cheese, or bacon and croutons

Fast-food restaurants

Although fast-food establishments often get a bad rap for unhealthy options, belly-flattening choices hide among the higher-calorie dishes. One of the biggest issues with fast-food is that even seemingly healthy choices can be loaded with sodium. And sodium can hold onto water weight, bloating your belly. So if you do eat at fast-food restaurants, be sure to keep your sodium intake limited the rest of the day to help compensate.

Another belly-bloater that commonly lurks in fast-food restaurants is refined carbohydrates. It can be hard to find a 100 percent whole-grain bun for your sandwich or a food that's breaded with anything but white flour. Some places do offer whole-grain options, but they're few and far between. So just be sure to limit your intake of refined carbohydrates as much as possible when selecting off the menu, and be sure to fit in whole grains at your other meals during the day.

Here are some basic tips to help keep your fast-food choices belly-friendly:

- **Avoid fried options.** Instead choose grilled, broiled, and steamed items whenever possible.

- **Watch out for condiments.** Mayo, special sauces, and even barbeque sauce and ketchup can provide you with a significant source of fat and sugar if you don't watch the quantity you use. Always order sauces on the side so you can monitor how much you use. Chapter 6 provides portion sizes of some common condiments.

- **Although it can be tempting, avoid supersizing your food.** Sure it seems like a deal — only an extra 50 cents — but you'll be bulking up your waistline if you give into this seeming value. Try downgrading instead. For instance, switching from a large fry to the child's size can save 500 calories or more!

- **Watch your drink choice.** Sodas, fruit punch, sweetened teas, and, worst of all, milkshakes can add hundreds (and even thousands!) of calories to your meal. And watch out for diet soda, too. It has few calories, but the carbonation can instantly bloat your belly as it fills it with air. Choose water, lowfat milk, or unsweetened iced tea instead.

Belly-friendly foods

At fast-food joints, look for the freshest items on the menu and those with the fewest unhealthy fats and refined carbs. Here are some possibilities:

- Apple slices (often offered as a French fry alternative on kids' menus)

- Baked potato with a small dab (1 tablespoon or less) of sour cream

- Chili (a small cup)

- Dishes made with grilled chicken or grilled fish

- Grilled chicken salad with lowfat dressing and a small pinch of cheese

- Lowfat yogurt with fruit

✔ Sandwiches made with lean protein, such as turkey breast or ham, on whole-grain bread (Ask for other condiments, such as mayo, on the side.)

✔ Small 3- or 4-ounce hamburger or cheeseburger

✔ Soft-shell tacos with limited cheese and small quantities of sour cream

✔ Vegetable burger on a bed of lettuce or a whole-grain bun

✔ Water, lowfat milk, or unsweetened iced tea

Belly-bloating foods

If you're heading to a fast-food establishment, try your best to ignore those foods that scream fat, sodium, and calories. Here are some of the worst offenders:

✔ Baked potato loaded with butter, sour cream, and bacon

✔ Crispy chicken or crispy fish sandwiches

✔ French fries, onion rings, and potato cakes

✔ Jumbo or super-sized burgers

✔ Milkshakes

✔ Salads topped with fried meats and large amounts of cheese, dressing, and croutons

✔ Sandwiches or burgers topped with high-fat proteins, such as cheese, bacon, and ham

✔ Tacos stuffed with ground beef, cheese, and large amounts of sour cream

Asian restaurants

If you love Asian food, you have so many restaurants to choose from. You can select anything from Chinese and Japanese to Thai and Vietnamese. The great news about Asian dishes is that they're often filled with vegetables. However, increased oils in cooking, refined carbohydrates like white rice, and high-sodium sauces can make some menu options major belly-bloaters. Some easy changes to make Asian dishes more belly-friendly include the following:

✔ **Ask for brown rice in place of white rice, if available.** If the restaurant doesn't offer brown rice, just eat a small amount of white rice, or skip it and eat more vegetables instead.

✔ **Request sauces on the side.** For dishes that come with sauces high in sodium or fat, ask for your protein and vegetables to be steamed separately with the sauce served on the side. Doing so allows you to dip each bite into the sauce so you consume less, meaning you get less sodium and fat.

✔ **Watch out for crispy, fried, or tempura dishes.** These dishes are high in fat and refined carbohydrates. Aim for steamed or lightly stir-fried options instead.

✔ **Choose lean proteins.** Ask for steamed, grilled, or broiled seafood, chicken breast, or even tofu as a great source of protein that contains little fat.

Belly-friendly foods

If you opt for Asian cuisine, try those dishes that contain the most veggies and lean proteins and those that are simply cooked. Consider the following:

✔ Bo Xa Lui Nuong (grilled beef with vegetables)

✔ Canh Chay soup

✔ Egg drop soup

✔ Dumplings, steamed (because these are typically made with refined grains, limit to one or two)

✔ Fresh (soft) spring rolls

✔ Hibachi vegetables and lean protein (fish, poultry, or beef)

✔ Miso soup

✔ Moo Goo Gai Pan

✔ Seafood kabobs

✔ Shrimp and snow peas

✔ Steamed or lightly stir-fried lean protein and vegetable entrees (like steamed chicken and broccoli or steamed tofu with vegetables)

✔ Sumashi soup

✔ Tom Yam soup (vegetarian or with fish)

Belly-bloating foods

Even though Asian dishes can be a healthy choice when eating out, you do have to watch for some pitfalls, such as heavy fat- and sodium-laden sauces and breaded meats and sides. Steer clear of these:

✔ Chawan mushi

✔ Deep-fried dishes

✔ Dishes made with high-fat sauces, such as lobster sauce

✔ Dishes smothered in high-sodium sauces, including soy, teriyaki, and oyster sauces

✔ Fried rice

- Fried sides, such as fried eggrolls, spring rolls, dumplings, shrimp toast, and wontons

- General Tso's chicken

- Kung Pao chicken

- Mu Shu pork

- Pad Thai

- Tempura dishes

- Vit Quay (roasted duck)

Italian restaurants

The good news is that Italian restaurants often offer many seafood and poultry options. They also tend to cook entrees in olive oil, which you know is a belly-friendly fat option. However, many pasta dishes are served with large quantities of pasta, mainly refined pasta, which isn't only a significant source of calories but also a major belly buster. However, you can avoid these belly-busting refined starches when eating at your favorite Italian eatery. You just have to remember the following few tricks when ordering:

- **Ask for your pasta on the side.** Many entrees are served over a bed of pasta, so it can be difficult to tell how much pasta you're actually eating. When you request it to be served on the side on a smaller, separate plate, you can monitor the portion size better.

- **Request whole-grain pasta.** Many Italian restaurants now offer whole-grain options, so make sure you ask when ordering.

- **Opt for marinara sauce.** Marinara sauce is typically low in fat and isn't a major source of calories, but other sauces, such as Alfredo, vodka, pesto, or cream sauce, are loaded with belly-busting fat.

- **Look for the words "breaded," "crispy," "fried," or "parmigiana," and avoid those entrees.** These terms often indicate that the entree is fried.

Belly-friendly foods

If you and your family have a tradition of spaghetti night at your local Italian restaurant, don't worry. You won't have to skip out. You can fill up with any of the following options:

- Appetizers like roasted red peppers, fresh mozzarella with tomato, grilled calamari, steamed clams, and bruschetta on whole-grain toast

- Baked, broiled, or grilled seafood, poultry, or lean beef with a side of vegetables instead of pasta

- Baked poultry in marinara or wine sauce

✔ Caprese salad

✔ Chicken cacciatore

✔ Cioppino

✔ Minestrone

✔ Ravioli (Although it's difficult to find a restaurant that serves whole-grain ravioli, the cheese or beef filling cuts down on the amount of refined grain you're consuming. Just make sure it's topped with marinara sauce, not Alfredo or another cream sauce.)

✔ Steamed seafood in a wine or marinara sauce

✔ Whole-grain pasta mixed with vegetables and topped with marinara or wine sauce

✔ Whole-grain, thin-crust pizza topped with vegetables

✔ Whole-grain pasta sides topped with marinara or wine sauce

Belly-bloating foods

To avoid slowing down your weight loss success, be sure to steer clear of the popular creamy, fried, and butter-laden dishes when eating at Italian joints. The following are sure to add to your muffin top:

✔ Dishes with large amounts of added butter, such as piccata dishes or dishes made with lemon-butter sauces

✔ Entrees made with high-fat proteins, such as meatballs and veal cutlets

✔ Entrees made with high-fat sauces, such as Alfredo, vodka, or other cream sauces

✔ High-fat appetizers, such as fried calamari, mozzarella sticks, or antipasto with large amounts of high-fat meats

✔ Main pasta entrees (Try to keep pasta as a side dish to prevent overeating, and choose whole-grain varieties whenever possible.)

✔ Pan- or deep-fried entrees like chicken parmigiana

✔ Pizza with meat toppings and a white flour crust, including Sicilian pizza

✔ Refined flour bread from the bread basket (and the butter just increases the belly bloat)

Mexican restaurants

You can find many belly-friendly options in Mexican restaurants, but you also have to be careful in what you order. Many Mexican entrees are loaded with cheese, refried beans, and white rice or white flour tortillas, which all can be belly busters.

Because most restaurants make your entree to order and certain entrees like fajitas allow you to assemble your own dish, it's possible to make a few easy substitutions to turn any Mexican entree into a belly-friendly option.

Keep these tips in mind when noshing on Mexican food:

- ✔ **If your meal comes in a tortilla, opt for whole-wheat whenever possible.** If whole-wheat tortillas aren't available, choose the soft corn tortilla over the white flour tortilla.

- ✔ **Watch out for high-calorie sides.** Refried beans, which are typically fried in lard, are the worst offenders. Opt instead for cooked black or pinto beans.

- ✔ **Nix the cheese.** Many Mexican dishes contain large amounts of cheese. Ask for the cheese to be left out of your dish or for the restaurant to go light with the cheese to avoid added saturated fat and sodium.

- ✔ **Always ask for sauces, such as sour cream and guacamole, on the side.** Then be sure to go light when adding them to your entree.

- ✔ **Opt for the soft taco.** Crispy taco shells are often fried, so go for the soft taco instead to cut down on added fat and calories.

Belly-friendly foods

You don't have to stop having your monthly Mexican night with your friends just because you're on the Belly Fat Diet. Believe it or not, you can find some tasty meals that won't pile on the pounds. Try the following:

- ✔ Black bean soup or baked chips with salsa for an appetizer (Many Mexican restaurants serve chips and salsa, but these are often fried chips. If your restaurant doesn't offer baked chips, skip them.)

- ✔ Chicken enchiladas prepared without cheese and with the sour cream on the side

- ✔ Burritos prepared without cheese

- ✔ Fajitas with lean protein options (Choose whole-grain tortillas and go easy on the cheese and sour cream when assembling them.)

- ✔ Grilled or broiled chicken, seafood, or beef entrees with a side of cooked black or pinto beans and vegetables

- ✔ Pollo picado without rice, paired with a side of vegetables

- ✔ Soft vegetarian tacos (Ask for cooked black or pinto beans instead of refried beans.)

- ✔ Soft chicken tacos (Make sure it's chicken breast meat rather than fatty dark meat.)

Belly-bloating foods

Of course, Mexican restaurants have their share of belly-bloating foods, including creamy cheese sauces and fried everything. Watch out for these belly busters:

- Appetizers like nachos covered in cheese, creamy soups, and fried chips
- Burritos loaded with cheese
- Carnitas (fried pork or beef)
- Chimichangas
- Chorizo (Mexican sausage)
- Fried ice cream (If you want dessert, select just one scoop of regular ice cream instead.)
- Quesadillas
- Refried beans
- Tacos in crispy shells
- Tacos stuffed with ground beef, cheese, and refried beans
- White rice

Middle Eastern/Greek restaurants

Middle Eastern and Greek restaurants tend to offer a large variety of foods, meaning you can find both belly-busters and belly-burners on the menu. The trick is to know which is which.

Some tips for eating healthfully at Greek and Middle Eastern restaurants include the following:

- **Watch your protein sources.** Certain cuts of beef, lamb, and pork can be high in fat, and it's not uncommon for these fattier cuts to be used in Greek and Middle Eastern restaurants. Try selecting lean poultry and vegetarian dishes instead.

- **Ask for sauces to be served on the side to cut down on added calories and fat.** For instance, ask for tahini, hummus, and baba ghanoush on the side. These sauces are rich in healthy fats, but it's still important to watch your portions because even healthy fat can slow weight loss when consumed in excess. Tzatziki sauce, which is made from Greek yogurt, cucumber, and garlic, is a safe bet when eating in these establishments.

✔ **Steer clear of added saturated fat and calories from additives like feta cheese.** Ask for your meal to be prepared without cheese or have it served on the side so you can control the portion.

✔ **Keep an eye on the sides you order.** Sides often include white rice or pita bread made from refined flour.

Belly-friendly foods

When eating Greek or Middle Eastern food, focus on the veggies and the lean proteins. Here are some excellent choices:

✔ Dolmades (stuffed grape leaves)

✔ Greek salad without feta cheese and with the dressing on the side

✔ Grilled, broiled, or baked seafood, poultry, or lean beef dishes with a side of vegetables

✔ Hummus with raw vegetables

✔ Kakavia soup

✔ Plaki

✔ Salads or entrees topped with tzatziki sauce

✔ Souvlaki (made with chicken)

✔ Yogurt and cucumber soup

Belly-bloating foods

The following foods are high-calorie and high-fat items that you want to steer clear of when going for Greek or Middle Eastern food:

✔ Baklava (Try a fruit dish for dessert instead.)

✔ Greek salad topped with feta cheese and dressing

✔ Gyros

✔ Moussaka

✔ Souvlaki (made with pork or lamb)

✔ Spanakopita (spinach pie)

Special Occasions: Social Eating

Eating at holiday and social gatherings can offer unique challenges when you're trying to lose weight and keep it off. Some of the most common obstacles you may face at events and holiday parties include

- ✔ Less-than-belly-friendly food being served as appetizers and for the main course (and no other choices)
- ✔ Increased alcohol consumption, which adds empty calories and can stimulate appetite
- ✔ Pressure from others to try all the food that's available, have dessert, finish something off so they can wash the pan, and so on
- ✔ Having so many choices you feel compelled to sample a bit of everything, which may lead to eating beyond true hunger
- ✔ Long delays before food is served, which can lead to you eating too quickly and not recognizing your body's satiety cues
- ✔ Hidden calories in foods, such as from added sauces or added fat during cooking
- ✔ Mindless eating that may occur if you're sitting or standing next to food for long periods of time
- ✔ Increased temptation as you're surrounded by others eating large portions or eating less-healthy food

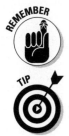

Allow yourself to enjoy a dessert or dish that you'd usually avoid, but keep the portion small. Eat it slowly so you can really savor it and feel satisfied.

For more helpful tips on sticking to the Belly Fat Diet at parties and while traveling, check out the articles at `dummies.com/go/bellyfat`.

Chapter 18

Belly Fat Maintenance Plan

*W*hen you reach your goal weight or are close to it, you may be asking what's next. After all, your Belly Fat Diet plan isn't a diet to go on and off; it's a lifestyle change, meaning that the habits and changes you have made throughout your Belly Fat Diet plan are things you want to stick with for life. Making lifestyle changes not only helps you lose weight, but also helps you keep it off for good. What's the point in losing weight if you're just going to regain it and be right back where you started? You want to make sure that your lifestyle changes are those you can stick with so you can stay at your goal weight for years to come, helping you continue to not only look great, but also feel great and stay healthy.

Throughout this chapter, I provide you with clear-cut guidelines and tips on how to maintain your weight for good. The Belly Fat maintenance plan shows you how to determine when you have reached your goal weight, how to break through plateaus if your progress stalls before you're at your long-term goal weight, and what you need to do to stay at this weight once and for all.

Why You Need a Maintenance Plan

If you want to be successful with long-term weight loss, you must have a maintenance plan. If you think that as soon as you get to your goal weight, you can just go back to your old habits, you're destined to regain the weight you have lost. After all, those old habits are what got you to your highest weight in the first place. Going back to those habits on a regular basis (and maintaining your losses) isn't a feasible option.

So you need to focus on making small, manageable changes over a period of time. This way you can lose weight while making these new behaviors a habit, which can help you stick with these new healthy changes and keep the weight, and belly fat, away permanently.

A maintenance plan doesn't mean you have to eat perfectly every day or measure every morsel of food that goes in your mouth. A maintenance plan is all about creating balance. You can eat any food you want, but some foods need to be consumed in moderation, whereas others can be enjoyed more regularly. After you find this balance, you'll realize that staying at a healthy body weight doesn't require a lifetime of deprivation. A healthy weight comes from a lifetime of listening to your body, making healthy choices, splurging on occasion, and staying active.

What is a maintenance plan?

Weight maintenance is basically upholding a consistent body weight over a period of months and years. Instead of reaching a goal weight only to start to regain weight, creating that yo-yo effect, weight maintenance means that you achieve a healthy body weight for you. You reach a weight that you can maintain without feeling the need to starve yourself and that you can stay at for a long period of time.

No one is the exact same weight every day. Weight can fluctuate on the scale for many reasons. So when it comes to weight maintenance, I recommend setting a weight range you're aiming to stay within rather than one specific weight. Try using a 3- to 5-pound weight range. So for instance, if your long-term goal is 135 pounds, your weight may fluctuate between 133–137 pounds. If your weight begins to slowly creep above this range, you can go back to Level 2 of your Belly Fat Diet plan until you're back within your goal range. (See Chapter 7 to read about the plans you can choose from.)

Deciding when to start

What was the main goal you set for yourself when you first started your Belly Fat Diet plan? Was it to reach a specific goal weight or body mass index (BMI)? Was it to reach a certain pant size or attain a certain healthy goal like having a normal blood pressure or reducing your blood sugar? After you've reached your long-term goal, you're typically ready to move into your maintenance plan.

Not everyone moves into maintenance mode at the same time or for the same reason. For instance, you may have decided to follow the Belly Fat Diet Plan to lower your risk of heart disease by shrinking visceral fat. If you haven't already met your goal of losing 5 inches around your waist, you may not be ready to transition to maintenance. Or, perhaps you were already at a healthy body weight but needed to lower your blood sugar levels. After those levels are remaining in the normal range, you may find that it's time to transition into your maintenance plan. The following questions can help you assess whether you're ready to transition to the maintenance plan:

✔ Are you at your goal weight?

✔ Is your BMI within the ideal range? (See Chapter 3.)

✔ Are your health goals, such as blood pressure, cholesterol, and blood sugar, within the normal range? (See Chapter 3.)

✔ Is your waist circumference within the ideal range? (See Chapter 3.)

Setting a Realistic Belly Fat Goal

When you begin your Belly Fat Diet meal plan and workout, you likely have a set goal in mind, whether that be a certain weight, a specific waist measurement, or a particular health goal, such as reducing your blood sugar or heart disease risk.

Although you may have set a goal in your mind, you need to make sure that it's not an unrealistic goal for your height and gender. If you set an unrealistic goal, you may feel like you have stalled or plateaued before reaching this goal, when in reality, you have actually achieved a healthy weight.

Body weight isn't the sole indicator of whether you've reached your goals. If your progress has stalled, but your waist circumference and health measurements (such as blood pressure and blood sugar) are all within the normal range, it's quite possible you're at your goal and should focus on maintenance.

In the following sections, I show you how to set your ideal goals based on your age, height, and gender.

Ideal weight goals

When setting weight loss goals for yourself, you must consider many factors, including your height, age, gender, activity level, and bone structure. Everyone's body is different, so you can't think of weight loss as a one-size-fits-all process.

For instance, are you athletic with a large amount of muscle mass? Do you have a large bone structure (usually evident by a large wrist circumference)? If so, you may be on the higher end of the healthy weight scale because muscle and bone mass weigh more on a scale than fat mass. If, on the other hand, you have limited muscle mass or a small bone structure, you want to aim to weigh toward the middle to lower end of the healthy weight range for your height.

If you're over age 55, you should aim to be in the middle to upper end of the healthy weight range for your height, because too low a body weight later in life can increase the risk of osteoporosis.

Use Table 18-1 to determine a healthy weight range for you if you're a female and Table 18-2 if you're a male.

Table 18-1	Healthy Weight Ranges for Women		
Height (Inches)	Healthy Weight Range (Pounds)	Height (Inches)	Healthy Weight Range (Pounds)
60	90–120	68	130–165
61	95–125	69	135–170
62	100–130	70	140–175
63	105–140	71	145–180
64	110–145	72	150–185
65	115–150	73	155–190
66	120–155	74	160–195
67	125–160		

Table 18-2	Healthy Weight Ranges for Men		
Height (Inches)	Healthy Weight Range (Pounds)	Height (Inches)	Healthy Weight Range (Pounds)
60	97–127	68	145–175
61	103–133	69	151–181
62	109–139	70	157–187
63	115–145	71	163–193
64	121–151	72	169–199
65	127–157	73	175–205
66	133–163	74	181–211
67	139–169		

Ideal waist measurement goals

A high waist circumference can increase your risk of many health problems, including heart disease and type 2 diabetes. (Check out Chapter 3 for details.) To help reduce your risk of medical complications, your waist circumference should be

✔ Less than 35 inches for women

✔ Less than 40 inches for men

Chapter 3 provides directions on how to accurately measure your waist circumference.

Achieving a waist circumference within the ideal range may be an indication that you have achieved, or are close to achieving, your ideal weight and health goals.

Ideal health goals

Some folks start the Belly Fat Diet plan in order to correct medical conditions they may be struggling with, such as high cholesterol, blood pressure, or blood sugar (glucose). Changing your diet and activity level with the Belly Fat Diet plan can reverse these high levels.

Having these health measurements within the normal range can also be an indication that you've achieved your ideal weight range.

Normal blood pressure is considered to be less than 120 mmHg systolic and less than 80 mmHg diastolic. A normal fasting glucose level should be 70–99 mg/dL. In Table 18-3, you can see the ideal range for cholesterol levels.

Table 18-3	Ideal Measurements for Cholesterol	
Blood Lipids	*Range*	*Risk Category*
Total cholesterol	Less than 170 mg/dL	Ideal
	Less than 200 mg/dL	Desirable
LDL cholesterol	Less than 100 mg/dL	Ideal
	100–129 mg/dL	Desirable
HDL cholesterol	40–59 mg/dL (men)	Desirable
	50–59 mg/dL (women)	Desirable
	Greater than 60 mg/dL (men and women)	Ideal
Triglycerides	Less than 150 mg/dL	Desirable

Breaking Plateaus

So what happens when you're doing your best and staying on track with your Belly Fat Diet plan, but all of a sudden you aren't seeing results? Is this a plateau? It depends. You first have to understand what a true plateau is. You aren't facing a plateau if your weight loss has dropped off for a week. It's normal to lose weight some weeks, not see any progress another week, and have a slight gain the following week. The number on the scale can fluctuate for many reasons, so one or two slow weeks don't indicate a true plateau.

A true plateau occurs when you have made no real progress for at least three or more weeks. And by no progress I mean

- ✔ No change in body weight
- ✔ No change in waist circumference
- ✔ No loss of inches (around the arms, thighs, and so on)

A true weight-loss plateau can happen for the following reasons:

- ✔ Weight loss progress may slow as your body adjusts to previous rapid weight loss.
- ✔ After a significant amount of weight loss, your meal plan may need a slight adjustment to continue to promote weight loss.
- ✔ You may have started to feel a bit too comfortable with your meal plan, and without realizing it your portion sizes may have slightly expanded.
- ✔ Decreased overall physical activity can slow or stall progress.
- ✔ Being less diligent with your Belly Fat Diet plan, such as limited food journaling, less planning, eating on the run, and so on, can stall weight loss efforts.

Be honest with yourself about your weight loss goals. Aiming for too low of a body weight may be unrealistic and unhealthy for your body. If you're aiming for an unrealistic weight, your body may resist your efforts and settle at a weight that's within a healthy range but not as low as your long-term goal. So don't just focus on the number on the scale. Keep in mind your waist measurements, body fat losses, and health changes, because these factors may give a more accurate representation of your overall progress.

At first, losing weight is always a bit easier and faster. As you get closer to your goal weight, however, your rate of weight loss naturally slows because you have less to lose. For instance, if you lose 2 pounds when you weigh 300 pounds, you only lose 0.6 percent of your body weight. But if you lose 2 pounds when you weigh 150 pounds, you're actually losing 1.3 percent of your entire body weight! So even though the pounds lost on the scale may seem to move a bit slower, you may still be losing the same percent of body weight or more!

If you're struggling with a true plateau, don't be discouraged. First, reevaluate your goals. Is it possible you're already at a healthy body weight? If so, you may not be experiencing a plateau. Instead your body may be trying to tell you that it's time to transition to a weight maintenance plan.

If you're struggling with a plateau and your weight isn't within the ideal range (see the earlier section "Setting a Realistic Belly Fat Goal"), you need to start making a few adjustments to break through this plateau. I explain the adjustments you can make to fight through plateaus in the following sections.

Adjusting your diet habits

If you've hit a true plateau in your weight loss, don't throw your hands up. Your diet habits may just need some adjustment to get back to losing pounds and body fat. Here are some suggestions to try:

- ✔ **Go back to measuring all your food portions.** I'm sure you think you're eating the correct portion size of all your food choices, but the reality is that anyone, even myself as a dietitian, can misjudge a portion size by view alone. If you're at a standstill with your weight loss efforts, go back to measuring out your serving size at all meals and snacks for at least one week to see whether it helps jump-start the scale a bit.

  Think about it this way: A teaspoon of oil is the size of the tip of your thumb. That's tiny! And it's easy to slightly underestimate how much oil you pour into a recipe. Just two extra teaspoons of oil a day can equal 1 pound of body fat you don't lose throughout the month. So clearly it can quickly add up.

- ✔ **Track your food intake.** Are you still keeping a detailed food journal? If not, flip back to Chapter 7 for a sample journal and instructions on how to keep it. Without journaling, you may be underestimating your food by as much as 40 percent! And that can greatly slow down or stall your weight loss efforts. A food journal helps you see whether you're on track with your meal plan or veering a bit off track.

- ✔ **Add variety to your meal plan.** Your body can become accustomed to the same meals and snacks day in and day out. Switch it up by varying your meals and adding a few new recipes. Doing so not only helps you break through the plateau, but it may also help keep you motivated to stay on track.

If you put the preceding tips into action and still aren't seeing much progress after a month in the way of inches or pounds being lost, you may want to go back to Level 1 of your Belly Fat Diet plan. However, it's important to only revert to Level 1 if you haven't seen any progress for at least four weeks. And you should only go back to Level 1 for two weeks. After these two weeks, proceed to Level 2, just like you've done in the past. Then stay at this level until you reach your long-term goals.

If you go back to Level 1 of the Moderation or Gradual-Change plan and still see no progress at all after a week, I recommend going to Level 1 of the Turbo-Charged plan for two weeks only. Then you can proceed to Level 2 of the Turbo-Charged plan until you achieve your desired weight.

As outlined in Chapter 7, the Turbo-Charged plan isn't appropriate for certain individuals. If you have any condition listed as inappropriate for this plan in Chapter 7, you may go back to Level 1 in only the Moderation or Gradual-Change plan.

Switching up your workouts

If you perform the exact same workout routine day in and day out, your body can become accustomed to it. When your body acclimates to your routine, your muscles aren't as challenged, meaning they require less energy to perform the same movements. And less energy equals fewer calories being burned.

So switch up your workouts on a regular basis to maximize muscle confusion. Doing so helps you burn more calories, promoting weight loss and a decrease in belly fat. The Belly Fat Diet workouts in Chapter 10 help you accomplish exactly that. These workouts provide you with challenging core exercises and give you a guideline for slowly transitioning to interval walking to help elevate your heart rate and maximize calorie burn.

If you don't follow the Belly Fat Diet workouts, make sure to include interval training on your own. For instance, if you bike ride for 30 minutes every day at the same speed, switch to a routine where you ride at one speed for 5 minutes, pedal as fast as you can for 1 minute, and then go back to the slower speed for 5 more minutes. Repeat this cycle continuously throughout the duration of your workout. Or incorporate increased resistance or incline during your cardiovascular workouts to challenge yourself and keep your workouts interesting. Just make sure to consult your physician before starting or changing any exercise routine.

You Reached Your Goal! Now What?

Congratulations on the fantastic progress you've made. It's a terrific accomplishment to reach your goal weight, and you should be so proud of yourself. All your hard work and dedication have finally paid off. And, because of your efforts, your body not only looks better, but it's so much healthier on the inside, too. Now you're ready to enter maintenance mode so you don't slowly creep back up to your highest weight. So in the following sections, I show you the key to maintaining your weight and staying motivated with your lifestyle change.

Maintaining your weight

After you've reached your goal weight, you're ready to switch gears. Instead of focusing on weight loss, you get to focus on maintaining your current body weight. A lot of people get thrown off at this point and ask questions like

✔ How much more food can I eat?

✔ Should I eat the same things I was when I was losing weight?

✔ If I change my meal plan or exercise routine, will the pounds pile back on?

The key to weight maintenance is all about moderation. It's important to continue to implement the healthy behaviors that have helped you reach your goal weight. Going back to old habits only causes the weight to come back. You want to slightly adjust your meal plan but continue to keep an eye on your portions. And don't forget that you need to splurge on occasion, because maintaining weight is a lifelong journey. You can't expect yourself to eat perfectly 100 percent of the time.

Weight maintenance is also a bit of trial and error. You can slowly increase your food intake, but to know exactly how much extra you can add, you need to keep track of what you're eating (so you know just how much more food you're adding) and keep careful track of your weight for a few weeks. (Chapter 7 shows you how to keep a food journal.)

I don't want you to get carried away with weighing yourself, but you should step on the scale at least once every week. This way, if your weight begins to creep up slightly, you can make a few small changes in your food intake and exercise level to get that extra pound or two off before they become 10 or 20 pounds.

Most people can maintain their weight by adding between 100–500 calories per day. The amount depends on your age, activity level, gender, height, and whether your weight loss progress slowed on its own or whether you were consistently losing weight until you decided you no longer needed to lose anymore. Here are some general guidelines:

- ✔ Add 100–300 calories per day for weight maintenance if you're

  - A woman over the age of 40 or a man over the age of 50

  - A woman who is less than 5 foot 7 inches tall (of any age)

  - A man who is less than 5 foot 8 inches tall (of any age)

  - A person of any age who performs less than 30 minutes of moderate exercise a day

  - If you hit a weight loss plateau at a desirable body weight

- ✔ Add up to 500 calories per day if you're

  - A woman under the age of 40 who is at least 5 foot 7 inches or taller

  - A man under the age of 50 who is at least 5 foot 8 inches or taller

  - If your weight loss progress never slowed or stalled while you followed the Belly Fat Diet plan

The next few sections provide weight maintenance meal plan guidelines that help you maintain your body weight. However, keep in mind that weight maintenance is very individualized. If you follow the maintenance plan and find after two to three weeks that you're still losing weight (and don't want to), add in an additional 100 calories per day for one week and monitor your weight. And if you're following the recommended plan and your weight is creeping upward slightly, cut back by 100 calories per day for a week and reassess your progress. Repeat either option until you're maintaining your weight for at least two weeks in a row.

To put it in perspective, 100 calories is generally equal to

- ✔ 1 starch serving
- ✔ 1 fruit serving
- ✔ 1 milk or yogurt serving
- ✔ 3 ounces of lean protein
- ✔ 2 fat servings

Maintenance meal plan guidelines for men

The maintenance meal plan I introduce in Table 18-4 is designed for most men. The average man tends to have a slightly higher metabolism than the average woman, due to increased muscle mass. However, if you find that you're following this maintenance plan exactly and your body weight is increasing slightly, try following the maintenance plan guidelines for women (in the next section), which may be better suited for a man of shorter stature, a man a bit older in years, or a man with limited physical activity.

Table 18-4		Maintenance Meal Plan for Men			
Vegetables	**Fruit**	**Milk/Yogurt**	**Starch**	**Protein**	**Fat**
4+	3	3	7	12 ounces	7

Maintenance meal plan guidelines for women

The maintenance meal plan in Table 18-5 is slightly lower in overall portions and calories than the men's plan because women generally have slightly lower metabolisms. It should work for most women, but, if you're following this plan and your weight continues to decrease, follow the maintenance plan for men in the preceding section to adjust your meal plan and maintain a stable weight.

If you find you're slowly regaining weight when following this plan, cut back by 100 calories per day for a week and reassess your progress. Repeat until you're maintaining your weight for at least two weeks in a row.

Table 18-5		Maintenance Meal Plan for Women			
Vegetables	**Fruit**	**Milk/Yogurt**	**Starch**	**Protein**	**Fat**
4+	3	2	5	10 ounces	7

Keeping your results with the 80/20 rule

If you want to keep your lost weight off, remember that you can't be perfect. No one is perfect, especially when it comes to food. And, if you try to be perfect 100 percent of the time with what you're eating, you're going to burn yourself out.

Part of healthy eating and weight maintenance is understanding that all foods have a place in your diet — some just more often than others. If you're a junk food junky, you can't expect to ignore chips or ice cream for the rest of your life. Doing so is just completely unrealistic. You shouldn't expect to eat chips every day, but an occasional splurge is fine. It's actually healthy.

Remember when you were back in school, studying for a huge exam? If you studied every waking hour, you started to forget what you were studying for in the first place and ended up doing worse on the exam, right? It's the same thing with healthy eating. If you obsess over your food choices and scrutinize every morsel that enters your mouth, you're going to eventually get so sick of doing it that you say "the heck with this" and shove whatever you feel like in your mouth. And that can put you right back to where you started.

Maintaining your weight loss is all about balance, which is why I want you to follow my 80/20 rule. I want you to focus 80 percent of the time on eating healthy, belly-friendly foods that shrink the waistline and fight inflammation. Then 20 percent of the time, you have room to veer off track a bit. This 20 percent is your splurge. You may choose to have one day a week where you have a splurge meal, or you may opt for a small snack twice a week where you don't exactly make the healthiest choice.

Splurging isn't a suggestion. I am making this a rule for a reason. If you don't follow this rule, you're either going to become too obsessive about what you're eating or you're going to burn out. Neither is a good option. So 20 percent of the time, relax a bit and have something that seems forbidden. Learning to enjoy and savor your food is part of mindful eating anyway!

This rule says to have a small splurge 20 percent of the time, but this splurge must be within reason. If every 5 days you eat an entire pizza and a gallon of ice cream, you're going to gain weight back no matter what you do the rest of the week. Splurging is fine, but binging or stuffing yourself until you feel sick is not. So just be reasonable about it. If you start to notice the numbers on the scale are creeping up a bit, just downsize the portions of your splurges a little bit.

Staying motivated with your workouts

In addition to keeping an eye on your portions to maintain a steady weight, you also need to stay active. In fact, regular exercise is more important during maintenance than in any point in your weight loss. It's even more important than when you're trying to lose weight. Research has shown the majority of people who have lost a significant amount of weight and have kept it off long term perform some form of physical activity or structured exercise on a regular basis.

Maintaining your weight is a lifelong process, which means you have to be active for life. And if you do the exact same exercise day in and day out, for years and years, you're likely to get bored with it. But exercise doesn't have to be boring! In fact, it should never be boring. Keeping it fun is what's going to help you stick with it.

Think back to when you were a child. What physical activities did you have fun doing? Did you love riding your bike? Shooting hoops on the basketball court? Or maybe playing tennis? These are all great forms of exercise. Regular exercise doesn't mean you have to be lifting weights at the gym or running on the treadmill. Don't get me wrong. These are terrific forms of exercise. But not everyone enjoys the gym. And if you're doing something you don't enjoy, you aren't going to stick with it.

So think outside of the box. Join a dance class, take up kickboxing, or start hiking in your local park. These are all fantastic forms of physical activity that can help keep the weight off. And the best part is that you'll have so much fun doing it that you won't even realize you're exercising.

It's also important to challenge yourself every once in a while too. Even if you're doing an activity you find fun, it's still easy to fall into a rut when doing the same thing over and over. So think of a way to push yourself a bit so you're always striving to get stronger and faster. For instance, consider the following:

✔ If you enjoy walking or running, sign up for a 5K or 10K race and work on improving your times.

✔ If you love swimming, join a Master's League where you can participate in races and challenge yourself against others.

✔ If you love to dance, try a variety of dance styles, such as ballroom and ballet.

Part V
The Part of Tens

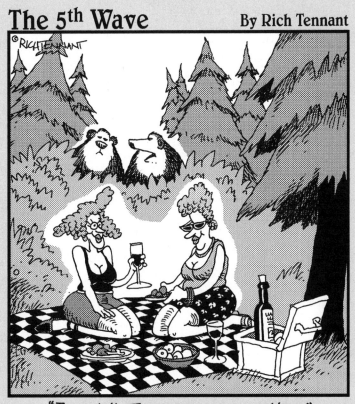

The 5th Wave   By Rich Tennant

"Forget it. Too many preservatives."

In this part . . .

There are many misconceptions about what really works in the fight against belly fat. That's why, in this part, I list the biggest belly-bloaters that you need to limit in your diet, and I provide an easy-to-read breakdown of nutrients that have been shown to help burn belly fat.

Chapter 19

Ten Belly-Bloating Foods

. . . .

In This Chapter

▶ Identifying foods that bloat your belly

▶ Understanding how certain foods can cause belly bloat

. . . .

*J*ust as many foods have the potential to shrink belly fat, quite a few others can bloat your belly. These belly bloaters work in different ways. Some can increase gas in your stomach, making your abdomen look and feel distended. Even though this bloating is only temporary, it can still be uncomfortable and make your pants feel quite snug around your waistline. Other foods, due to their nutritional content, can lead to long-term belly bloat from increased visceral fat storage. In this chapter, I show you some of the worst offenders to be aware of and avoid.

Bagels

Not every bagel is a belly bloater. However, the typical bagel is. If you go to the bagel store or a deli, you almost always get a huge bagel made with 100 percent refined flour. Even though it tastes good, that refined flour sets off the cascading events of elevated blood sugar, elevated insulin levels, and increased belly fat storage.

If you're a bagel lover, don't worry. Healthier options exist. Aim for a small bagel (the size of the palm of your hand), and make sure it's made with 100 percent whole grains.

Cabbage

It tastes great and is great for you, but cabbage may be tough on your belly! Cabbage is a vegetable known for increasing gas production in the gastrointestinal tract during digestion. And this increased gas production can bloat your belly. Gas-producing vegetables are often easier to digest and break down when cooked well. So if you do have cabbage, choose cooked over raw. And don't eat large quantities of cabbage on a day you want your waistline to look as slim and toned as possible.

Carbonated Water

How can carbonated water be a belly bloater when it doesn't have any calories or fat? Well, it certainly won't pack on the pounds, and it is hydrating, but the added carbonation can be quite bloating. This bloating is due to the gas from the air blended with the water. The bloating is only temporary, but for one to three hours after drinking carbonated water, you may feel as though your belly has expanded. The carbonation can make your stomach look distended and cause clothing to fit more snuggly around your midsection.

If you really love carbonated beverages, aim to drink just one glass per day. Also, avoid carbonated beverages a few days before an event or outing where you want your belly to look as flat as possible.

Cola (Including Diet Cola)

Cola is a staple at many restaurants and homes, but it can be a huge belly bloater. In addition to the carbonation that increases gas in the stomach (which causes immediate belly bloat), the sugar in cola can make that temporary bloat turn into a permanently larger belly! Depending on the cola, it may contain sugar, corn syrup, or another liquid sweetener. All of these sweeteners have the same long-term effect: increased fat storage right in your abdominal area. High sugar content, especially in liquid form, immediately raises blood sugar, which in turn spikes insulin levels. This elevated insulin level signals your body to begin storing the excess sugar as fat. And, of course, your body places it in the easiest and most convenient location: your belly.

Diet soda isn't the answer. It doesn't contain sugar, but it still contains carbonation, which is an instant belly bloater. Diet sodas are also packed full of artificial sweeteners. These sweeteners are foreign chemicals to your body, so when they're consumed in excessive amounts, they may increase inflammation, which in the long run can increase health risks and belly fat. Your best solution is to try a naturally flavored seltzer or a glass of water with a splash of lemon or lime juice for added flavor.

Fried Foods

Deep-fried foods, including French fries, can cause you to feel heavy and sluggish because the high levels of fat in these foods slow digestion. In addition, the fat used to fry your deep-fried snacks and meals isn't the healthy fat that flattens your belly. In fact, commercially fried foods often contain the most dangerous of all fats: trans fats. These fats in even small amounts have been linked to many negative health effects (such as heart disease). They can also significantly elevate inflammation in your body.

If you love fried foods, try breading the foods in whole-grain flour and pan-frying them in a small amount of olive oil (or baking them instead). The foods will come out crispy and delicious without all the dangerous fat.

Ice Cream

Ice cream can be a belly bloater in a couple of ways. First, it contains a large amount of sugar, and food high in sugar causes both blood sugar and insulin levels to rise, resulting in the storage of more belly fat. Because ice cream is a milk product, it also contains high levels of lactose, the sugar found in milk. Many individuals have lactose intolerance, which causes them to have trouble breaking down lactose and leads to increased gas production, bloat, and even diarrhea. Extreme temperatures in foods, such as very cold (like ice cream), can also stress the gastrointestinal tract and lead to cramping and bloating.

Ice cream's belly-bloating characteristics may disappoint you, but you don't have to completely disown this cool treat. Just keep your intake within moderation, and when you do splurge, keep your portion to ½ cup to 1 cup. If you're lactose intolerant, choose a soy-based ice cream or a lactose-free variety.

Sausage

Sausage is a fatty meat that's loaded with unhealthy saturated fat. This fat clogs arteries and may also increase inflammation, which has a direct link to belly fat storage. Sausage is almost always high in sodium as well. And food high in sodium causes your body to retain water, giving your belly a bloated look and feel. And lastly, don't forget that sausage, due to its high fat content, is high in calories. So consuming it on a regular basis can lead to weight gain.

If you love sausage, make the switch to a leaner, more belly-friendly option. Sausage made with leaner meats like turkey, chicken, or venison contains less saturated fat and fewer calories. Even leaner options can be high in sodium, so save them for occasional treats rather than meal staples.

Sugar Alcohols

Sugar alcohols are sugar substitutes that can only be partially digested by the body. Many times you see these in foods like sugar-free candy, gum, and snacks. They're often listed as xylitol, sorbitol, and maltitol. Because they're only partially digested in your body, they provide fewer calories per gram than actual sugar, but they also can cause gastrointestinal side effects, such as bloating, gas, and diarrhea. And all that bloat and gas can cause your abdomen to look distended. So you're better off avoiding these or consuming them in small quantities to prevent belly bloating.

Sugar-Free Gum

Sugar-free gum is virtually calorie free, so how can it possibly bloat your belly? Let me explain. Chewing gum, in general, while fine to do, can lead to the swallowing of air. The more air that you swallow, the more this air accumulates in your gastrointestinal tract, which can cause bloating, pressure, and belly expansion. In addition, the sugar alcohols (discussed in the preceding section) in sugar-free gum have some side effects. They can increase gas and cause bloating, abdominal pain, and even diarrhea. However, gum containing sugar alcohols can have some health benefits, such as helping to prevent dental cavities. It also has no impact on blood sugar and insulin levels due to the low glycemic index of sugar alcohols.

If you love gum, you don't need to give it up. Just aim for only a few pieces per day.

White Rice

Rice can be a healthy grain but only when it's in its natural form (such as brown rice or wild rice). White rice, on the other hand, has been refined and stripped of the outermost and innermost layers of grain, removing most of the fiber, nutrients, and proteins. In fact, it's one of the most processed grains and has a high glycemic index. As a result, white rice digests rapidly in your body, creating that cascading effect of increased insulin levels, increased fat storage, and an increased waistline over time. Also, as a refined grain, white rice offers a low level of satiety. So you'll eat it, won't feel very full, and then eat more. This cycle can lead to an excessive calorie intake and increased weight gain.

If rice is a staple in your diet, you can keep it that way. Simply choose a less-processed option instead. Brown rice and wild rice can be substituted for white rice in almost any recipe and are much friendlier to your waistline!

Chapter 20

Ten Nutrients That Shrink Your Belly

In This Chapter

▶ Looking at some nutrients that can promote fat loss

▶ Identifying the health benefits of certain compounds and nutrients

*H*ealthy eating and exercise can shrink your waistline and blast away belly fat. But certain nutrients also have the ability to help you burn belly fat faster and more effectively. Incorporating the ten nutrients in this chapter on a regular basis through seasonings, food choices, and supplements may help you shed fat, especially around your midsection, more productively, helping you to reach your weight loss goals even faster!

Calcium Pyruvate

Calcium pyruvate is a substance that occurs naturally and is made in your body during digestion and metabolism. This nutrient's main role is to make energy and fuel your cells. Some new research, however, indicates that it may also be a powerful fat fighter.

A study done by the University of Pittsburgh found that obese women lost 48 percent more fat when following a calorie-restricted diet with supplemental calcium pyruvate than those women following the diet alone. It appears that calcium pyruvate can get into the fat cells and help them burn energy more effectively, promoting more weight loss.

Calcium pyruvate occurs naturally in foods like red apples, red grapes, red wine, and cheeses. It can also be taken in supplemental form. If supplementing with calcium pyruvate, take 1,000 milligrams on an empty stomach before each meal up to three times per day. Taking too much of this supplement may cause nausea, however.

Caraway Seeds

Bloating and gas can occur in your gastrointestinal tract for a number of reasons. And increased gas can cause your belly to bloat. To help get rid of gas, try snacking on caraway seeds. Eat a small handful (about 1 tablespoon) after meals, especially meals that contain gas-producing foods.

Caraway seeds are effective at reducing gas and bloating because they're a powerful digestive aid. They help to expel and eliminate gas due to their carminative properties. Caraway seeds are also beneficial at keeping bloat away because they help the good bacteria in your gastrointestinal tract digest and break down food while inhibiting the growth of the bad bacteria.

Cinnamon

Research has found that the active compound methylhydroxy chalcone polymer (MHCP) in cinnamon makes fat cells more receptive to insulin. When cells are more receptive to insulin, they allow the insulin to transport sugar into the cells for energy, thus keeping insulin levels in the bloodstream low. High insulin levels trigger the body to store more fat, especially in your midsection. So consuming a seasoning like cinnamon that helps maintain healthy levels of insulin is a great way to combat belly fat.

Try sprinkling cinnamon on everything from oatmeal to apples to popcorn! Cinnamon supplements are also available and may help provide belly-slimming benefits.

Epigallocatechin Gallate (EGCG)

The main polyphenol, epigallocatechin gallate (EGCG), in green tea has been shown to have thermogenic properties and to help increase fat oxidation. In fact, one study found that when overweight individuals consumed the same number of calories and performed the same amount of exercise, those drinking green tea lost more weight, especially weight from the abdomen. Green tea is also loaded with powerful antioxidants, which help decrease inflammation (another belly-fat contributor) and fight off disease and infection. Aim for brewed green tea over powders and supplements.

Fucoxanthin

Fucoxanthin is a carotenoid found in brown seaweed. Research on this compound suggests it may be a powerful fat fighter. In animal studies, overweight and obese mice were found to lose 5 to 10 percent of their entire body weight when consuming fucoxanthin. Although research is still unclear as to exactly how fucoxanthin promotes weight loss, it may be due to its ability to target a specific protein that increases the rate at which abdominal fat is burned.

Edible brown seaweed is available in Japanese specialty stores and health food stores under the names *wakame* and *hijiki*. Fucoxanthin is available as a nutritional supplement, but more research is still needed in humans to see whether this compound is as effective in promoting weight loss as it is in animals. Until more research is done, I recommend adding brown seaweed into recipes, such as miso soup, rather than consuming it as a supplement. If you do choose to consume supplemental fucoxanthin, don't exceed 500 milligrams per day.

Omega-3 Fatty Acids

Omega-3-rich foods been shown to help reduce abdominal fat storage. Studies have also shown that they keep the stress hormones cortisol and adrenaline from peaking, helping to prevent damage to your body from chronic stress and also helping prevent increased fat storage caused by elevated cortisol levels.

Fatty fish, such as salmon, is a great source of omega-3 fatty acids. However, plant-based sources, such as chia seeds, walnuts, and flaxseed, are terrific sources as well. Supplemental omega-3 fatty acids are also fine. If you do take a supplement, an appropriate dosage is 1,000–2,000 milligrams per day. Omega-3 fatty acids can act as a blood thinner, so make sure to discuss with your physician whether this supplement is appropriate for you.

Quercetin

Quercetin, a powerful flavonoid, has been shown to not only improve the immune system and promote cardiovascular health but also fight belly fat. Research has shown that this flavonoid can block baby fat cells from maturing and is more effective at inhibiting the rate of new fat cell formation than any other flavonoid. Quercetin also is effective at decreasing inflammation in the body.

Large amounts of quercetin are found in apples, onions (especially red onions), and green tea. Red grapes, tomatoes, broccoli, cherries, raspberries, and leafy greens are also excellent sources. Aim to take in quercetin from foods rather than supplements, because foods rich in quercetin contain many additional health benefits.

Resveratrol

Studies have indicated that high levels of resveratrol in your diet may boost metabolism, helping you to burn more calories (and more belly fat) throughout the day. Resveratrol has also been shown to suppress levels of the hormone estrogen. High levels of estrogen in your body promote increased fat storage, so suppressing these levels may decrease body fat while helping to increase lean muscle mass.

Resveratrol is found in red grapes, red wine, peanuts, and dark chocolate. Supplements are available, but make sure to consult your physician before increasing your intake of resveratrol in a supplement form, especially if you're taking any hormone-based medication.

Vitamin C

When the stress hormone cortisol is chronically elevated in the body, you can experience increased fat storage in the abdominal area. However, research has shown that vitamin C helps reduce stress hormone levels and return the stress hormone cortisol to normal levels after a stressful situation. This reduction in cortisol may help to prevent increased belly-fat storage.

Aim to consume at least two foods rich in vitamin C each day. Options include oranges, kiwis, and green peppers. Vitamin C is available in supplement form, but taking in nutrients through food is always the best option. If you do opt for a supplement, keep your dosage to 500 milligrams per day and choose a time-released formula for the best benefit.

Water

How much simpler can it get? Just drinking water may shrink your belly! A study from the Journal of Clinical Endocrinology and Metabolism showed that individuals increased their metabolic rates by 30 percent after drinking approximately 17 ounces of water. Other research indicates that increasing fluid volume in the body may help to promote the breakdown of fat. And because dehydration can suppress metabolism, you have even more reasons to drink up! Aim for at least 64 ounces of water daily.

Index

Apple & Mac

iPad 2 For Dummies,
3rd Edition
978-1-118-17679-5

iPhone 4S For Dummies,
5th Edition
978-1-118-03671-6

iPod touch For Dummies,
3rd Edition
978-1-118-12960-9

Mac OS X Lion
For Dummies
978-1-118-02205-4

Blogging & Social Media

CityVille For Dummies
978-1-118-08337-6

Facebook For Dummies,
4th Edition
978-1-118-09562-1

Mom Blogging
For Dummies
978-1-118-03843-7

Twitter For Dummies,
2nd Edition
978-0-470-76879-2

WordPress For Dummies,
4th Edition
978-1-118-07342-1

Business

Cash Flow For Dummies
978-1-118-01850-7

Investing For Dummies,
6th Edition
978-0-470-90545-6

Job Searching with Social
Media For Dummies
978-0-470-93072-4

QuickBooks 2012
For Dummies
978-1-118-09120-3

Resumes For Dummies,
6th Edition
978-0-470-87361-8

Starting an Etsy Business
For Dummies
978-0-470-93067-0

Cooking & Entertaining

Cooking Basics
For Dummies, 4th Edition
978-0-470-91388-8

Wine For Dummies,
4th Edition
978-0-470-04579-4

Diet & Nutrition

Kettlebells For Dummies
978-0-470-59929-7

Nutrition For Dummies,
5th Edition
978-0-470-93231-5

Restaurant Calorie Counter
For Dummies,
2nd Edition
978-0-470-64405-8

Digital Photography

Digital SLR Cameras &
Photography For Dummies,
4th Edition
978-1-118-14489-3

Digital SLR Settings
& Shortcuts
For Dummies
978-0-470-91763-3

Photoshop Elements 10
For Dummies
978-1-118-10742-3

Gardening

Gardening Basics
For Dummies
978-0-470-03749-2

Vegetable Gardening
For Dummies,
2nd Edition
978-0-470-49870-5

Green/Sustainable

Raising Chickens
For Dummies
978-0-470-46544-8

Green Cleaning
For Dummies
978-0-470-39106-8

Health

Diabetes For Dummies,
3rd Edition
978-0-470-27086-8

Food Allergies
For Dummies
978-0-470-09584-3

Living Gluten-Free
For Dummies,
2nd Edition
978-0-470-58589-4

Hobbies

Beekeeping
For Dummies,
2nd Edition
978-0-470-43065-1

Chess For Dummies,
3rd Edition
978-1-118-01695-4

Drawing For Dummies,
2nd Edition
978-0-470-61842-4

eBay For Dummies,
7th Edition
978-1-118-09806-6

Knitting For Dummies,
2nd Edition
978-0-470-28747-7

Language & Foreign Language

English Grammar
For Dummies,
2nd Edition
978-0-470-54664-2

French For Dummies,
2nd Edition
978-1-118-00464-7

German For Dummies,
2nd Edition
978-0-470-90101-4

Spanish Essentials
For Dummies
978-0-470-63751-7

Spanish For Dummies,
2nd Edition
978-0-470-87855-2

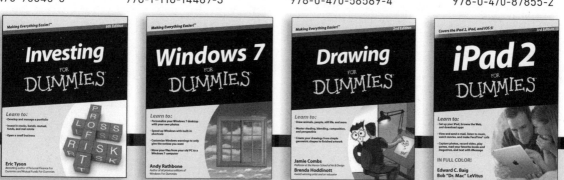

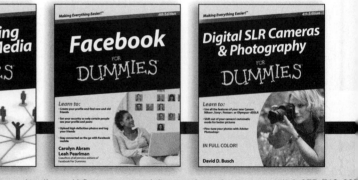

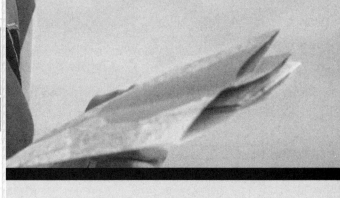

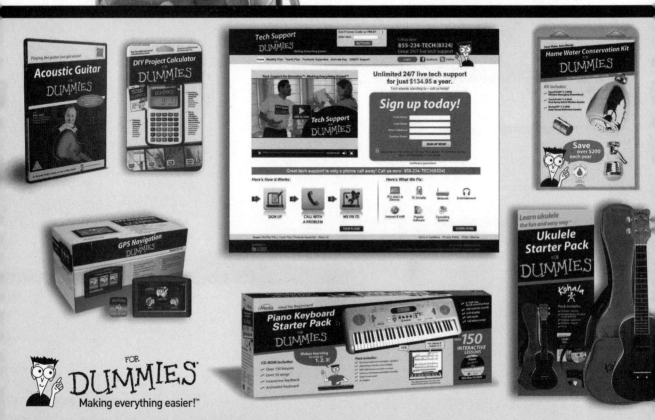